CLEMENTS
HIGH SCHOOL LIBRARY
P.O. BOX 1004
SUGAR LAND, TEXAS 77478

THE STARS OF STAND-UP COMEDY

GARLAND REFERENCE LIBRARY
OF THE HUMANITIES
(VOL. 564)

The Stars of Stand-up Comedy

A Biographical Encyclopedia

Ronald Lande Smith

Garland Publishing, Inc.
New York & London 1986

© 1986 Ronald Lande Smith
All rights reserved

Photos on pp. 8, 31, 70, 79, 102, 118, 144, 171 © Ronald L. Smith
Others courtesy: Warner Bros. Records, Columbia Records, Atlantic Records/
Patty Conte, NBC, ABC, CBS, PBS, New York Public Library, Jerry Ohlinger,
Rogers & Cowan, The Shefrin Company, Gerard W. Purcell, Pete Barbutti,
Orson Bean, Bob and Ray, George Burns, Red Buttons, Bill Cosby, Shecky
Greene, Will Jordan, Eddie Lawrence, Stiller & Meara, Photo Archives,
Universal Studios, Elektra Records, MCA Records, author's collection.

Library of Congress Cataloging-in-Publication Data

Smith, Ronald Lande, 1952–
The stars of stand-up comedy.

(Garland reference library of the humanities ; vol. 564)
Bibliography: p.
1. Comedians—United States—Biography—Dictionaries.
2. Comedians—United States—Bibliography. I. Title.
II. Series: Garland reference library of the humanities ; v. 564.
PN2285.S547   1986   792.7′028′0922 [B]   84-48408
ISBN 0-8240-8803-4 (alk. paper)

Interior book design by Jonathan Billing
Printed on acid-free, 250-year-life paper
Manufactured in the United States of America

THE COMEDIANS

Abbott and Costello 1
Don Adams 3
Allen and Rossi 5
Steve Allen 6
Woody Allen 9
Morey Amsterdam 12
Pete Barbutti 14
Belle Barth 15
Orson Bean 16
Jack Benny 19
Milton Berle 21
Shelley Berman 24
Bob and Ray 27
Victor Borge 30
David Brenner 32
Lenny Bruce 35
Lord Buckley 38
Burns and Schreiber 40
George Burns 42
Red Buttons 45
Godfrey Cambridge 47
George Carlin 49
Johnny Carson 52
Jack Carter 55
Dick Cavett 57
Cheech and Chong 60
Myron Cohen 62
Cook and Moore 64
Irwin Corey 67
Bill Cosby 69
Norm Crosby 72
Bill Dana 74
Rodney Dangerfield 76
Phyllis Diller 78
Flanders and Swann 81
Frank Fontaine 83
Redd Foxx 85
David Frost 87
David Frye 88
Brother Dave Gardner 90
George Gobel 91
Shecky Greene 93
Dick Gregory 94
Buddy Hackett 97
Homer and Jethro 99
Bob Hope 100
George Jessel 103
Will Jordan 105
Jackie Kannon 107
Gabe Kaplan 109
Alan King 111

George Kirby 113
Robert Klein 115
Eddie Lawrence 116
Tom Lehrer 119
Jack E. Leonard 121
Sam Levenson 123
Joe E. Lewis 124
Rich Little 126
Paul Lynde 128
Moms Mabley 131
Charlie Manna 133
Pigmeat Markham 134
Martin and Lewis 136
Steve Martin 138
Groucho Marx 141
Jackie Mason 144
Vaughn Meader 147
Moran and Mack 150
Martin Mull 151
Eddie Murphy 153
Jan Murray 156
Bob Newhart 157
Nichols and May 160
Richard Pryor 162
Reiner and Brooks 166
Don Rickles 168
Joan Rivers 171
Will Rogers 174
Rowan and Martin 177
Anna Russell 179
Mark Russell 181
Nipsey Russell 183
Mort Sahl 184
Soupy Sales 187
Jean Shepherd 189
Allan Sherman 191
Red Skelton 194
Smith and Dale 197
The Smothers Brothers 199
David Steinberg 202
Stiller and Meara 204
Lily Tomlin 206
Jackie Vernon 209
Charlie Weaver 211
Weber and Fields 213
Pearl Williams 216
Robin Williams 218
Flip Wilson 220
Jonathan Winters 222
Henny Youngman 225

PREFACE

This is, actually a post-face, since you've probably browsed through the book, already. In fact, you've probably read a few of the biographies, too. It's the logical thing to do. This book really needs no preface or introduction—it's obviously an encyclopedia of stand-up comedians, their lives and the way they produce laughter. And all I can add is, it's about time.

There's no need to use this space to acknowledge the secretary who made the coffee, the typist who typed or the researchers who researched. To paraphrase Groucho Marx in his autobiography, I sweated out every word of this thing myself: the interviews, research, screening films, listening to monologues, transcribing, typing, etc. It became such a full-time job I even decided to stick my full name on it instead of just plain Ron Smith.

For curious readers or scholars, I should at least define "stand-up" as a term, and explain who is in the book and who isn't.

"Stand-up" here applies to the art of getting up in front of people and being funny—one of the easiest sounding, most difficult things in the world.

The image of the stand-up comic is a guy in a tuxedo telling mother-in-law jokes in front of drunks. But as this book demonstrates, stand-up comics come in many styles, and some even sit down (Victor Borge at the piano), do sketch material (Nichols and May), use free-form (Mort Sahl) or even read comic letters out loud (Charley Weaver).

Steve Allen once said there are perhaps only 300 comedians in the world. That's quite an endangered species. Only half that number do stand-up, and fewer than that do it exclusively. To whittle the number down to 101, I've excluded such comedians as Jackie Gleason, Sid Caesar and Danny Kaye, who have performed monologues or solo sketches on occasion, but are not stand-up specialists. W. C. Fields performed a "Temperance Lecture" monologue, but he too rarely performed solo concerts. Some, such as Andy Griffith, Jimmie Walker and Freddie Prinze, began in stand-up but achieved greater fame in situation comedy. Most talk-show hosts, for example, Jack Paar and David Letterman, have done monologues but few of us could quote a memorable line from them.

When an included comedian has worked at stand-up as well as other kinds of comedy (Woody Allen, Jack Benny, Abbott & Costello, etc.) my profile has largely confined itself to the solo work, rather than to film, radio or television.

Some readers will probably note some glaring (or at least squinting) omissions. The average reader may agree with 90% of my selections (and I'll take an "A" anytime) but recall a few comics who deserve mention over some others. They have a legitimate case.

This is an encyclopedia not only of comedians, but of stand-up styles as well. I've tried to include all types of comics: regional performers, risqué acts, lounge acts, Vegas types, one-liner gag men, sketch artists, journeymen, slapsticks and sophisticates. There was no room to include *every* Vegas comic, or regional comic, etc., so where I had to choose among several of equal stature, I picked the one I considered best. If two were equal, I chose the most accessible. That may help to explain Brother Dave Gardner over Jerry Clower, or Pearl Williams over Rusty Warren.

Ultimately, the major considerations were: Did this comedian contribute something unique to stand-up? Is the comedian famous now, or famous enough at one time to be included for historical reasons? Is the material funny? Is the comedian influential?

Every effort has been made to make this book as complete and factual as possible. Since this is a pioneering effort, and some comics or their managers were either wary of revealing biographical material or didn't give a damn about posterity, it was not always possible to recheck every fact with the ultimate source.

In fact, the ultimate source was often unreliable. Performers are notorious for changing birthdates, forgetting career details and embellishing anecdotes. Often advancing years affect the memory. Smith and Dale, for example, named many different streets as the one they "met" on. In such cases, I located the oldest extant newspaper clippings and interviews (which would be freshest in terms of memory) and assembled as many references as possible, picking the truth from the most often repeated information or the most reliable sources.

Even so, spellings of real names become mangled by typographical errors, apocryphal anecdotes are reprinted as fact, and one writer's mistake becomes another's source. Printing Soupy Sales's real name as Hines is an example of an erroneous report that was reprinted as fact in every major reference book.

This book is intended both for general readers and scholars, balancing interesting biography, jokes and fun with facts, insight and evaluation. The list of credits are thorough without being fanatical: they are intended to list major film and television credits, but not all minor ones. Major long-playing record albums are included (with serial numbers for collectors), but not 45's or 78's. The reader should also be advised that with video cassettes becoming increasingly popular, more "lost" material should be available in the coming years than ever before.

I have interviewed many of the performers in this book, but not all of them obviously, some quotations are from print, radio or television interviews. In the interests of space and fluidity, I've not prepared a detailed source bibliography.

I've resisted including obscure or unnecessary factual detail in the biographies. A comedian's wife's name, the name of his elementary school or the call letters of the radio station that first played his record are rarely vital. And for a book on comedians, nothing could be more boring.

I'd like to avoid trivial detail in information about the author, too. But on a personal note, I hope I share with the comedians included their creativity and sensitivity. Like taking to the stage, taking to the typewriter is fraught with doubt, work, worry—as well as fun and a sense of accomplishment. Getting a line just right is similar to perfecting the phrasing of a joke. If comedians are basically serious, so was my intent in re-writing, re-typing and digging up as many facts as possible, in addition to quoting jokes correctly from the television and radio shows I've taped for 20 years, and the 600 or more comedy albums I've accumulated.

Finally, having performed on television and radio, performing comedy from "Let Peas Be With You," my book of comic verse, I think I have some empathy for the strange art of getting up in front of strangers and being funny—getting laughs where they were expected, not getting laughs where they were expected and getting laughs where they weren't expected.

Like the comedian who constantly wonders if he's going to be funny, I spent a long time with each biography, trying to be as fair and as true as possible. It's an incredible responsibility, I feel, to distill someone's life in a few pages, bumping over traumas, sliding past years of struggle, neatly categorizing and analyzing each fateful twist. Along the way in my interviews and attempts at interview, some comics showed their dark sides of suspicion, shyness and insecurity. And others showed their good humor, warmth, sensitivity and gentleness. I expected both sides, even from the same individual.

If there had been enough space and time (the time to find the people and pry out the information), this book could have included perhaps another 50 comics. Happily, this book is not the only testament to stand-up comedians. The most crucial is laughter, and the comedians—the great ones—get their reward every time they perform.

The Encyclopedia

ABBOTT AND COSTELLO

Considered primarily film comedians today, Abbott & Costello gained fame first as a stand-up act in vaudeville and on radio. Most of their movies were generally highlighted by stand-up wordplay routines or classic burlesque sketches lifted almost verbatim from the stage.

Abbott worked behind the scenes as a theater cashier and producer before becoming known as one of the best straight men in the business. Costello, once an amateur boxer, drifted through many odd jobs, including movie stuntman, before taking a gamble as a comedian. Broke, he saw an advertisement for a Dutch comedian, and ad-libbed his way through the part. Gradually he perfected his craft working in burlesque houses with various partners.

In 1936 they teamed up. Legend has it that Bud substituted when Lou's straight man failed to show up, but the mundane truth is that the two men had worked with many other partners, became acquainted, admired each other's work and decided to take a chance together.

They probably didn't realize then just how perfect their "chemistry of opposites" was. It was more than Bud's being tall, thin and impatient, and Lou's being short, fat and incorrigible. They had a unique relationship, at times adversaries, at times partners, sometimes Bud the con man and Lou the pratfalling stooge. Accused of having little warmth or interpersonal contact (in one movie Bud gives Lou a gun to commit suicide with), the team often mirrored, if unintentionally and subliminally, the real love, hate and exasperation two intimates feel for each other.

It's this tension that propels a routine like "Who's on First" as much as Bud's underrated gruffness and Lou's comic perplexity. If Laurel and Hardy did the routine, it would be two idiots flabbily going through the motions, with Ollie assuming grandiose superiority. If Hope and Crosby did it, it wouldn't make sense, since neither is that bright or that stupid. But with Abbott & Costello, Abbott seems to enjoy his partner's helplessness, at times deliberately fueling it by offering one-word, ambiguous answers. And Costello, like a child always asking its parent, "but why . . .," keeps right on asking preposterous questions. And the routine itself is so contrived, jokeless and downright silly that only Bud and Lou could have made it the substantial, irrepressible laugh getter it is no matter how often it's heard.

"Strange as it may seem," Bud says, blithely tossing out the premise, "they give ballplayers peculiar names—nicknames. Who's on first, What's on second, I Don't Know is on third—"

"That's what I want to find out," Lou says with childlike expectation.

"I'm telling you. Who's on first, What's on second, I Don't Know is on third."

"You know the fellows' names?"

"Yes."

"Well, then, who's playin' first?"

"Yes."

"I mean the fellow's name on first base."

"Who."

"The guy on first base."

"Who's on first."

"Well, what are you asking me for?"

"I'm not asking you, I'm telling you. Who is on first."

"All I'm tryin' to do is find out what's the guy's name on first base."

"No, What is on second base."

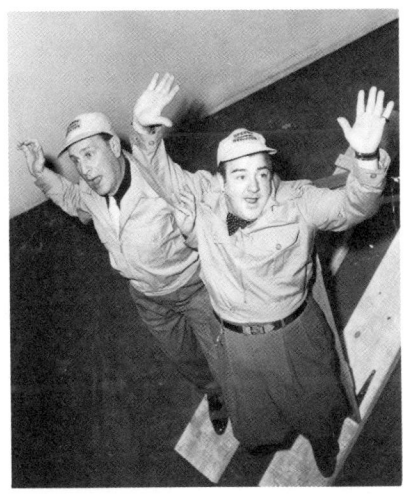

BUD ABBOTT b. William Abbott, October 2, 1895, Asbury Park, New Jersey; d. April 24, 1974
LOU COSTELLO b. Louis Francis Cristillo, March 6, 1906, Paterson, New Jersey; d. March 3, 1959

Records:
Abbott & Costello on Radio (Radiola MR 1038), Buck Privates (Radiola 1135), Abbott & Costello (Memorabilia MLP 731), Abbott & Costello Christmas (Holiday HDY-1939), Who's on First (Nostalgia Lane PB 0069), Abbott & Costello (Nostalgia Lane PB 7071, 2 lps), Best of Abbott & Costello and Amos & Andy (Radiex 6), Hey Abbott (Murray Hill 899981, 3 lps).

Compilations:
Golden Age of Comedy (RCA Victor LPV-580), Jest Like Old Times (Radiola #1).

TV:
The Abbott & Costello Show (CBS 1952-53).

Films on Video:
Buck Privates (MCA), Hold That Ghost (MCA), Abbott & Costello Meet Frankenstein (MCA), Abbott & Costello in Hollywood (MGM/UA), Africa Screams (Budget Video).

Video:
Hey, Abbott! (Vid-America, Vestron), Abbott & Costello Live (4 vols., SRO Video).

Bios:
Bud and Lou (Bob Thomas), Lou's on First (Chris Costello), Abbott & Costello Book (Jim Mulholland).

"I'm not askin' you who's on second."
"Who's on first!"
"What's the guy's name on first base?"
"What's the guy's name on second base."
"I'm not askin' you who's on second."
"Who's on first."
"I don't know."
"He's on third, we're not talking about him. . . ."

With split-second timing, steady characterization and perfectly polished edges, the routine goes on for five minutes or so, never once growing tiresome, going overboard or becoming predictable. At least, not predictable in the negative sense. Everyone in the audience knows exactly when Lou's about to get back on the word merry-go-round, although they're sometimes with him as Bud throws in the newest curve: a pitcher named Tomorrow, a left-fielder named Why.

It was this sketch that caused a sensation when the duo were booked on radio's "Kate Smith Show." But it was only one of many that Abbott & Costello had picked up in vaudeville, from standard wheezes like "The Lemon Sketch," "Crazy House" and "Go Ahead and Sing" to a variety of pun bits like "Watts Are Volts" and "Gold Ore What." No other comedy team had as many polished routines to offer, each one made a classic by *them* even though many were in the public domain. In fact, only one, "Slowly I Turned," has really been picked up by others after Abbott & Costello laid down their definitive version of it.

The difference between Bud and Lou could be seen offstage from the start. Bud was, by general consensus, the introvert; quiet, shy and amiable. Lou was the catalyst who stood up to studio bosses, had the ego necessary to negotiate tough deals and had the desire and drive to lead both men to fame and fortune. Lou was the gambler, and Bud the follower, usually with a slight grumble. Bud was against the team's moving out of vaudeville, even though vaudeville was dying. And it was Bud who had the most misgivings about trying movies. Lou was conservative too, but in more positive ways. He insisted on bringing their tried-and-true routines before the public, who "rediscovered" them and wanted them over and over in movie after movie.

Following "The Kate Smith Show" in 1938, the boys went to Broadway with *The Streets of Paris*, then tested films with *One Night in the Tropics*, containing a fragment of "Who's on First" and some other bits. By their next film, *Buck Privates*, they were a smash, and remained a top box-office attraction throughout the 1940's.

Buck Privates is essentially "The Best of Abbott & Costello's Stand-Up Routines" with some songs added. In it they performed many of their radio favorites. (In radio, incidentally, the team had remedied one defect: they sounded alike. Costello adopted a higher-pitched voice, and Bud got a bit gruffer.) In subsequent movies, the team always included a set stand-up bit such as "Floogle Street" or "The Horse's Fodder," although they developed more visual comedy as well, with Costello proving to be a master at spontaneous-looking slapstick.

The duo developed an almost unlimited supply of word-confusion routines. It's easy to remember Lou jumping off in frustration and hysteria when Bud started in with "We must take a U-drive. It's Hertz," or "When the flu flies we must flee," or "I'll get you a loan in the bank."

"It's gold ore," Bud begins one routine. "Gold or what? It's gotta be gold or something," Lou shouts.

"It was made by a smith," Bud continues.

"Couldn't a Jones make it?"

"You take a shovel and you go down into the mine. You locate the mother lode. Then you strike the vein. . . ."

"When you say to me that I have to go into a mine with a shovel and hit my mother in the vein while she's carrying a load—that's going too far!"

Sometimes they went pretty far with the concept, doing bits about Mrs. Pike's Pekingese dog ("Get me Pike's Peke") or getting into an argument about a girl who lives in a flawless room ("Don't she fall through?") and eats her board three times a day ("Where does she get all that lumber?"). But they attacked each routine with freshness and enthusiasm, and audiences roared over these snappy quickies, and over the more involved bits in which sly Bud would dupe his pal into loaning him $50, or eating mustard, or playing a radio loud enough to get himself into trouble with the police.

Lou would get into wild ad-libbing, and Bud, the perfect straight man, knew exactly when to cuff him back with a "talk sense, Costello" or "get serious." Or perhaps Costello would end things with his long, wistful "I'm a baaaaaaad boy."

The team feuded during the mid-40's, with Lou demanding a larger percentage for his role as star comic. The rift could easily be seen in movies like *Little Giant* and *Time of Their Lives* where Abbott is a supporting player only. On radio Bud was sometimes the butt of the joke: "Heyyyy Abbott! Where do all the little bugs go in the wintertime?" "Search me." "No thanks, I was just askin'!" The rift was eventually smoothed over and Abbott & Costello continued on into the 1950's.

As the 50's wore on, Abbott's health began to deteriorate. He suffered from epilepsy, and the terror of sudden seizures and his anxiety over these attacks drove him to alcohol. He was having some trouble keeping up with his partner. The team split up officially on July 14, 1957. Costello made one film on his own, but died suddenly just two years after the break-up.

Abbott, driven more by the demands of the I.R.S. than anything else, briefly teamed with Candy Candido to perform the old routines, but was too ill to handle the rigors of a demanding performance schedule. In 1967 he played himself and Stan Irwin played Lou in a cartoon series.

In later years, he had nothing but kind words for the memory of Lou Costello, passing over any controversy by insisting there were "never any arguments." However, Bob Thomas's controversial biography described not only intense drama in the duo's lives (Costello's year-old son drowned in his swimming pool, yet the team went on radio that night with their routines) but also Costello's intense drive. The book incensed relatives of both men, and Chris Costello's *Lou's on First* came up with tempering evidence often contrary to reports from Thomas's sources.

DON ADAMS

More famous now as a TV comedy actor, Don Adams started in stand-up and still performs routines in Las Vegas from time to time. In the late 1950's he was good enough, and bad enough, to be ranked with Lenny Bruce, Tom Lehrer and Shelley Berman in *Time* magazine's infamous attack on "Sick-Nik" comics.

Back then, Adams would open his act with something like this: "I

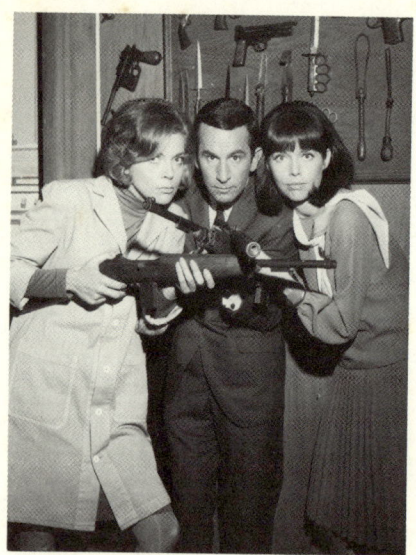

b. Donald Yarmy, April 13, 1926, New York, New York

Records:
Don Adams (Signature SM 1010), The Detective (Roulette R 25317), Roving Reporter (GNP–Crescendo s-91), Get Smart (United Artists UAL 3533), Don Adams Live At the Sands? (United Artists UAS 6604).

TV:
The Bill Dana Show (NBC 1963–65), Tennessee Tuxedo (syndicated 1963), Get Smart (NBC 1965–69; CBS 1969–70), The Partners (NBC 1971–72), Don Adams' Screen Test (syndicated 1975), Inspector Gadget (syndicated 1983–); Check It Out (1985, Cable).

Broadway:
Harold.

Films:
The Nude Bomb (aka: The Return of Maxwell Smart), Jimmy the Kid.

Video:
Inspector Gadget (Family Home Entertainment).

read an article in the paper today which I think is quite important. It's about the new Russian atomic submarine. And it says that the new Russian atomic submarine set a new world's record, two minutes, forty-eight seconds for submerging, surfacing, firing and submerging again. This cuts two minutes off the previous world's record and I think that these men deserve a lot of credit—especially the ones that were left on deck."

Acknowledging sick humor, he had a popular routine in which he told an airline crash joke and then added, "Sitting in the audience tonight are some relatives of the victims of the last terrible plane crash at La Guardia . . . Mr. Thompson who lost a wife and two children—Mr. Thompson, would you stand up and take a bow please . . . let's give him a nice hand, folks. No tears . . . just take your bow and shut up . . . and here's the man who owns the garage where the bodies were stacked. Nice of you, sir, to give up all that garage space. . . ."

Years later he enjoyed keeping an edge to his humor, adopting dashes of the Don Rickles approach (to a ringsider: "Do the words 'get out' mean anything to you, sir?") along with a hip bit on his half-German wife, who "still gets mail from a cousin in Argentina." At the wedding, he said, "My wife was so nervous her monocle kept falling off. And then after the wedding my side of the family signed the wedding book—and her side of the family burned it . . . not the wedding book . . . they burned my side of the family. The reception was great. Her father was a lot of laughs once we got him away from the machine gun. . . . His idea of a good time is a forced march to Milwaukee."

Adams's real family life has had its share of storminess. He's been married three times and has four children. He grew up on 93rd Street on the Upper West Side of Manhattan, remembering, "My mother was an Irish Catholic and my father was a Hungarian Jew. When they married, both families disowned them."

As a kid he tagged along after a rowdy crowd that included Larry Storch and James Komack, who both started their careers in stand-up. After attending DeWitt Clinton High School in the Bronx, Adams spent four tough years in the Marines, and suffered a bout of black water fever at Guadalcanal. In 1948 he teamed up with Jay Lawrence. As "The Young Brothers," Adams recalls, "We did over 100 impressions in 20 minutes in our act."

As a solo he found the nightclub atmosphere stifling: "I worked in saloons and hated it. I'm a non-drinker for one thing, and I loathed getting to bed at six in the morning, getting up at 2 in the afternoon and spending my day in dark holes. . . . In nightclubs or theaters a comedian never knows what sort of audience he'll face. A routine can slay one group but die before another audience a few hours later. It's nerve wracking."

In 1954 he crashed an "Arthur Godfrey Talent Scouts" audition and won. On the TV shows of Garry Moore and Perry Como he developed such safe routines as "Bengal Lancer," "The Umpire" and "The Prosecuting Attorney," and began to hone a specific character—a straight, short-sighted authority, a know-nothing who thought he knew everything; he could be a blindly efficient soldier, a lawyer or a detective.

The general public got its first long look at this Adams character when the comic played Glick, the house dick, on "The Bill Dana Show" in 1963. Dana had written for Adams years before.

With a pompous facade of dignity, the little comic made self-deception funny. He showed the insecurity and doubts behind the bravado. In fact, an early catch-phrase Adams used in his variety show days, and repeated on the series, was the vulnerable, "You sure know how to hurt a guy," uttered when deflated by little things like the truth.

In addition to continuing club work, Adams discovered that his unique speaking voice offered comic possibilities in another field: he became the star of a Saturday morning cartoon show, as a penguin named Tennessee Tuxedo. The show had a respectable run. A Broadway try, *Harold*, didn't.

Glick the Detective was spun into Maxwell Smart, Agent 86 of Control ("86" being a bartender's term for a drunk who's had enough). "Get Smart" was a hit from the start. With his beady eyes narrowed into a steely squint of confidence, his posture cocky, his voice a high-pitched nasal sneer, Adams comically exuded self-made cool.

He could tell his enemies, "I'm a well-trained agent and I can withstand eight hours of torture!" But when his bluff was called, that hint of human frailty and chagrin entered Adams's voice: "Would you believe . . . six hours of torture?" Finally, barely holding onto his tattered bravado, "How about five minutes of spanking?"

The "Would you believe" phrase had emerged years earlier in a sketch written by Bill Dana. "As a matter of fact," says Adams, "I dropped the line from the skit. I just had no idea of its potential."

Like Dana, Adams builds comedy around catch-phrases ("Sorry about that") and solid jokes written by formula. A typical "Get Smart" set-up and punchline: "In a minute a dozen agents will break in here with guns and knives and kill me. Well . . . it could be worse. At least I have my health."

Adams won three Emmy Awards for "Get Smart," and became a more frequent, welcomed guest in Las Vegas. The best example of his stand-up work is his last album, 1968's "Live at the Sands." In recent years the "Get Smart" image has stuck: he's done movies, print and TV ads, and recently a cartoon series, all with secret agent themes.

ALLEN AND ROSSI

Considered the logical successors to Dean Martin and Jerry Lewis, Italian singer Steve Rossi was smooth if not suave, and Jewish comic Marty Allen was the child-like troublemaker. They were super-hot in the early and mid-1960's, burning up nightclubs across the country with their interview routines (Steve as straight man to Marty the astronaut, mechanical man, Playboy bunny, Oriental ball player, etc.).

Their humor was more gag-oriented than that of Martin and Lewis, mostly because Allen was a different breed of man-child from Lewis. While Lewis was a manic little monster, Allen, with his mournful nasal voice, mass of jet black cotton candy hair and saucer-sized eyes, looked like a kid with stage fright. As the act warmed up, Marty would get more impish, spouting smart answers and wisecracks, but basically there was surprise humor in Rossi's attempts to handle a wayward boy capable of saying almost anything that came to mind.

Typical of their patter is this fragment—Rossi interviewing Allen as Richard Burton's stand-in during the filming of *Cleopatra*: "I hear it cost $40 million to make *Cleopatra*." "Yeah, some girls are more expensive than others." "*Cleopatra*'s a mummy!" "No wonder, the way she fooled around."

Like the Smothers Brothers, the team could often get very silly (Allen:

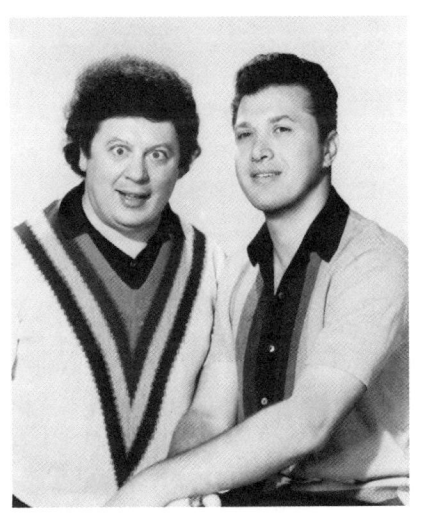

MARTY ALLEN   b. March 23, 1922, Pittsburgh, Pennsylvania
STEVE ROSSI   b. May 25, 1932

Records:
Hello Dere (Paramount 2270), One More Time: Hello Dere (ABC-Paramount 445), Too Funny for Words (Reprise R 6104), Great Society (Mercury 61015), In Person (Mercury SR 60979), Batman and Rubin (Mercury 11077), The Truth About the Green Hornet (Roulette 507). Rossi with Slappy White: I Found Me a White Man, You Find Yourself One (Roulette 42065). Bernie Allen and Steve Rossi (Laff Records).

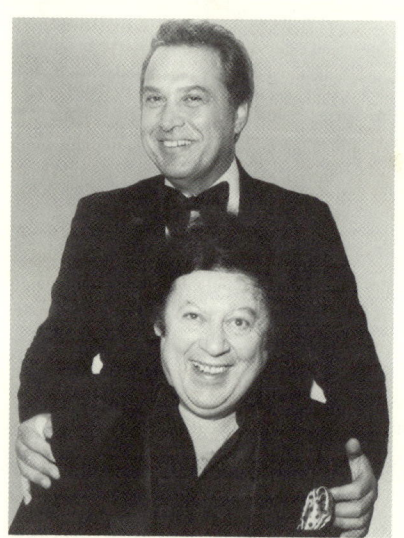

"I feel like a dog." Rossi: "How long have you felt like a dog?" Allen: "Since I was a puppy."). But in deference to the nightclub audiences that "discovered" them, they could also be pleasantly blue. Talking about Playboy bunnies, Allen opens his eyes wide and says, "Are they voluptuous!" Rossi: "Have you seen anything like it before?" Allen: "Not since I was a baby."

The lovable, rotund Marty Allen, so much the child, got away with a lot of very infantile one-liners ("Oh give me a home where the buffalo roam—and I'll show you a house full of dirt.") and grade-school comebacks ("What do you think about the Taft–Hartley Bill?" "I think we oughta pay it."). He made a catch-phrase out of a shy, New York–accented "Hello dere," the traditional opening line for any character Rossi was about to interview.

The "Hello Dere" album went gold in 1962, although their best effort was "Too Funny for Words," released the next year. The team appeared on "The Ed Sullivan Show" 40 times, including, coincidentally, all the shows on which The Beatles appeared, prompting Sullivan to remark, "If you can follow The Beatles, you can do anything."

In 1968, after a healthy run, the team amicably split up. Marty Allen continued as a solo, appearing in clubs and becoming a regular on TV game shows. Steve Rossi needed a new partner, and in rapid succession made show-biz news with his unusual choices. First came Rossi and Ross, with the aging Joe E. Ross. Ross had his own famous catch-phrase, or rather, catch-gasp: "Oooh! Oooh!," an excited ejaculation usually signalling the dawning of a brilliant (but ultimately silly) idea. He'd perfected it while co-starring with Fred Gwynne on "Car 54, Where Are You?"

The next combination was black and white, the interracial teaming of Rossi with veteran Slappy White, who had once been teamed with Redd Foxx. It was another interesting notion that didn't quite succeed. The public evidently wanted Allen and Rossi—and got it: *Bernie* Allen. Confused fans were not amused, nor was Marty Allen, who contemplated a lawsuit. Rossi eventually supplemented his singing engagements with work as a Las Vegas show producer and manager.

On October 7, 1983, Allen and Rossi reunited on stage for a weekend at an Atlantic City resort. Months before, Rossi caught Allen's solo act and was cajoled by the audience to come up on stage.

"People started yelling, 'Get him up on stage,'" Allen recalled. "To tell the truth, I didn't know Steve had so many relatives. So I brought him up and it was fun. Later the hotel management said that since nostalgia was in, would we consider coming back together." The team has made successful appearances since at many Vegas/Atlantic City resorts.

STEVE ALLEN

A "Steve Allen Encyclopedia," and a thick one, is needed to list all the accomplishments of this modern Renaissance man. A jack of all trades—and a master of them, too—Allen has made an indelible mark in music, literature and comedy.

The son of comedienne Belle Montrose (Milton Berle once called her the funniest woman in the world) and vaudevillian Billy Allen, Steve's early life was marked by a lot of travel, colorful "backstage" excitement and enough trauma to leave him a rather shy, sickly youth. His mother's mood swings following his father's death were bewildering. So were the unusual show people who sometimes took care of him.

"When other children were in kindergarten," he recalled, "I was sitting in theaters, either watching comedians perform or seeing early Laurel and Hardy, Charlie Chaplin, Charlie Chase and Buster Keaton movies."

He grew up in Chicago but, when his asthma grew worse, settled in Arizona. It was while a student at Arizona State Teacher's College that the journalism major became interested in radio: "I started as a comedian in radio and I sort of came out of that rather than nightclubs or vaudeville. Consequently much of my early radio comedy was sort of loosely in the Fred Allen/Henry Morgan tradition."

He dropped out of college to become a disk jockey in Phoenix. He was in the Army briefly, but his asthma problems led to an early discharge. By 1948, Allen was in Los Angeles, doing a free-wheeling music and talk show, demonstrating his ability to ad-lib and fill the time with witty conversation. At the time he was also flexing his creativity in other ways, writing magazine columns, doing the commentary for a film called *Down Memory Lane* and composing a hit song, "Let's Go to Church Next Sunday."

He quickly transferred his radio show to television, and a 1950 local late-night variety show in New York blossomed into the legendary "Tonight Show," where Steve Allen dazzled the nation with his humor and inventive stunts.

Allen not only created the first successful national talk show, he also introduced many of the "bits" that have become comedy staples. He joked with people in the audience, played "Stump the Band" with them, conducted put-on phone calls to strangers and performed stunts (he dove into a tub of Jell-O and once festooned himself with tea bags and was dunked into a giant cup).

He gave audiences "The Man in the Street" interview with up-and-coming comics such as Don Knotts, Louis Nye and Tom Poston. The list of comedians he discovered is a lengthy one. And there was a favorite comedy character, "The Question Man."

The Question Man was able to figure out the question to almost any answer. Like these: "The answer: Butterfield eight three thousand. The question: How many hamburgers did Butterfield eat?" "The answer: Frankincense and Myrhh. The question: Name an obscure comedy team." "The answer: 33 1/3, 45 and 78. The question: What are the measurements of your unmarried sister?"

He could draw belly laughs by simply reading, with appropriately outrageous emphasis, the hot-headed "Letters to the Editor" appearing in New York's *Daily News*. He was capable of great charm, wit and whimsy, and his hip bits of silly improvisation made him cool enough for a young generation to want to imitate.

"I always manage to see something ridiculous in whatever matter I have under consideration," he once said, although his serious side caused second wife Jayne Meadows to describe him as "not subdued but silent, gentle, pre-occupied." Lenny Bruce put it more simply: "He's very aware of societal problems . . . the most literate comic I ever met . . . and the most moral."

Once asked if he worried about his ratings, he said, "Good God, no, I am worried about mankind's rating." He said, "Man was not put on this earth primarily to have hit record albums, to be utterly irresistible to the opposite sex, to use cocaine or to wear the tightest possible jeans." He insisted that people who employ words like "bleeding hearts" and "do-gooders" were "dry-hearted do-nothings."

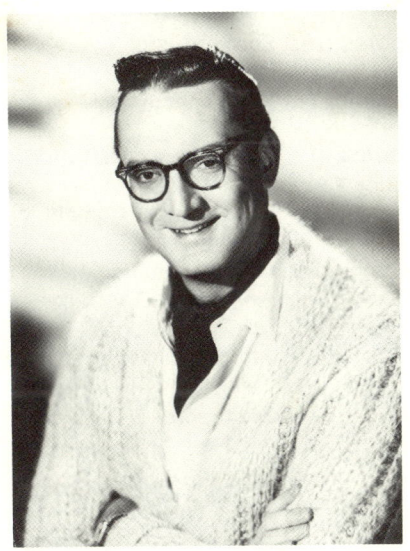

b. December 26, 1921, New York, New York

Records:
Funny Fone Calls (Dot 3472, reissued as Casablanca 4228113661), More Funny Fone Calls (Dot 3517, reissued as Casablanca 4228113671).

Compilations:
Laugh of the Party (includes "Very Square Dance"; Coral CRL 57017), Fun Time (includes "What Is a Freem?"; Coral CRL 57072).

TV:
Tonight! (NBC 1954–57), The Steve Allen Show (CBS 1950–52), The Steve Allen Show (NBC 1956–60; ABC 1961; syndicated 1962–64, 1967–69), I've Got a Secret (CBS 1964–67), Steve Allen's Laugh Back (1976), The Big Show (1979–80), The Steve Allen Comedy Hour (CBS 1967), Meeting of Minds (PBS 1980), The Music Room (Disney Cable 1984), The Comedy Room (Disney Cable 1984), The Start of Something Big (syndicated 1985).

Films:
Down Memory Lane, I'll Get By, The Benny Goodman Story, The Big Circus, College Confidential, Warning Shot, Where Were You When the Lights Went Out, The Comic, The Sunshine Boys, Heart Beat.

Songs:
This Could Be the Start of Something Big, Picnic, Houseboat, On the Beach.

Scores and Show Music:
A Man Called Dagger, Sophie, Seymour Glick Is Alive and Sick.

Books:
Funny People, Funny Men, More Funny People, Fourteen for Tonight, Mark It and Strike It, Curses, Schmock! Schmock!, Meeting of Minds, Explaining China, The Talk Show Murders, Beloved Son: A Story of the Jesus Cults, Ripoff: The Corruption That Plagues America, Not All of Your Laughter Not All of Your Tears, A Flash of Swallows.

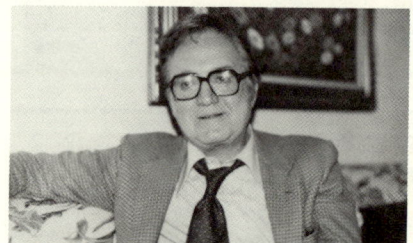

The man with "a relaxed amusement with life itself" has a Groucho Marxian genius for interrupting himself to attach a joke to a sentence, or inserting a parenthetical pun. Refusing membership in an organization he remarked, "I was invited to sit on the committee—and if there's anything I'd like to do to that committee it's sit on it." His ad-libs come quickly off-stage, too. Once a waiter spilled hot coffee on his head. "I'm terribly sorry, sir, is there anything I can do?" the waiter asked. "Yes," Allen answered, "would you please drop a little cream and sugar up there, too?"

While he was giving breaks to new comics, and to old ones out of favor, and in between shows where he was covered by red ants or driving cars into solid blocks of ice, Allen was active writing books of short stories and poetry and dozens of serious nonfiction works. He made 30 record albums, composed his theme song ("This Could Be the Start of Something Big") and is listed in the Guinness Book of World Records as the "most prolific composer" in modern times, with over 2,000 tunes to his credit.

Over the decades he's had several talk shows in many formats, conducted one-man jazz shows, wrote the Broadway musical Sophie and many revues and—one of his proudest achievements—created the "Meeting of Minds" series for PBS.

Yet despite the awards and accolades, Allen remains self-effacing, with a shy sense of humility. And although he has impressive credits, he does not have the appearance of a "driven" person. He gets 10 to 12 hours' sleep and mentions, "I have a lot of mental energy, but not any more physical energy than anyone else (never having been anyone else, I can only conjecture about that)."

"In the typical day I'm likely to touch on several if not all of the creative areas. Literally every day I write a few jokes, or funny thoughts—ideas for comedy plays or monologues, material I might create and send some other comedian if it's not my style of performing humor. And I carry a little tape recorder at all times."

Allen is of course a capable stand-up comic when he finds the time, and is one of the premiere speakers at public functions, roasts and charity events. The Allen wit as a master of ceremonies, after-dinner speaker and stand-up star was the subject of the book Schmock! Schmock! (the title is based on his popular nonsense catch-phrase). It included many gems:

"On this show tonight for the National Association for the Advancement of Colored People we also have in the audience some Negroes, as well as a few blacks. It's admirable that Negroes, blacks and colored can come together and work out their differences."

Following up a prune whip commercial, he observed, "A man would have to be pretty low to whip a prune. Think of it, my friends, a prune is little, it's old, wrinkled, defenseless. You show me a man who would whip a prune and I'll show you a man who would beat an egg."

He wondered aloud how an educational toy company could spell its name "Playskool," and riffing on baseball, he noted, "new teams have names with a terribly commercial ring to them. Like Houston Oilers . . . Milwaukee Brewers. If that's the way it's going to be, they should rename all the old teams so that the names correspond to the image of the city . . . the Chicago Gangsters beat the Boston Stranglers today . . . and on the international sports scene, the Paris Peace Talkers won a close one over the Philadelphia Cream Cheesers. . . ."

Allen's always been adept at audience participation, too:

"How can I win at blackjack?" someone asked.
"Use a real blackjack."

"Do you believe in reincarnation? What would you like to come back as?"

"I'd like to come back as fast as I can."

"Where were you and what were you doing when you thought of that great song 'Gravy Waltz'?"

"I was sitting at my piano, writing a song as I recall."

Witty, hip and flippant, but never cruel in his humor, Allen remains one of the most admired, respected and *liked* comedians in show business.

"My dominant gift is for the composition of music," says Allen. "I write several songs a week and I have done that for a half a century." His current workload usually involves tours in which he plays jazz piano (alone and with bands), book projects, TV specials and comedy writing. The flow is unending.

Allen once commented philosophically on the flow of life: "No matter how unhappy you are at the moment, you can be absolutely certain that before the passage of much time, you'll feel quite happy. Unfortunately, the other side of the coin is also true. No matter how much fun you're having this afternoon you can be certain before the passage of many days, you'll feel quite depressed about one thing or another. So it's an endless cycle that stops only with your death. It's not particularly cheering when you're having a good time, but then one never tends to think of such things at such times."

Recently Allen commented on his own career. Noting the ease with which he was able to write songs, do sketches and find an audience for his comedy, he said, "the world has patted me on the head and said, 'that's nice, you can do that, we'll put you on the air. We buy that.' And I don't think that's how it's supposed to be. You're supposed to work in an attic, and slave, or sleep with the producer—something you've got to suffer and give up. And I never had to do any of that. It's all been fun." He chuckled and added, "Thank you, world."

WOODY ALLEN

"Woody Allen, Stand-Up Comic 1964–1968." Although the title of the reissued records of the era sounds like an obituary, Allen's short life as a nightclub comic produced some of the funniest and most influential monologues of all time.

"A nightclub act is really murder to write," says Allen. "You can only perfect it by performing it long before it's ready. You know you're going to go up there and die for a while." Of his first year in the business, he adds: "It was the worst year of my life. I'd feel this fear in my stomach every morning, the minute I woke up, and it would be there until I went on at 11 o'clock at night."

Most people think every year is traumatic for Allen, and that neurosis and fear are constantly with him. The premiere comedian of modern-day anxiety grew up with myriad insecurities and received mediocre grades in school, but contrary to his image, little red-headed Allen Konigsberg was not a complete disaster. He was a solid second baseman for a Police Athletic League team (and dreamed of becoming a Brooklyn Dodger), was good at track and even qualified for the Golden Gloves boxing tournament (his parents ultimately cancelled his fighting ambitions).

"I was not a good student," Allen recalls, "no good in math, Spanish, history or anything. I didn't study . . . I lived in the movies. I'd go seven

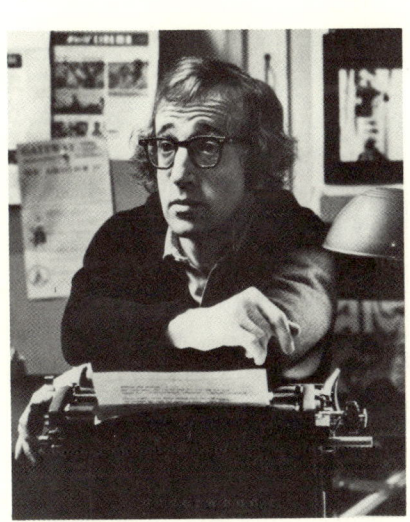

b. Allen Stewart Konigsberg, December 1, 1935, Brooklyn, New York

Records:
Woody Allen (Colpix SCP 488; once rereleased on Bell as "The Wacky World of Woody Allen"), Woody Allen II (Colpix CP 488), Woody Allen III (Capitol ST 2986). His three albums were reedited and reissued on a two-record set known as: The Nightclub Years: 1964–1968 (United Artists UAS-9968). A slightly different version came out as: Woody Allen Stand-Up Comic 1964–1968 (United Artists UA-LA 849, reissued as Liberty LWB 00849, reissued as Casablanca 2-7145).

Films on Video:
What's Up Tiger Lily (Vestron), Take the Money and Run (CBS/Fox), Love and Death (CBS/Fox), Sleeper (CBS/Fox), Everything You Always Wanted to Know About Sex (Warner), Zelig (Warner), Annie Hall (CBS/Fox), Manhattan (MGM-UA), Broadway Danny Rose (Vestron).

Plays:
Don't Drink the Water, Play it Again Sam, Floating Light Bulb.

Books:
Getting Even, Without Feathers, Side Effects, Four Film Scripts.

Bios:
Woody Allen (Adler & Feinman), Films of Woody Allen (Myles Palmer), On Being Funny (Eric Lax), Loser Wins All (Jacowar), Woody Allen (Lee Guthrie), But We Need the Eggs (Diane Jacobs), Love, Sex, Death . . . Woody Allen's Comedy (Foster Hirsch).

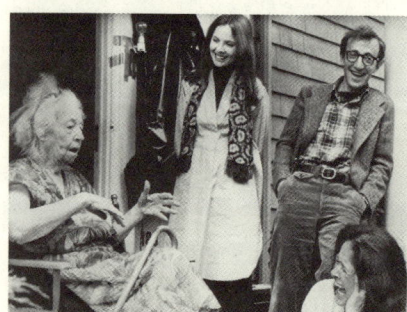

days a week and sometimes sat through two or three shows. The movies served as my education."

Allen started his career writing one-liners for such newspaper columnists as Earl Wilson. The first to make it into print—when Allen was 15—read "Woody Allen says he ate at a restaurant that had OPS prices—over people's salaries."

From writing quickies for columnists, Allen found employment working for a publicist. Bon mots in the papers attributed to such stars as Guy Lombardo or Arthur Murray were not "overheard at" a movie premiere or star party: they were scribbled on the subway by Midwood High Schooler Allen, who got $25 a week for his work.

At 17 he became a full-time comedy writer, joining NBC's staff at $175 a week. He wrote for Peter Lind Hayes, Herb Shriner and others. In 1957, his work for Sid Caesar won him a Sylvania Award, and the following year he was nominated for an Emmy. Ultimately he made $1,700 a week as a staffer for "The Garry Moore Show." Allen, who'd developed a reputation as the shy kid with weird ideas, couldn't get many through with Moore: "They preferred to do sketches where Carol Burnett falls down."

Allen's major influence in stand-up was Mort Sahl. It must have been immensely encouraging to him to see someone step up dressed in ordinary clothes, using a therapy-style delivery, loading his jokes with hostility, psychological jargon and spontaneous wit. In 1960, Allen put together his own act. Shelley Berman, the first new-wave neurotic comic, was one of the earliest to give Allen a break, introducing him to a club audience, letting him go on after his own show.

The following year, Allen's agents, Rollins and Joffe, secured work for him at The Duplex in New York's Greenwich Village. Painfully nervous, Allen went through a torturous period, encouraged by his agents, propelled by his innate competitive drive. At the Hungry i he was so unhinged by hecklers he turned his back on the audience, mumbling and plodding along in a daze until the club owner mercifully put the spotlight out.

At first some of the one-liners were similar to other comics' conceptions, especially those of such childhood influences as Bob Hope. Of his tough neighborhood, Allen cracked, "the kids stole hubcaps—from moving cars." But soon the 5'6", 125-pound comic developed his persona as the mousey, weak, intellectual loser with an underlying streak of fight and fantasy.

As "Heywood Allen," he recounted his neurotic boyhood ("I used to steal second base, and feel guilty and go back"). He couldn't have a dog, but his parents got him an ant. He trained it ("Kill!") only to encounter Sheldon, a bully: "Spot was with me. I said KILL! And Sheldon stepped on my dog." He described the warmth of family: "This is an antique pocket watch . . . my grandfather, on his deathbed—sold me this watch."

"Paranoia, anxiety, alienation, insecurity, these have always been very pregnant sources of comedy, you know? Sure I've used them," Allen says, "but the way you present yourself, comedically, just happens . . . you develop your own style instinctively, without, I think, a lot of calculation. And ineptness is simply one of the great comic traditions."

Allen's monologues struck a chord with many. He became the personification of the stepped-on, anxiety-ridden urbanite, too civilized for a brutal world, fearful of crime, women, men and almost everything else. He lived in fantasy and shared it with his fans: the story of aliens who come to earth to bring us their laundry, a squad from the public library surrounding Allen's house to get their books back, a moose who fights a married couple in a moose suit for first prize at a costume party. The fantasies were agonies (a talking elevator that turns anti-Semitic) and ecstasies ("It so happens on my honeymoon night my wife stopped in the middle of everything and gave me a standing ovation").

His potent one-liners, the pain and pathos he delivered in a throw-away line, his persona and his ability to time and phrase a joke to perfection amazed even veteran comics like Groucho Marx. Critics loved to quote Allenisms: "I was caught cheating on a metaphysics final—I looked within the soul of the boy sitting next to me.... I have an intense desire to return to the womb—anybody's.... My one regret in life is that I'm not somebody else."

By 1963 the young comic was successfully touring the chic nightclubs. The following year he was getting $10,000 for a concert. He was approached to do the screenplay for *What's New Pussycat*, and ended up with a small part as well. More movies followed. He began writing plays. By 1968 Allen had phased out his stand-up comedy, although he made occasional appearances in the early 1970's, and even showed enough confidence by that time to face an audience for a "question and answer" segment. Allen has always been quick with an ad-lib: "What is one of your biggest thrills in life?" he was once asked. "Jumping naked into a vat of cold Roosevelt dimes."

At first Allen's movies were filmed versions of stand-up material. His fantasy of chain-gang workers escaping "posed as an immense charm bracelet" turned up visually in the gag-filled *Take the Money and Run*. One could easily imagine Allen spinning the plot of *Bananas* or scenes from *Everything You Always Wanted to Know about Sex* into short stories like his earlier "Moose" routine.

Allen progressed with each film, scoring meaningfully with *Sleeper* and *Love and Death*. He also produced short comic magazine pieces which were collected into books. Here Allen could satisfy his need for quick creative gratification in the midst of a long movie project. Unlike monologues, these pieces could be embroidered with more lasting images, deeper wit. One-liners appeared in print form: "Not only is God dead, but try getting a plumber on a Saturday night."

Allen won an Academy Award for his most ambitious blend of comedy and characterization, *Annie Hall*, a film about which he had doubts each day of shooting. "I have, I think, an appropriate amount of self-loathing," he says, "and I think that's important for everybody. I don't trust people who are too confident about themselves . . . but to not take yourself seriously is important, to not think you're so hot because you're not."

Many films have followed, with intentionally and unintentionally varying amounts of humor. Most have been interesting, rewarding and challenging ("If you're succeeding too much, you're doing something wrong," says Allen). Each experiment has been greeted with detailed analysis by critics.

Allen was married twice: to Harlene Rosen (1954–58) and Louise Lasser (1966–70). He's remained a very eligible bachelor since.

Over the years Allen has retained a frenzied cult following. The man who has captured modern-day problems of confusion, anxiety and anhedonia so well is admired by some, identified with by others and sought out as a kindred spirit by a variety of mentally uneasy people. Allen's simultaneous need for a certain amount of attention and legitimate anxiety and revulsion toward pesty, well-meaning fans has led to mutual ill-feeling and paradoxical pictures of him in public places muffled in oversized hats. A peak in lunacy was the appearance of an entire book devoted to fans' dreams about Woody. Allen's views on the subject were expressed in *Stardust Memories*, which foresaw, with shocking irony, the tragedy of John Lennon's death.

Fans still seek out the man who has been so obsessed with questions of life and death, and who has gone through two decades of psychoanalysis. They figure he's gotten through so much, he must have an answer for them. To Natalie Gittelson in *The New York Times* he explained part of his philosophy:

"There's such widespread religious disappointment, a general realization about the emptiness of everything that's very hard for the society to bear . . . a society with so many shortcomings—desensitized by television, drugs, fast-food chains, loud music and mechanical sex. Until we find a resolution for our terrors, we're going to have an expedient culture—directing all its energies toward coping with the nightmares and fears of existence, seeking nothing but peace, respite and surcease from anxiety . . . we've got to give up the immediate, self-gratifying view. We've got to find the transition to a lifestyle and a culture in which we make tough, honest, moral and ethical choices simply because—on the most basic, pragmatic grounds—they are seen to be the highest good."

It's a speech that recalls Chaplin coming through the make-up to deliver a message in *The Great Dictator*. As to his day-to-day amusements, he says, "I get fun out of a few diversions. Basketball. Playing the clarinet. And other foolish things, like going for walks, drifting in and out of revival houses, buying records, sitting on park benches . . . what I'm doing for a living is what I would do for amusement . . . I write."

Allen's current work continues to veer between comedy and deep psychic grappling, and his persona remains a fascinating set of paradoxes: loser and Lothario, angst-ridden weakling and angry, persistent anarchist, cynic and idealist, pessimist and optimist. And paradox often shows up as a device of his comedy: "I don't believe in the afterlife . . . although I am bringing a change of underwear."

While he continues to write plays and make films, there remains, on a few records, the sharp, rich and well-constructed legacy of his stand-up act. This material would be considered a pinnacle for anyone—but it was only the beginning for Woody Allen.

MOREY AMSTERDAM

"The Human Joke Machine," Morey Amsterdam differs from the other one-liner specialist, Henny Youngman, by letting the customers choose their own poison. He often calls out to the audience for topics and then fires back the jokes. Between patter he'll saw a few notes on his cello. Like Youngman with the violin, Amsterdam found this prop a good way to punctuate punch lines and space out the laughs.

For the times when there wasn't a friendly voice out in the audience, Morey didn't hide behind the cello. He simply became his own friendly voice. Turning his head slightly to one side, he'd call out, "Hey, why don't you tell some drunk jokes!" And without missing a beat, he'd reply with a deadpan, "Funny you should ask," and go right into them. It was a cute bit of business that worked well for the cute (5'6") little comic.

While Amsterdam seemed in size and attitude like an affable, good-natured and harmless jokester, he proved he had the stamina and guts for stand-up work by appearing at Colosimo's, one of the most notorious speakeasys in Chicago. It was there that the fledgling comic entertained some of the toughest gangsters around.

"Maybe they thought I had a machine gun in my cello case," he told *TV Guide*, "but the racket guys loved me. Al Capone called me 'Kid.' He'd pick me up and drive me out to his home in Cicero. He'd cook spaghetti for me and I'd play Italian songs for him."

Charles G. Dawes, then the Vice President of the United States, once caught Amsterdam's act and was so impressed he invited Morey to dinner. Later that night, Morey turned up at Capone's home: "It was the one night in my life that I had dinner with both the Vice President and the president of vice."

An accomplished cellist, Amsterdam grew up in San Francisco: "My father was concertmaster of the San Francisco Symphony Orchestra. We had guests in our house like Caruso, Lily Pons and Paderewski." Not only was Morey a quick study with the cello, he was a superior student, graduating from high school at 15.

Morey first appeared on radio as a boy soprano, but within a few years he was disappointing his father and delighting radio audiences by his switch from classical music to comedy. At first he wrote for such performers as Jack Benny, Robert Benchley and Bob Hope. For Will Rogers he penned, "Our congressmen are the finest body of men money can buy." Amsterdam was soon a star on radio himself. He never forgot the cello—or his father's wishes—and when he eventually played a concert with the Los Angeles Philharmonic, it was his father's proudest moment.

Amsterdam combined comedy and music, writing several novelty songs including his signature tune, "Yuk-a-Puc." "Yuk-a-Puc" was a nonsense word chorus that divided comedy stanzas. A typical line went: "I got an aunt named Minnie, weighs 264. When she sits on the chair, there's so much of her there, most of her sits on the floor." Chorus: "Yuk-a-puc, yuk-a-puc, yuk-a-puc, yuk-a-puc, yuk-a-puc." Few songs had so many built-in yuks!

"The only thing we can turn on in our house without getting Morey Amsterdam is the water faucet," said Fred Allen. And he was right. In the late 1940's and 50's, Morey was all over the dial. He was a pioneer in television, starring in his own show in 1948. "The Morey Amsterdam Show" was set in a nightclub, allowing for both comedy and variety acts. His nightclub staff included a waiter played by Art Carney and a cigarette girl played by aspiring author Jacqueline Susann.

Amsterdam was also a regular on many quiz shows, and the co-star with Jerry Lester of "Broadway Open House," NBC's first try at a late-night variety program. But his "five happiest years in show business" were the ones spent on "The Dick Van Dyke Show." As comedy writer Buddy Sorrell he was a natural, playing the seasoned veteran whose sharp one-liners added punch to Rob Petrie's cerebral comedy and visual humor. His easy one-liners spiced up almost every script. "I am Buddy," Amsterdam recalled. "Buddy is not only a comic, but an experienced writer, a fellow who knows timing and funny situations." He was nominated for an Emmy in 1966.

Morey appeared often on TV after "The Dick Van Dyke Show" ended, played dinner theater and nightclubs, and toured in a topless "This Was Burlesque"-type review, which was produced as a special for cable TV. Long married to Kay Patrick and father of two children, at age

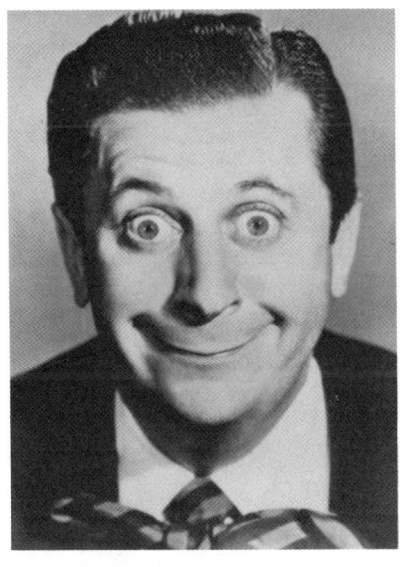

b. December 14, 1912, Chicago, Illinois

Records:
Funny You Should Ask (Marsh MLP 101M), The Next One Will Kill You! (Roulette R 25196).

TV:
The Morey Amsterdam Show (CBS 1948–49; Dumont 1949–50), Broadway Open House (NBC 1950–51), Battle of the Ages (CBS 1952), The Dick Van Dyke Show (CBS 1961–66), Can You Top This (syndicated 1970).

Songs:
Rum and Coca Cola, Oh My Achin' Back, Why Oh Why Did I Ever Leave Wyoming, Yuk-a-Puc.

Books:
Keep Laughing, Morey Amsterdam's Book for Drinkers—or Betty Cooker's Crock Book.

69 Morey was temporarily stalled by a triple-bypass heart operation. He came back several months later and resumed his career. "I am a very, very lucky man. God was with me," he said, "and I give Him thanks." Letters from his fans poured in, giving him their thanks too, for so many memorable moments of comedy.

PETE BARBUTTI

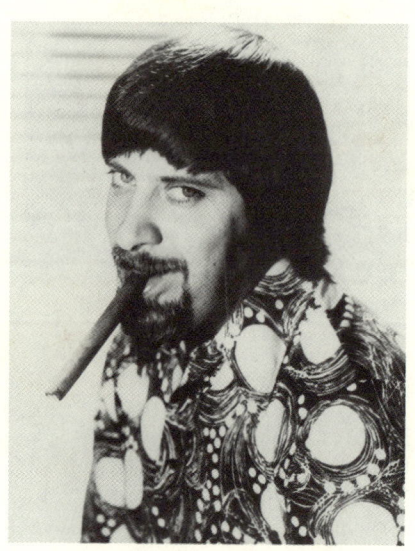

b. May 4, 1934, Scranton, Pennsylvania

Records:
Here's Pete (Vee-Jay VJ 1133), The Very Funny Side of Pete Barbutti (Decca DL 5008), At the Sahara (Contrast).

"Jazz and comedy are alike," says Pete Barbutti, "you take a basic premise and do different things with the idea, making it fresh and new each time." A successful jazz pianist, he "gradually, over the course of a light year, slipped into comedy full time. Although I've always been relatively uninhibited, the class clown and all that in school, my career was always in music."

Barbutti took accordion lessons when he was 11 and within a year was picking up spending money playing at Polish and Italian weddings. In high school he studied percussion, sat in with the University of Scranton's band and was selected "first chair" percussionist by the Scranton Philharmonic Orchestra.

He supported himself by operating accordion schools in Carbondale and Honesdale, Pennsylvania, and after service in the Army Reserves (he became assistant conductor for the 79th Division Band) he played in several groups including "The Millionaires," which toured the country for six years and was a Las Vegas attraction.

"I was the least inhibited member of the group and I would announce the songs," he recalls. "Eventually I got bored and the introductions got more important than the songs." In 1962 he became a full-time stand-up comic, and to get away from Vegas, where he was known as a musician, Barbutti took a few gigs in Spokane, Washington. After a few months of playing American Legion halls and small clubs, his manager got him a job writing and starring in a special for a local TV station.

"He told me I'd have to write all the music, all the comedy, and even rehearse the singers. He also told me there was no pay—but we'd get the tape."

With some misgivings, Barbutti went through with the deal and the tape was duly given to his manager, who literally haunted "The Steve Allen Show" trying to get someone to watch his client's work. "He went to their office every day. Finally as a joke they got one of their go-fers, just a kid, to watch the tape. He got one of the writers, the writers watched, they got Steve, they got the producers, and two hours later they called me. It happened out of nowhere."

A set of tours with Nat King Cole further advanced Barbutti's reputation. With his background in jazz, Barbutti demonstrated an easy-going hipness, a sly, offbeat style.

Many of Barbutti's early routines had to do with music. He did routines satirizing the different styles of singers, including amateurs who can't find the right key and after charging high up the scale suddenly end up sinking low when they can't hit the notes. He did a whimsical bit on a back-up singer who breaks out on his own, only to baffle audiences by singing nothing but the "ooooh, aahhhh" harmony parts and none of the lyrics. He did riffs on sound-alike pop tunes and pop disk jockeys, and a music and comedy routine on an "Accordeen School" where students are suckered into buying accordions. In between he did light, conversational bits about semantics, jazz lingo and cool vs. straight folk, which recalled the ad-lib sound of Mort Sahl and Lenny Bruce. Like Bruce, he often played to the band, comfortably encouraged by their laughter:

"I've been advised against that all my life, playing to the band, but in any legitimate art form you should never pursue the common denominator. If the public likes it and buys it, that's all well and good, but if they don't at least you've been honest about what you're doing. So I always worked to the band, and if the public catches on, and they usually do, all the better. I prefer to work quasi-hip clubs, jazz clubs, but I work other ways too."

Through the 1960's, Barbutti became known as a "comedian's comedian," and audiences loved being in on the jokes. But he had accessible silliness for all, including a routine on bullfights:

"Let's talk about the land of dignity, passion and romance, the land of the bullfight. ("Ireland!" a heckler shouts out.) Ireland? No sir, the word was bull *fight* . . . there's only one country this romantic: Passionate Poland! Have you ever seen a Polish bullfight? The big difference is in the attitude of the bull. The Polish bull is well adjusted and doesn't want to fight. There are several ways to arouse a bull. Number *two*. . . ."

As the fight gets underway, "the arena becomes very solemn, for the local clergy appears, and he consecrates the animal. And everyone stands up and shouts 'Holy Cow!' Wanna hear something worse? Then the people complain, because no matter where you put them, they're sitting behind a Pole!"

Barbutti's made over 500 TV appearances, including "The Tonight Show" which he continues to do a dozen times a year. He's achieved a comfortable balance for himself, touring when he wants to, turning down sit-com roles ("I have a tough time doing something that's bad without saying something about it—how many sitcoms around are any good?") and lately doing a few TV shows in Canada, his own humor show ("Pete's Place") and a loose-formatted celebrity cooking series.

He is still a favorite of other comics, many of whom come to see Barbutti when he performs in his hometown of Las Vegas. In the audience during the taping of his last comedy record were such diverse stars as Shecky Greene, George Carlin, Don Rickles and Chevy Chase. Although the image of comedians is a frantic, hyped-up one, Barbutti is one of many popular "low-profile" comedians who aren't driven, who can enjoy life without a constant spotlight. And here's one who has no aspirations to "serious" movies, either: "The way I see life I'm not sure I could do a serious part," he says, " 'cause life is so wacky to me."

BELLE BARTH

"The Hildegarde of the Underworld," as Walter Winchell dubbed her, Belle Barth was originally a singer-pianist who had successes with such standards as "You're Nobody Till Somebody Loves You." By the 1950's and 60's she'd become more of an entertainer in the tradition of Sophie Tucker, a woman Belle very much admired. She found risque, burlesque-style material suited her, and the songs became incidental to the jokes.

A fixture for decades in the Catskills and later Miami Beach, she became notorious for a series of comedy albums released and re-released on several minor record labels. Over three million copies were sold of these "Not for Air Play" lps, every one loaded with bawdy, "Over Sexteen"-type humor. For adults, and for the children who snuck the

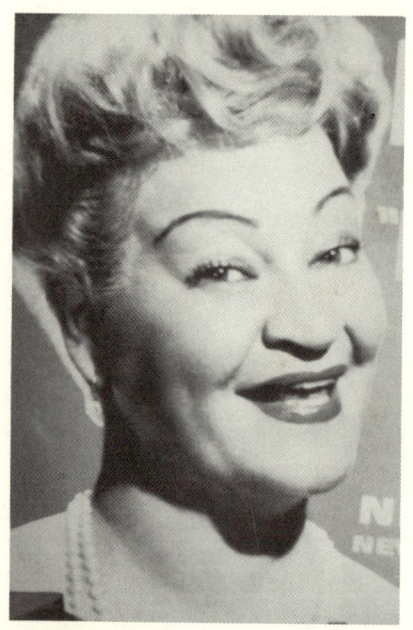

b. Belle Salzman, April 27, 1911, East Harlem, New York; d. February 14, 1971

Records:
In Person (Laugh Time LT 901), If I Embarrass You Tell Your Friends (After Hour Records LAH 69), Her New Act (Riot R 301), Wild Wild World (Record Productions LP 14,000,001), Belle Barth in Las Vegas (Record Productions LP 14,000,002), Hell's Belle (Laff A 115), The Customer Comes First (Laff A 109), I Don't Mean to Be Vulgar, But If It's Profitable (Surprise 169), Book of Knowledge "Memorial Album" (Laff 180).

albums out and listened to them as well, Barth offered cracks that were hip enough at the time to stop people cold, then heat them up.

It took a few moments to get some of Barth's one-liners: "Remember that song 'I used to kiss him on the cheek but now it's all over'?" "Two women were at a Mau-Mau feast. One says, 'Oooh, the food is so yummy.' The other says, 'Yeah, I'm having a ball.' " "Hear about the French diplomat who kisses babies before they're born?" Belle also gave her listeners a crash-course in Yiddish and Italian pseudonyms for private parts. She could take some of the vulgarity out of a joke by couching the four-letter words in colorful Yiddish slang. And like the best madam, she had a cute and condescending way about her as she guided her eager novices through then-unfamiliar slang words and actions—like "69."

"My next story is a little risque," she would say with all the innocence of a kindergarten teacher. And then, when the audience was leering, laughing and loving the shock of their raunchy roller-coaster ride through sexuality, she'd become bolder and bolder: "Hear about the girl who couldn't join the Key Club 'cause she didn't have a key—so she joined a country club . . . hear about the girl who swore she was a virgin, sat on a fire hydrant and slid right down?"

And true to form, the audience revelled in it, calling out jokes till Belle would squelch 'em with a line like "Hey! Shut your hole, girlie, mine's makin' money." It was all a rather innocent form of vulgarity, and quite acceptable in its proper place. The problem for Belle Barth was drinking. As one insider remembers, "When she drank, she got really dirty, and she'd get busted. She'd always go too far with four-letter words."

Barth, like Mae West, was never inconvenienced for long in her bouts with the authorities. After all, she was basically just offering a good time, with risque stories and funny songs. "I don't sing sad songs," she'd say, "people come to a nightclub to laugh. They wanna cry—they stay home."

Eventually Barth was able to hold forth at her own Belle Barth Pub in Miami, exchanging ad-libs with ringsiders, quick stories and swiftie parodies with a radical turn: "The Farmer in the Dell, The Farmer in the Dell . . . I had a cherry once but now it's shot to hell!"

To those who expressed indignation, she'd simply say, "If you're so refined, how come you know what I'm talking about?" Not as complex a philosophy as Lenny Bruce's, but an effective one. "If I embarrass you," she'd smile, "tell your friends!"

Barth's albums hold up fairly well, and, proving that times haven't changed that much, some of these jokes still turn up today, spoken by Vegas shock comics like Buddy Hackett, indicating there's still a market for vulgarity—as long as it's coming from somebody physically cute and nonthreatening.

ORSON BEAN

Broadway actor, author, frequent TV game show panelist, magazine columnist, founder of The Fifteenth Street School, Orson Bean is a man of many accomplishments. The first of these was stand-up comic, and in the 1950's he was one of the nation's best.

"I started as a magician," Bean recalls. He made trees out of paper, made a birdcage disappear and "hypnotized" members of the audience. The act was a fake, but Bean discovered that once on stage, and scared, audience volunteers did whatever they were told, even if it was a whispered "pretend you're hypnotized."

"A lot of comedians—W.C. Fields, Johnny Carson, Fred Allen and many others—started out with another skill like juggling or magic which they could use while you built up enough jokes and routines," says Bean.

Many comics share another trait: a scarred childhood. "My mother and father's marriage was, to say the least, tempestuous. She began to threaten suicide when I was about six years old. 'If your father ever leaves me, I'll kill myself,' she'd say. 'If you want me to stay alive, it's your job to keep him around.'"

The woman made some harrowing bluffs at taking her own life. Meanwhile, Bean immersed himself in learning magic tricks of illusion and escape, and was rebellious at school. When he was 16, Bean's father took a job in Alaska, leaving son and wife behind. Bean couldn't cope with his mother, who was now drinking heavily. He moved into a furnished room with the money he was making as a bus boy.

A week later, his mother killed herself. The suicide note read: "My husband has left me and my son won't come to visit."

It was after a hitch in the Army that Bean seriously began his performing career, and took his un-serious name: "I was working in a nightclub in Boston and I had an opening line—My name is Dallas Burrows, Harvard 48, Yale 0. And it never got anything. And the piano player in the band said it was because I didn't have a funny name. So every night he gave me a different funny name to use, like Roger Duck. And one night I used Orson Bean and it got a laugh so I kept it. Upon such tiny turns of fate. . . ."

Bean's sophisticated humor and ingratiating, whimsical shaggy dog stories initially didn't go over as well as his magic, but when he reached New York, he finally found his audience. He told of his Vermont heritage ("My grandfather hates Southerners. Stay away from Hartford, he used to say") and did a good-natured sketch about a man on trial for having sex with an ostrich.

He was invited to perform his material in a Broadway revue, John Murray Anderson's *Almanac*. At the same time he was appearing as a headliner at The Blue Angel. He was the first comedy lp star for Fantasy Records (to be followed by Lenny Bruce) and was often on "The Ed Sullivan Show." He studied acting, anticipating more varied roles on the stage. And it was a good thing he did, for suddenly he couldn't work on television.

"I got blacklisted. Not because I was a communist, but because I was horny for a communist girl; I went to a few meetings with her. Then I stopped working on TV as a comic and I worked in theater because the blacklist never had any influence in the theater because there weren't any sponsors."

Looking back, Bean characteristically views the experience as "interesting . . . the non-survivors became bitter or in certain cases committed suicide or gave up the business. But the survivors' lives took very interesting turns. I went into theater. So did Zero Mostel, who was a character man in movies. He was completely blacklisted and took off-off Broadway jobs which he never would've done because the money wasn't right. He took risks, and that led to *Rhinoceros* and *Fiddler on the Roof* and he became a major stage star because he was blacklisted. Jack Gilford, too. And there are many, many cases of people who went on to do fascinating and interesting work because their lives had to change.

"I was annoyed at the time—I knew there was a blacklist around and I was playing with fire—all I'm saying is that I went into it with my eyes open. Not that they weren't bastards, the blacklisters, they were. But it's

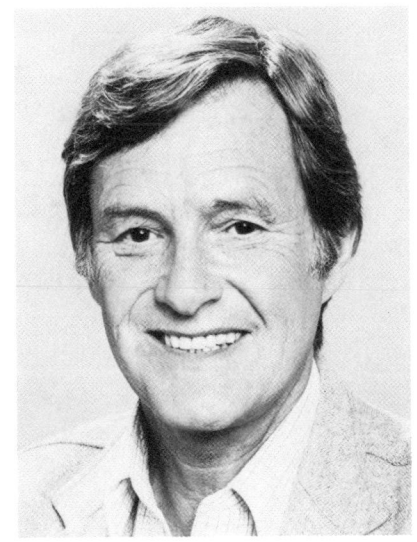

b. Dallas Frederick Burrows, July 22, 1928, Burlington, Vermont

Records:
At the Hungry i (Fantasy 7009), I Ate the Baloney (Columbia CS 9743).

Broadway:
Men of Distinction, Almanac, Will Success Spoil Rock Hunter, Subways Are for Sleeping, Never Too Late.

Book:
Me and the Orgone.

an interesting and totally unknown part of the blacklist that prior to the McCarthy days, large parts of Hollywood were controlled by members of the Communist party or extreme leftists.

"In some cases you had to be a left-winger to get into a movie where the writer and director were Communists. This went on for a period of years. And there were a group of right wing or reactionary actors who were furious about this, and when the McCarthy period came, they were only too happy to get their revenge . . . so it's all interesting. . . . If you're gonna be pissed off about it, well, that's dumb. I thought it was interesting to be blacklisted, to stop working for a year. I'm not saying I wasn't pissed off, but—what the hell. Learn what you can from it."

Bean also was interested in the kind of learning that came only from self-analysis. He was in therapy for 10 years, followed by studies in Reichian psychiatry and Orgonomy.

Politically, Bean turned from being a campaigner for John F. Kennedy in 1960 to campaigning for Richard Nixon in 1968. Professionally, he hosted "The Tonight Show" 100 times, and worked on game shows, but never returned to stand-up. One of his early jokes was about a town so small "the tide came out . . . and never came back." For a time, Bean left show business and wasn't coming back.

He's writing a book, "Love Letter to an Ex-Wife," about his "dropout" period from 1970 to 1979: "I entered into a period of being an old hippie and not pursuing a career but making a living doing talk shows and game shows." He confounded Johnny Carson by describing transcendental experiences communicating with butterflies. Young fans, unaware of his accomplishments in stand-up, knew him for his wacky ad-libbing on "To Tell the Truth."

"I stopped doing the talk shows and game shows about 4½ years ago because I really felt like getting back to work on the stage," he says. "I started paying my dues, working on the road. One day I was doing 'To Tell the Truth' and I just said 'Number Three,' and there was a long pause. And then I thought I really don't want to know if he's the real goat milker or not. So I just stopped doin' it. I had enough." He appeared on tour in *Mass Appeal* and *A Life in the Theater*. He presented his own adaptation of *A Christmas Carol*, *40 Deuce* and *The Show Off* with Jean Stapleton in New York.

While many comics draw their humor from hostility, Bean will always be remembered as one of the few "likable" comics who jested from the gentle side. When questioned about his stance as one of the first "nice" comics, Bean mused for a moment and said, "I think it just has to do with your character. The most important thing in my life has always been to be happy. I spent most of my life trying to find out how to be the happiest bastard who ever lived. And I spent years in analysis, all kinds of therapy to get there, but I think that just shows in your work. I have no interest in being dour, or unhappy. I don't mean that I've always been happy, but when I wasn't I wasn't satisfied with that. It wasn't the way I wanted to present myself. I never consciously thought about it, but I think that's true . . . it has to do with who you are and your attitude."

Bean's attitudes in comedy also come from his major influence, Stan Laurel. He corresponded with Laurel and was co-founder of "The Sons of the Desert," the fraternal Laurel and Hardy organization: "Whenever I get caught in traffic, or some stupid ridiculous thing happens to me, and I start to get pissed off, I say to myself, I would be laughing if this thing were happening to Stan and Ollie. Then I start laughing about it."

Now that Bean has left his whimsical sad-funny poems, Eucalyptus tree making and monologue sketches behind, one wonders what the quintessential Orson Bean stage role would be. Bean doesn't hesitate for a moment. The character he most enjoys playing on stage is Elwood P. Dowd, the fellow with the giant invisible rabbit in *Harvey*.

JACK BENNY

"Hello everybody, this is Jack Benny. There will be a slight pause for everyone to say 'Who Cares.'"

With that line Jack Benny made his radio debut in 1932. He stayed on radio for 23 years, starting his first series that season. He then starred on television in a long-running, classic program, and did occasional specials thereafter. By the time of his death he was probably the best-loved comedian in show business, viewed almost as a member of the family.

"I try to make my character encompass everything that is wrong with everybody," he once said. "On the air I have everybody's faults. All listeners know someone or have a relative who is a tightwad, show-off or something of that sort."

Almost from the start he pioneered a new type of humor, self-effacing, filled with human foibles, based not on "Top Banana" bombast and vaudeville pratfall but on characterization, timing and subtle inflection.

Benny studied the violin as a child. One of his first jobs in show business was as a violinist in the orchestra of a theater in Waukegan, the Chicago suburb that had become home. Today, the Jack Benny Junior High School stands there.

He met pianist Cora Sadisbury there, and the two got an act together. Other partners followed. When Benny joined the Navy during World War I, the seasoned performer was part of a traveling show that raised money for Navy Relief. Benny did more than play the violin and tell a few deprecating jokes before each number. He turned up in vaudeville skits, playing such characters as "Izzy, the Disorderly Orderly." He developed skills as a comedy actor and, in the hectic, slap-dash world of the revue, an ability to ad-lib. One time the lights failed while he was on stage, and he and pianist Zev Confrey kept the audience amused by a steady stream of improvised gags. Such experience helped make the young comic confident and poised as a stand-up star.

At first he was known as Ben K. Benny, but that name was a little too close to that of Ben Bernie. A sailor friend, using the then-popular catchphrase introduction, "Hiya Jack," gave Benny an idea for a likable new first name. By 1921, "Jack Benny: Aristocrat of Humor" was making $450 a week for his monologues. As George Burns recalls, "Even back then he did stingy jokes. Like the one about taking his date to dinner—and she got so excited she dropped her tray."

In 1926 he was on Broadway in *The Great Temptations*, and the following year he married the tempting Sadie Marks, later known to fans as Mary Livingstone. In 1932 he brought his low-key comedy to radio: with his sponsor's obvious influence, he was billed as "The Canada Dry Comedian."

Much has been written about that mysterious thing called "timing," maybe too much, since a great joke can withstand an indifferent or at least an unpolished delivery. But for those looking for a definition of "timing," it can be found in studying Benny. Like most comics who have a background in music, he knew the cadence and rhythm of a line and

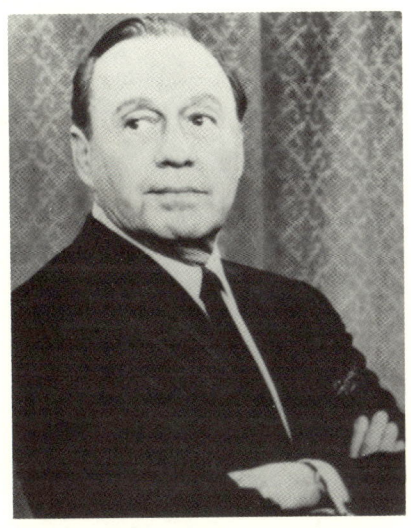

b. Benjamin Kubelsky, February 14, 1894, Chicago, Illinois; d. December 26, 1974

Records:
Jack Benny 1933 (Mark 56 #764), Jack Benny 1936 (Mark 56 #765), Jack Benny 1940 (Mark 56 #766), The Jack Benny Story (Radiola MR 4546), The Feuds of Jack Benny and Fred Allen (Radiola MR 2930), The Feud Continues (Radiola MR 1111), The Horn Blows at Midnight (Radiola MR 1068), Conversations in Hollywood #2 (Citadel CT 6029).

Compilations:
Son of Jest Like Old Times (Radiola #2), Golden Age of Comedy (Evolution 3013), Magic Moments from the Tonight Show (Casablanca SPNB 1296), The Minstrel Men (Colpix CL 434).

TV:
The Jack Benny Show (CBS 1950–64; NBC 1964–65).

Films:
Buck Benny Rides Again, Charley's Aunt, To Be or Not to Be, The Meanest Man in the World, George Washington Slept Here, The Horn Blows at Midnight.

Video:
Jack Benny Program 1958, 1959 (Video Yesteryear), The Big Time Variety Show (Video Yesteryear), Milton Berle Spectacular (Video Dimensions), The Jack Benny Show 1952 (with You Bet Your Life) (Video Yesteryear).

Bios:
Jack Benny (Mary Livingstone Benny), Jack Benny (Irving Fein), The Jack Benny Show (Milt Josefsberg).

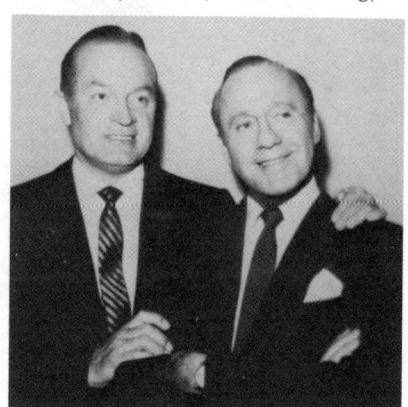

where to apply the emphasis. But also, like a master composer, he knew the value of silence.

Benny's personality encouraged this attention to timing. Sometimes bewildered or vacillating, he got giant laughs just by pausing and muttering "hmmmm." He also evinced the helpless frustration of the middle-class everyman with his pauses and then an irritated but hopeless "Now cut that out!"

One of the classic jokes on Benny (and few comics ever were the butt of so many so often) involves a thug approaching the comedian on the street: "Your money or your life!" he growls. After a pause, Benny says, "I'm thinking it over!"

That key joke evolved out of a very real situation of exasperation, and out of a hunt for the properly timed gag.

Two of Benny's writers, Milt Josefsberg and John Tackaberry, were trying to get that sequence down. Josefsberg thought he had it. "Your money or your life. . . . You mean I have a choice?"

It was a reasonable laugh-getter, but Tackaberry didn't like it. The irritation began to build. When Josefsberg demanded a smarter line from his smart-guy partner, Tackaberry snapped, "I'm thinking it over!" And that, unintentionally, was that. With . . . a pause.

By 1945 Benny's radio program was practically an institution, and other comics adopted humor based on character, sophistication and wit. At the time Benny wrote, "In the past 20 years, American humor—accelerated by radio—has come out of the barnyard . . . the public today demands more of its humor than a laugh at any price. It resents too much insulting, too much cynicism. In short, the public likes good comedy but it likes good taste even better." He went on to proclaim, "Nobody gets hurt on our program. It's all in the spirit of fun. We try to follow one simple rule: if it hurts it isn't funny."

The Benny character was so popular that the comedian couldn't get away from the jokes. When he visited President Harry Truman, carrying his violin case, a White House guard said, "What have you got in that case?" Benny shot back, "A machine gun!" The guard answered, "Thank God. I thought it was your violin."

Actually Benny made good use of his Stradivarius, helping to raise millions of dollars for charity, for Israel Bonds and for symphony orchestras. And he liked to spread his money around, but in ways that didn't "hurt" his stingy character. Once he hired out the Automat and gave each of his 400 guests two dollars worth of nickles for the machines.

Benny made a gradual crossover into television, wary at first of overexposure. But just as he had proved to be a welcome change from the vaudevillians, he contrasted well with the frantic, gag-oriented comics of early TV. When many ran dry, Benny was still around, still a top attraction.

He found that he was even more successful on TV, where audiences could see his "Hmmmm" accompanied by a hand raised whimsically to his chin, his long pauses accentuated by a flattened mouth and rolling eyes, his "stuck-up" comic egotism enhanced by his mincing gait. His relaxed monologues delighted audiences, as did his sketches. The program is still rerun, and episodes are available on videocassette. While it's true that, like Laurel and Hardy's, Benny's style is perceived as "slow" (it was, ironically, Laurel who criticized Benny for "holding his takes" too long), most audiences can still easily appreciate the foibles and catchphrases that made Benny such a beloved star for so long.

"We've never tried to be flashy," Benny said, "to dazzle the public each week with some new and tremendous spectacle. During my show business career I learned that people like to laugh at familiar things.

That's why we don't change too many things on our show. We know people like to share a joke—and that's our show—we share our jokes with them in the comfort of their home."

Benny, who prided himself on being a "good editor," knew how to pick excellent gags. He always shared the credit with those who came up with them. In the midst of his comic feud with Fred Allen, he parried an Allen insult with, "You wouldn't have said that if my writers were here."

Off camera Benny was something of a loner, a worrier who fretted to make sure his show went along perfectly. He was enough of a perfectionist that when, in later years, he did a sketch with George Burns in which he played Gracie Allen in drag, Benny shaved his legs for the part.

If he was not the type to be witty and "on" all the time, neither was he the stereotyped "morose" comic. Most found him to be kind and gentle, a low-key star. He could also be quite candid and surprising. To columnist James Bacon he nostalgically recalled his vaudeville days in San Francisco, when he finally had the money to afford clean clothes and attract showgirls: "My happiest days were putting on a pair of clean socks and then getting a blow job."

George Burns loved to tell of Benny's unusual "put-on" sense of humor. Once Burns called up just to say hello. "So hello," Jack said, hanging up. When Burns and Allen played London, Benny called Burns, ostensibly from California, said, "Hello, George. Sorry I can't be there," and hung up. A few moments later, Benny topped the put-on by strolling into Burns's London suite.

As Burns recalls, "Jack was a quiet riot. He stood there quietly and he'd kill the audience. I once saw him do something I don't think any other comedian could do. He walked on stage at Caesar's Palace, and he stood in the center of the stage, folded his arms and looked at the audience for practically a minute—and that's a long time. And the audience laughed, and they laughed loud. And he finally looked at them and said, 'What are you laughing at?' That was his opening. I don't think any other comedian around today could do that."

Benny was always working, playing nighclubs, doing concerts, raising money for charity. At 80 he said, "Age is a matter of mind over matter—if you don't mind, it doesn't matter." He was scheduled to star in *The Sunshine Boys* with Walter Matthau, but two months before the start of filming, he fell ill. He had cancer of the pancreas, and the end was quick.

Many fans were shocked at his passing. Although 80, he looked closer to his fabled 39, and he had been making public appearances regularly. "He was stingy to the end," Bob Hope said at the funeral. "He only gave us 80 years and it wasn't enough. . . . How do you say goodbye to a man who is not just a good friend but a national treasure. . . . No one will ever replace Jack Benny."

MILTON BERLE

"Good evening ladies and germs. I mean ladies and gentlemen. But why should I call you ladies and gentlemen? You know what you are. I just want to (burp) . . . I don't remember eating that. I just got back into town from Florida. I flew in. My arms are very tired. . . . These are the jokes! What is this, an audience or an oil painting?"

This is vintage Milton Berle, to the point of stereotype. But Milton Berle is more than "the thief of badgags" (to use Walter Winchell's

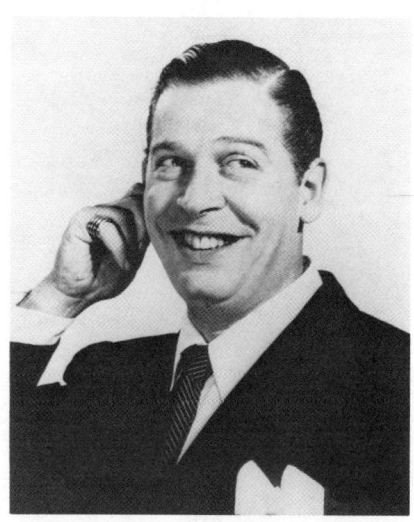

b. Milton Berlinger, Harlem, New York, July 12, 1908

Records:
Uncle Miltie on Radio (Radiola MR 1064), Starring Milton Berle (Mark 56 #778).

TV:
The Milton Berle Show (NBC 1948–56), Kraft Music Hall (NBC 1958–59), Jackpot Bowling (NBC 1960–61), The Milton Berle Show (ABC 1966–67).

Films:
Sun Valley Serenade, Tall, Dark and Handsome, It's a Mad, Mad, Mad, Mad World.

Broadway:
The Goodbye People.

Off-Broadway:
Goodnight, Grandpa.

Video:
Milton Berle Show 1963 (Video Dimensions), Buick-Berle Show 1954 (Video Dimensions), Milton Berle Spectacular 1962 (Video Dimensions), Texaco Star Theater 1951 (Video Yesteryear), Milton Berle Show 1963, 1966 (Video Yesteryear), Kraft Music Hall 1955 (Video Yesteryear).

Book:
Milton Berle: An Autobiography.

nickname for him). He's a consummate pro at stand-up, and rather than considering him an "anything for a laugh" comic, critics have come to realize that his art is in making anything *get* a laugh. Calling on his memory of over 50,000 jokes, utilizing brawling ad-libs, audience shpritzes and a barrage of physical comedy bits, Berle can devastate an audience in a way few can. He can overpower almost any crowd and make it his.

His talent was evident when he was only a child. He won a local talent show doing a Charlie Chaplin routine and from then on his stage-struck mother made sure he became a star in show business.

The woman saw more than a chance for fame. Milton's success meant a change in the family's finances. The Berlingers lived in poverty in Harlem, sometimes went hungry, and once were even thrown out into the gutter. Berle never forgot the feeling when "everything you own in the world is vomited out onto the street."

As a youngster Berle made many silent films, appearing in Chaplin's *Tillie's Punctured Romance* and *The Perils of Pauline* (in which he was tossed from a moving train). His mother tried all the old tricks to get young Milton on the stage and she made up new ones. Once she snuck the boy backstage, hoping to push him before the audience while Al Jolson was performing. The idea was to show how cleverly he did a Jolson impression. Instead, the boy was summarily bounced out of the theater. Another gambit was more successful. After he won a job in the chorus, Milton's mother ordered him to dance out of step with the others. He got big laughs for this, and fortunately, the director kept the bit in the show.

"When I stopped doing kid acts and started out on my own as a stand-up single," Berle recalled, "my mother would be out in the audience for every show, laughing hysterically, getting the crowd started." One of Berle's earliest ad-libs, to the sound of one voice laughing, was "Thanks, Mom."

The versatile performer was an emcee at Loew's State at 17, and learned juggling and card tricks as well as jokes. He would later display musical talent, too, writing dozens of songs including "Sam, You Made the Pants Too Long." As an emcee and comic, he developed a brash style that kept the show going under any circumstances. "The Milton Berle image I made up myself: the brassy, wise-cracking drugstore cowboy, streetcorner comic. The put-down artist: these are the jokes, folks."

Berle was aggressive, and he also had the attitude that he was tops at delivering jokes. Some comics resented the nonchalance with which he would make a joke his own, and his idea that these jokes were not told best until told by him. Fred Allen once approached him with a stack of photos, saying, "You're using my act, you might as well put my photographs in the lobby, too." Decades later, at a roast, Jackie Mason cracked, "We're all here paying tribute to our own material."

Of course, a simple joke thief could not have risen to the stardom Berle attained. He made $10,000 a week in vaudeville, and in 1929 made his first television appearance—over experimental closed circuit in Chicago. By 1931 he was soloing at The Palace, and was a popular face in the Ziegfeld Follies.

Berle was a colorful character offstage, noted for his prowess with women and his ineptitude at gambling. One of his famous comic shticks, dressing in drag, had its origin in a real-life episode where Berle had to be a girl to get a girl.

His latest lady friend lived at The Barbizon, a strictly women only residence in New York. Berle dressed up as an elegant Barbizon deb and effortlessly slipped through the lobby. Once in his lady's room, he slipped off the drag and spent the night.

Berle shook up audiences with his drag humor: "Before television when Gypsy Rose Lee became popular, I was doing my nightclub act.... I'd start with my street clothes and take off everything down to a bra with tassels and a gold thing on my crotch with a heart right in the middle."

The top banana personality, bombastic jokes and wild visual antics were often in evidence offstage. He once said to Christine Jorgensen, "I'll show you my old nose if you show me your old cock." Sometimes, Berle paid for his brashness. A gangster-type, who didn't like to be kidded, had his own way of silencing a wiseguy. He grabbed Berle, hauled him up by his tie, and stuck a fork into his neck.

Berle began making movies in 1938, but it was in 1948, as the first major personality to move into television, that he made his greatest mark in show business. He became "Uncle Miltie" to millions, the rollicking star whose live Tuesday night show at 8pm caused many to buy a TV set for the first time. So many people stayed transfixed, staring at the tube, that at 9pm water companies actually charted drops in water pressure—as people turned off their sets and went to the bathroom.

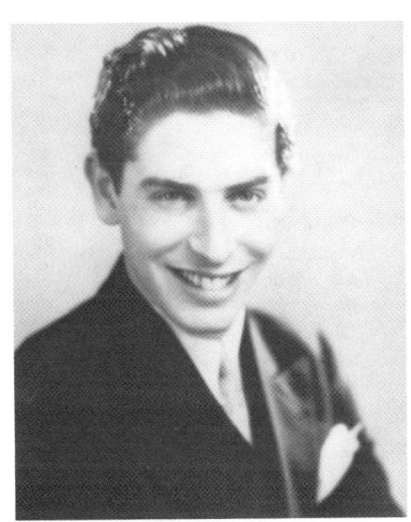

"I never used a cue card," Berle said. "Trying to remember was difficult, but by *not* remembering and mixing up and getting stalled and fluffing, the next line became funnier because of my ad-libs. Now where did I get the ad-libs? Only from the background of paying my dues and doing my homework in prior years in vaudeville and nightclubs. So if I forgot my monologue which wasn't on cards I'd go into what I remembered from Newark or San Francisco."

Berle signed one of the most talked-about deals in TV history, a contract with NBC guaranteeing $200,000 a year for 30 years. "The six million was considered a lot of money in those days," Berle recalls, "but it wouldn't seem like so much for stars now."

The symbol of the golden age of television, Berle remembers, "We did everything live. It was real, it was fun. You screwed up, tough. You had egg on your face. Now it's all tape and retakes and canned laughter. It's robbed TV of its spontaneity."

Berle was a sensation from his September 21, 1948, debut right through to the end of the 1950's. He was a frequent guest star on both comedy and drama series in the early 1960's, and starred in the movie *It's a Mad, Mad, Mad, Mad World*. Following another variety series in 1967, he pursued not only comedy dates but serious stage work. He turned in a brilliant performance in *The Goodbye People* on Broadway, and to perform in an off-Broadway play he turned down $70,000 a week in Vegas and accepted $1,000 a week. But despite the critics' raves for his serious acting, Berle remains the irrepressible comic.

He once organized a vaudeville tour with George Jessel. Asked why, in his 70's, he was doing such a thing, he said, "I do it because I'm hammy. You know what I say? Get this: Berle'd ham!"

"I don't think you should quit working, ever," he says. "If you do have to retire, find something else to do. You've got to keep your mind busy or you'll spend too much time dwelling on unpleasant things." He reflects, "It is quite sad when you see that here's a guy who makes people laugh and he doesn't get many laughs out of his own life. But that's the real story. I must say that's the truth.... I've got to hear them laugh. It's hammy, it's corny, but it's true."

His autobiography caused a stir, with its account of many sexual exploits with such women as Marilyn Monroe, Betty Hutton, Dorothy Kilgallen and Aimee Semple McPherson. It also contained this evaluation amid the laughs and the good times: "I have a lot of regrets about things I did and said, for the way I pushed and shoved and bullied during those hysterical years. My only defense, which is no defense, is the pressure. . . . You take a kid, make him a star . . . it's a miracle if that kid doesn't grow up to be a man who believes he's Casanova, Einstein and Jesus Christ all rolled into one."

Berle continues to delight fans with his fast, frantic comedy and heartfelt dramatic performances. There are many movies, recordings and TV kinescopes of past glory, too. But another legacy is yet to come. Berle has willed to the Library of Congress perhaps the most mammoth gift anyone has ever offered to the cause of laughter: his file of over five million jokes, carefully catalogued, "cross-indexed by subject, by comic, who did them first and where." Of course, five million index cards probably can't generate the laughter that an evening of Berle live can.

"You want to know my favorite thing to do after all these years?" Berle asks. "Anything where I can use make-up, take a bow and hear laughs and applause."

SHELLEY BERMAN

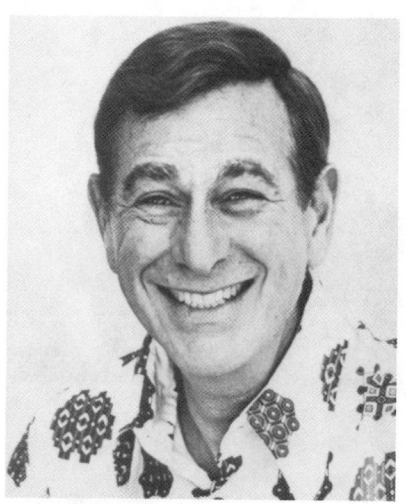

b. February 3, 1924, Chicago, Illinois

Records:
Inside Shelley Berman (Verve MGV 15003), Outside Shelley Berman (Verve MGVS 6107), Edge of Shelley Berman (Verve MGVS 6161), Personal Appearance (Verve V/V6 15027), New Sides (Verve V/V6 15036), Sex Life of the Primate (Verve V/V6 15043), Let Me Tell You a Funny Story (Metro M 546; a "best of" with new introductions).

The frustrations, neuroses and hang-ups of modern living ate up Shelley Berman, so he spat them back into society's face. It was a losing battle and his brilliant star faded, but at one time Berman was the top comic in the land, his finger gripping the weak pulse of the average besieged little man. The proof is still around on his many classic albums.

"I'm not a sick comedian," Berman would say, "I'm a healthy actor." But he couldn't make a healthy living as an actor. He joined the Woodstock Players in 1947 but struggled for ten years in a variety of odd jobs. Working with Chicago's improvisational Compass Players, he made the transition to stand-up comedy, but with an actor's sensibilities. He popularized the concept of the "comedy concert," where, in a nightclub setting, he would offer one-act miniatures and comic lectures.

Berman would portray Franz Kafka thwarted by a legion of long-distance telephone operators stealing his dimes and making him repeat names and numbers constantly. He gave a dissertation on the din made by an air conditioner. He created a vivid (but totally fictional) account of his father's wary but compassionate views on his entering show business.

Berman crafted his sketches with a poet's care, altering words and phrases for maximum effect. Basically shy and nervous on stage, he compensated by adopting a rigid, somewhat officious style of delivery. He also expected the crowd to be well-mannered, attentive and quiet. "If anyone breathes too heavily he gets a coronary," Lenny Bruce mocked. Berman's insistence on as much decorum as possible, and little noise (including "limited" bar service to avoid the sound of whirring blenders), added to his image as a finnicky perfectionist. But club owners didn't mind; not when Berman's comedy brought in huge crowds.

"Inside Shelley Berman" was the first comedy album ever to achieve Gold Record status. Berman almost formally introduces each sketch, including the brilliant "Morning After the Night Before" in which a man learns, slowly and painfully, of the havoc he caused at a drunken party the previous night. It's a telephone monologue, a device Berman discovered while doing improvisations: "I couldn't find a partner to work with one night, so I simply used the telephone—that's how the telephone began."

This led to another trademark: the bar stool. "When I began, all I had were telephone calls, and I can't imagine anyone doing ten-minute phone calls standing up, so I wanted to sit down. If I sat in a chair I couldn't be seen, so I borrowed a stool."

Berman's targets were almost always the agonies of everyday existence, small things that make pressure build: TV commercials, specks in milk, getting spinach between your teeth on a date, losing a burning cigarette while driving, trying to remove pins from a new shirt or keep a paper napkin on your lap. Small points they were, but not trivial ones, not when handled by someone so keenly aware of perverse human nature.

The infamous "Buttermilk" routine on his first album is typical. In private life, Berman could easily get upset with the lack of quality in workmanship, the lack of courtesy in sales help, the noisy degeneration of a peaceful environment and, manically and humorously taken to an extreme, the "ugly white map" left behind after the buttermilk has been enjoyed. Lenny Bruce seemed particularly awed and/or jealous over Berman's ability to wring laughs from such a slender topic. His capsule impersonation of Berman consisted of him muttering two words: "Buttermilk. Freud!"

Berman had more traditional routines, too, including an extended airplane routine lacerating stupid stewardesses, the negativity of plentiful air-sick bags and the general hysteria of crash jitters (a topic most 1950's comics seemed obsessed with). But Berman's sensitivity not only produced a clever monologue, but also led to its demise. When on December 16, 1960, a mid-air collision between two planes scattered 134 bodies across Queens, New York, Berman was shaken. The routine tasted like ashes in his mouth and he refused to perform it ever again. This was typical of the man Mort Sahl described as "a perfectionist who worries about everything, serious about his work, a method comedian." Today Berman does a more general routine on airplanes, with lines such as this: "Have you ever been frisked on a plane trip? They frisk you and then, on the plane, they serve and everybody has a steak knife!"

In the early 60's Berman was making $500,000 a year. His routines continued to blend gentle neurotic dementia with more hysterical concepts, like a man bleeding profusely and unable to find a doctor (he deliriously calls a gynecologist, assuring him his cut finger is on a "rather feminine" looking hand). Beginning another bit, Berman insults his audience as "well intentioned people who only want to help—and don't." He then launches into a morbidly funny sketch about a woman hanging off the ledge of a department store and one man's futile attempts to get help.

For material like this, Berman was awarded second place, behind Lenny Bruce, on most critics' sick comics list. *Time* magazine, running short of epithets in attacking the new-wave comedians, simply announced that Berman's face resembled "a hastily sculpted meatball."

Poet Louis Untermeyer hailed Berman: "He makes his audiences forget the cost and calamities of modern life by recognizing and, what is more, responding to its absurdities. He projects everyday occurrences so persuasively that, little by little, line by line, laugh after laugh, they become excruciating. This is Berman's prime gift: a way of turning ordinary happenings into extraordinary situations, of transforming personal mishaps into universal experiences. This is the role of the great comedians, to make one laugh, and think, and turning the thought over, to laugh again."

Around 1963 Berman perversely began bucking his successful image of the cerebral comic: "It was okay at the beginning, but after a while you grow out of that. I'm fed up to the chin with this so-called intelligentsia. When I began to be the darling of a certain select cult . . . I improved and enlarged my comedy devices." The result was the creation of a new character, the schlemiel, a goofy guy who can't get a date and is surrounded by fairweather friends. In a way, this was a natural evolution for Berman, who in conversation actually sounds closer to this character than to the intellectual lecturer of his first albums. But this delving into pathos blunted "The Edge of Shelley Berman," his third lp.

His fourth album, though, was a reversal, a hyper live performance, a "Personal Appearance" of raging intensity that blended all elements of his style: absurdity, real characters (the conventioneer calling home) and, in one masterful bit, dark comedy (a man calls the hotel desk clerk to complain there is no window in his room . . . no light switch . . . and now, no door).

Berman's compassion and pain were released with pinpoint sharpness in his pieces, but as might be expected, in private the comedian possessed some of the same characteristics as his thwarted, miserable characters. He appeared as a miserable man in an episode of "The Twilight Zone," grumbling because the rest of the world was not like him. Unfortunately, in the public mind the performer and the man held the same image exactly, and one incident served to drive the point home like a nail in a coffin.

As amazing as it seems, Berman insists his career was punctured by one vignette on a TV documentary. "Comedian Backstage," aired on NBC in 1963, offered Berman in concert. During his long, serio-comic "Father and Son" routine, a telephone rang offstage. Berman ignored it, but it was clearly audible.

Just a few days earlier he'd expressly insisted that the backstage telephone be removed from the hook during performance to prevent just such a problem. After the show, the cameras followed Berman backstage, where he erupted. Seizing the wall phone, Berman petulantly dashed the receiver down, to show that this was how it was supposed to be: receiver *off* the hook, dangling by its cord. On camera, staring in bewilderment, was Berman's agent, young Marty Klein.

Viewers didn't see all the stagehands, just the one man. "It looked like I was yelling at the kid," Berman recalled. Twenty years later he was still ruefully describing himself as "arrogant, a child, an idiot, a fool" in the eyes of viewers. He insisted his reputation for being demanding dogged him after that.

Allen and Rossi had a joke: "I was Shelley Berman's manager." "What happened?" "The phone rang!" It got a laugh from a general audience, more proof the problem wasn't all in Berman's imagination. As strange as it seems now, this was "scandal."

Still worse for Berman was what happened after his first surge of popularity. He was #1 in 1960, but now club owners could choose someone else, like the new #1, Bob Newhart (coincidentally another telephone comic). Coming up fast for the intellectuals was neurotic Woody Allen. The year Allen arrived, 1964, was the year Berman recorded his last album.

Allen's neurosis was visceral. Sexual frustrations were more universal than buttermilk woes. With people cynically ingesting carcinogens, who cared about oatmeal specks? The fastidious, uptight, proper, older comic with his brilliant bits that required some concentration was up against fast-paced, gag-oriented Allen, and the new wave of easy-going people like Newhart and Bill Cosby. And there was the bad rep rap, even though Berman was never late for a show, never drunk, never refused to go on, etc. etc.

"Little by little I tried to phase myself out of comedy," says Berman. He toured in stock productions of *Two by Two*, *The Odd Couple*, *The Rothschilds* and *Fiddler on the Roof*. He worked, but things weren't pleasant. The nadir came in 1978 when his son died of a brain tumor at age 12.

But over the years, the clouds began to lift. Berman began doing more and more comedy concerts. It may be a combination of a new audience unaware of dim scandal and rediscovering great comedy, and an old audience realizing that Berman's bits are better on the rerun than those of most new comics fresh from "The Comedy Store." Once again Berman is being recognized for his momentous achievements in stand-up decades ago, and for his continued talents, newer material and reliable ability to make audiences laugh when he makes personal appearances today.

BOB AND RAY

Some odd things were coming over the air at Boston's WHDH in 1946. There were strange commercials, like this one for sweaters, with an announcer saying, "We have two styles: turtle or V-neck. State what kind of neck you have." And sometimes it seemed another station drifted in, a bizarro, mirror-like duplicate that played short, enigmatic episodes of "Mary Noble, Backstage Wife" and "Mr. Keen, Tracer of Lost Persons," only they came out "Mary Backstayge, Noble Wife" and "Mr. Trace, Keener Than Most Persons."

What it was, was Bob and Ray.

Robert Brackett Elliott had always been a fan of radio, from Fred Allen and Stoopnagle and Bud to Raymond Knight. He and his parents sometimes went to New York and invariably they would visit one of the radio stations and sit in on a broadcast. Bob emulated these shows while still at Winchester High School, entertaining classmates with mini radio productions in which he played all the parts.

He attended the Feagin School of Drama, where his classmates included Angela Lansbury and Jeff Chandler, and after returning home got a job on WHDH. After World War II, he resumed his duties there, meeting up with recently hired newsman Ray Goulding.

Raymond Walter Goulding's father was a textile mill supervisor and the first man in the neighborhood to own a radio. Young Ray couldn't get enough, and so at 17, he landed an announcer's job on WLLH, a local station. The station was so small Ray eventually assumed a variety of responsibilities, from handling live broadcasts of high school basketball games to rewriting news copy on a quick deadline. Ray moved on to bigger radio stations, and then after the war turned up at WHDH where he did the news broadcasts during the morning show of Bob Elliott.

"I began staying in the studio and bailing him out with some chatter, what with all the awful records he had to play," Ray recalled. Tall, hefty, hearty-voiced Ray and mild-mannered, slight, sandy-haired Bob were an odd combination, and their style of humor was odd too.

Perhaps they developed their subtle humor by trying to slip jokes past sponsors who didn't like to be overtly kidded about their products. Bob and Ray's tongue-in-cheek parody was often right on the edge of reality, with only slight humorous inflection and exaggeration. Hip listeners became attuned to such "public service" announcements as:

"The National Parks Association reminds you not to throw things into

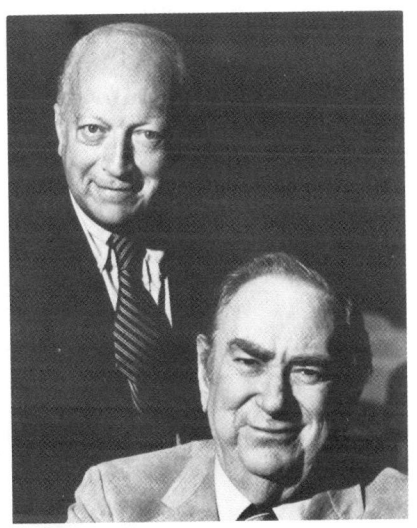

BOB ELLIOTT b. March 26, 1923, Boston, Massachusetts
RAY GOULDING b. March 20, 1922, Lowell, Massachusetts

Records:
Stereo Spectacular 1958 (RCA Victor LSP 1773), Bob and Ray on a Platter (RCA Victor LSP 2131), Vintage Bob and Ray (Genesis 1047), The Two and Only (Columbia S 30412).

Compilations:
Laff of the Party (Coral CRL 57017), Fun Time (Coral CRL 57072), Golden Age of Comedy (Evolution 3013), Golden Age of Comedy (RCA Victor LPV 580), Mary Backstayge (Radiola–Bob and Ray Productions).

Video:
Bob and Ray and Two Others (Pacific Arts).

Broadway:
The Two and Only.

Books:
Write If You Get Work: From Approximately Coast to Coast It's the Bob & Ray Show, The New Improved Bob & Ray Book.

the Grand Canyon. The Grand Canyon is your canyon. It's the deepest canyon we have. But it will cease to be the deepest canyon we have if tourists and campers keep throwing things into it. If you want to help this great campaign to preserve our national wonders, use the litter cans on your city sidewalks. Don't throw things into the Grand Canyon."

The duo had their own show, "Matinee with Bob and Ray," and began developing a set of weirdly named stock characters: Elmer W. Litzinger, Augustus Winesap, Mug Mellish, Mary McGoon and Ramses Fletch. They began to perform comedy sketches lampooning still-popular radio shows, and broadcast such mock special reports as the live remote from Utah where railroad workers connected track from the East and West coasts—only to witness a huge crash as the trains met head on.

Bob and Ray moved their skits, patter and fearless commercial parodies to New York in 1951. Before long they were literally all over both the radio and TV dials, credits including a WNBC radio show, a 15-minute TV show on WABC, an eight-year series for the "Monitor" radio show, and eventually programs on WINS and WOR. In the midst of this (1952 and 1957) they received Peabody Awards. Although mostly apolitical, they boldly took on Senator Joseph McCarthy as a satirical target. Along with Stan Freberg, they were really the only comedians still active in radio.

In 1955 the team formed their own ad agency, Goulding-Elliott-Graham (now Goulding-Elliott-Greybar) so they could produce the kind of humorous, interesting commercials that never seemed to appear on their shows. They had a hit almost immediately when they played Bert and Harry Piel for a series of beer commercials. They also made some records for RCA Victor which today are among the most expensive and sought-after rare comedy albums, often fetching $40 a copy.

The unusual team of two straight men appeared on television through the 1960's, but it was still in radio that they flourished. Even today, on National Public Radio, they amuse fans with their "Finley Quality Network" of programs and with such favorite characters as nasal-voiced newsman Wally Ballou and the McBeebee brothers who speak in mind-numbing near synchronization. Of course, being fraternal twins, full synchronization is obviously impossible.

In 1970 they starred on Broadway in *Bob and Ray, the Two and Only*, which was a huge success although their subtlety sometimes mystified elderly women at Wednesday matinees who would wander out at intermission and neglect to return.

The show offered viewers a variety of quirky stand-up routines. One of their finest and most inexplicable bits involves an exasperated interviewer and a representative of the "Slow Talkers of America." Bob, with elephantine pauses, asserts that "We . . . the slow . . . talkers . . . of America . . . believe in . . . choosing . . . our . . . words . . . carefully." Ray frantically tries to speed up the interview by trying to anticipate what Bob is about to say:

"We are . . . here . . ."
"In New York City—"
"In . . . the city of . . . New York . . . attending . . ."
"A convention!"
"Our . . . annual . . ."
"Convention—"
"Membership . . ."
"*Convention!*"

Ray's comic frustration and Bob's slow determination are in perfect counterpoint as the routine builds to . . . at last . . . the conclusion.

Equally memorable is the simple conversation between an interviewer and an authority on the Komodo dragon. Here the conversation constantly twists back on itself as a careless, uninterested interviewer and a dull guest repeat each other ad nauseum:

"The Komodo dragon is the world's largest living lizard. . . ."
"They're of the lizard family, aren't they?"
"Yes. They are the world's largest living lizard. There are two Komodo dragons at the National Zoo in Washington. The former President of Indonesia, Sukarno, gifted us with them."
"Well now, if we wanted to take the kiddies to see a Komodo dragon, where would we go to take the kiddies to see a Komodo dragon?"
"The National Zoo in Washington has two Komodo dragons. There is a stuffed Komodo dragon at the Imperial Palace in Nepal."
"I heard a foreign potentate gave us two Komodo dragons. . . ."

And on it goes. In cases like this, Bob and Ray's humor is like a slow-motion Abbott & Costello routine. The audience sees the frustration and confusion—and laughs all the more. Other times Bob and Ray material seems sublimely subliminal—fans who look deeply find satires of man's enigma and ennui. Sometimes it's the realistic parody that does it, or simply a whimsical, inexplicably funny concept, like the man who annoys his waiter by asking to order from a kiddie menu, because "I like children's portions, and I like to have my meat cut up for me." Typical of their radio work was an appearance by a "Food and Drink Imitator" named Fentress Synom:

"His shirt sleeves are colored like a skinless frankfurter . . . he is putting his arms simulating hot dogs at his sides, and it really resembles a pair of franks on either side of a plate piled high with beans! Wonderful. . . ."

In introducing a book of Bob and Ray scripts, Kurt Vonnegut, Jr. wrote that they feature "Americans who are almost fourth-rate or below, engaged in enterprises which, if not contemptible, are at least insane. And while other comedians show us persons tormented by bad luck and enemies and so on, Bob and Ray's characters threaten to wreck themselves and their surroundings with their own stupidity. . . . Man is not evil, they seem to say. He is simply too hilariously stupid to survive."

Typically, Bob and Ray are a comedy team that have a perfect chemistry on stage but seldom meet socially. There's no reason to, since they put in full days at their agency, on radio, and are together on performance tours. Bob is married (his wife was formerly married to Raymond Knight, who eventually was a Bob and Ray writer until his death) with three daughters and two sons. Ray has four sons and two daughters.

And the duo use these classic lines to end their shows: "This is Ray Goulding reminding you to write if you get work . . . And Bob Elliott reminding you to hang by your thumbs."

VICTOR BORGE

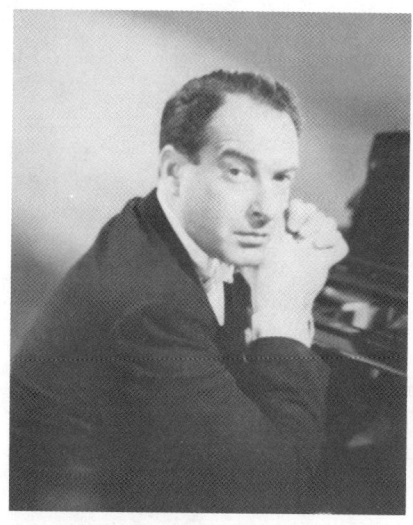

b. Borge Rosenbaum, January 3, 1909, Copenhagen, Denmark

Records:
Caught in the Act (Columbia CL 646), Comedy in Music (Columbia CL 554), Borge's Back (MGM 3995; aka: Great Moments in Comedy [Verve V 15044]), Piccolo, Saxie and Company (Columbia CL 1233), Hans Christian Andersen (Decca 734406).

TV:
The Victor Borge Show (NBC 1951).

Video:
Hollywood Palace 1968 (Video Yesteryear).

Books:
My Favorite Intermissions, My Favorite Comedies in Music.

There probably hasn't been an article about Victor Borge that hasn't included some reference to his being the "unmelancholy Dane." But Borge takes that in stride: "There is a bit of Hans Christian Andersen in every Dane. This gloomy Hamlet stuff is for the bards."

Borge's whimsical humor at the keyboard and his stand-up routines about oddities in the English language have kept audiences laughing for more than 40 years. Most of the incidental sight gags (adjusting the piano stool, playing the sheet music upside down, snapping the piano lid down on his fingers) were based on the mannerisms of a nervous recitalist. That man was Borge.

Although he made his orchestral debut at age 10 playing Rachmaninoff's Second Piano Concerto with the Copenhagen Philharmonic, these performances were always a trial: "I would live a year in a half hour. A mistake could ruin your career. I was scared. I was frightened. Around my 20th year I knew that if I had to go through this for the rest of my life I wouldn't last very long."

As a comedian in concert, Borge says, "I am my own master. I decide the tempo. I don't have to do anything that's given. I do whatever I feel at the moment. Nobody interrupts me, and all that I ever hear is civilized laughter. How can you ever tire doing this? Even when I go on with a heavy cold when I'm not feeling well, it takes over. It is relaxing."

Borge was a big star in Denmark, and he speaks Swedish and German as well. He made his first movie in 1936, *Miss Muller's Jubilee*. But within a few years, everything changed. Adolf Hitler came to power. Borge aimed some of his satire at Germany. "What's the difference between a Nazi and a dog?" he asked on stage. "The Nazi usually lifts his arm."

The comedian was relentless. So was the SS. "I was on the Führer's most wanted list because of my satires. I was able to catch the last troopship to leave Petsame, Finland, with only five minutes to spare."

Arriving penniless in America, Borge performed as a straight pianist. "Borge is good," a critic wrote, "but he's no Horowitz." Borge shrugged that off: "That should come as a relief to the parents of Horowitz."

He went to the movies every day, and learned English from watching the films over and over. He learned his jokes phonetically at first, and easily found humor in learning the language. Once he mused, "I don't understand some phrases. Take 'I look forward to seeing you.' Why don't you *listen* forward to *looking* me?"

"One night a woman came to me after a concert and said, 'I haven't laughed so much since my husband died.' My own English isn't too good. Somebody remarked to me, 'Spring in the air, Mr. Borge,' and I jumped eight feet."

He got his big break on Bing Crosby's radio show and became a weekly guest, performing over 50 times. He enjoyed even greater success on television. In 1953 he was calculated to have been the highest paid performer for what amounted to $2,917 a minute.

When Borge had his own TV show, he proved to be a conservative boss. His writers had to stay within a certain framework. He felt his audience wanted to see a certain thing from him, and in general, he didn't divert from his basic gentle piano fun and quirky monology. He evidently knew best, because he honed his routines until they were classics.

"If what a performer possesses is valuable, it shouldn't be changed for change's sake. Let him repeat his best stuff. Let new generations see it." He has hours and hours of classic bits which he chooses spontaneously.

Borge did "the same thing" 849 times, and it put him in the Guinness Book of World Records. He starred in the longest running one-man show in Broadway history, Comedy in Music, from October 2, 1953, to January 21, 1956. Theater critic Brooks Atkinson called him "the funniest entertainer in the world."

The balance of comedy and music is a difficult one. He says, "Some want music, some don't need music, some are bored when there is music, and some have come to laugh. There has to be enough musical content and humor to satisfy everyone." At times Borge has been asked to take an entirely serious route, but aside from his nervousness about performing "straight," he notes, "Humor looks at things both seriously and humorously. Seriousness has no other side. It is just serious."

Touring constantly, Borge has never worn out his welcome. Audiences are still eager to see his classic bits whenever he comes to town. He remains a very skillful monologist; even his accent and stop-start cadence are amusing. He knows how to use deadpan throw-away lines and sly understatement. When he goes to the piano, the audience remains guessing, thrown off by each offbeat bit of pantomime and foolery. As he adjusts his chair, stop-starts different pieces and tosses off ad-libs, the audience shares a mutual befuddlement, a good-humored euphoria and the knowledge that they're in on the put-on. An entire evening of false-starts, recognition humor in melding classical tunes with pop standards, or mild jokes about the English language could be wearying, but Borge's sparkling quirkiness and the audience's eagerness to aid and abet his parlor games always make for a satisfying performance.

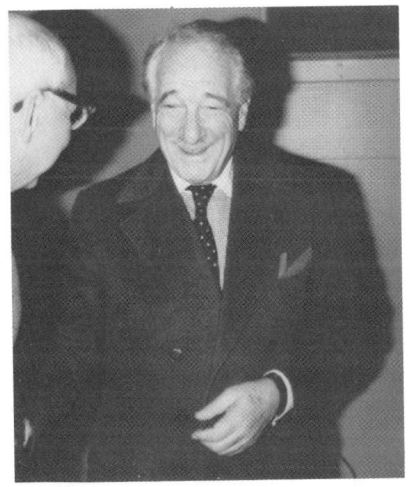

Borge wrings laughs from some very simple premises, like his delirious bit that raises the *number* in words, so that one becomes two, two becomes three "and so-fifth," through an entire comic lecture. He also delights with his equally popular punctuation lesson, where the "silent" punctuation marks of everyday speech (commas, periods, quotation marks, exclamation points, etc.) are brought to life with pops, clicks and other zany sounds.

Borge is also a deft monologist, not given enough credit for the artistry of his gags. Here, talking about Las Vegas room service, he triple-tops himself.

"My wife called down and asked for room service and a half hour later they sent up a table and a dealer (laughter) . . . of course, my wife doesn't gamble, so she sent the table back (laughter) . . . and then just before I left the apartment I sent the dealer back (laughter) . . . I don't gamble either (laughter, applause)."

Analyzing jokes is generally a fruitless procedure, but a student of comedy will note not only that Borge builds gag on top of gag, but keeps the listener off-balance too. The listener isn't expecting any of it. The audience is laughing when he mentions room service taking a half hour. Perhaps they expect a time joke, like "a half hour later they sent up a three-minute egg." They're off-balance again when Borge's wife sends the table back, but not the dealer. Is Borge the fool? Well, they laugh again when they realize he isn't and he sends the dealer away, and ties it off neatly with his own joke about gambling.

Borge's act is laced with ad-libs and asides. He might pause, asking, "Did you know that Mozart had no arms and no legs? I've seen statues of him on peoples' pianos." Or he'll say, "I want to thank my parents for making this possible—and I want to thank my children for making this necessary."

Offstage the ad-libs don't stop. To a bellhop carrying in his large wardrobe case he whispered, "That is my wife. Put her down please, I'll unpack her later." He enjoys light, off-the-cuff remarks and personalizes things for the audience, commenting on the town, the parking lot, the concert hall, all with a local slant. Spontaneously he chooses which of his many classical routines he'll do for the show. Only one part of his stage presence is carefully pre-planned:

"Once at a Florence Foster Jenkins recital I looked up and her accompanist's fly was open. I have ever since been terrified and I have my zippers sewed in backward so the flap will cover any failure to zip up."

In 1963 Senator Abraham Ribicoff said, "His skill is that of an expert, but his languages are the universal languages of music and laughter." Says Borge in performance, "A smile is the shortest distance between people." Knighted by Denmark, Finland, Sweden and Norway, Borge remains a beloved, honored performer the world over, one with a great sense of decency and sensitivity, who even strives to make sure his jokes are all inoffensive.

In recent years he has performed his concerts abetted by a dual pianist-stooge, or a pretty soprano for a segment parodying opera recitals, but even in his mid-70's he hasn't slowed his 200-concerts-a-year pace. He has also served as a conductor with the major orchestras of the world and has presided over "Pops" concerts.

He enjoys vacations in St. Croix, and makes his home in Greenwich, Connecticut, where he can be close to the sea: "With me the three B's are Bach, Beethoven and Boats." Of his adopted land he says, "From the beginning, I sensed that this would be a wonderful place to live. I remember being astonished by a headline in an American newspaper which said 'To Hell with Hitler!' Finally somebody was not afraid. It was like a breath of fresh air." He continues, "Nobody seems to have the Americans' enormous capacity for unselfish charity. Wherever there is a famine, flood or earthquake, America is always there with massive assistance. Twice your young men plunged themselves into the holocaust of war to save Europe and preserve human dignity."

The serious side of Borge emerges when discussing his flight from the Nazis, and there is a touching end to the tale of his departure from his homeland. "I was able to sneak back to Copenhagen for a final visit with my mother, dying of cancer at 94. The hour she was buried, I alone played the organ in a church in Stockholm."

Of his faithful audience, he says simply, "It's always a tremendous lift when you see a sea of people who welcome you warmly. It's the same feelings when children approach you to see what you have in your pocket or your bag, a surprise for them. An audience also must not be disappointed." They never are with Borge.

DAVID BRENNER

A throwback to the kind of nameless, faceless stand-up comics Ed Sullivan used to book in the early 1960's, David Brenner gets solid laughs, but neither he nor his jokes are remembered by audiences in the morning. But in an era when most young comics work dirty or act crazy, he's found a niche for himself as a very reliable Vegas performer and a ubiquitous variety show personality. More comfortable than distinctive, Brenner is nevertheless one of the most successful comedians around.

Brenner's attitude toward comedy reflects his workmanlike stance: "Comedy for me is just a means to an end, a way of reaching my financial goals . . . when something unexpected happens on stage and I begin to ad-lib, it's like I'm a plumber. You know, you're working on the elbow joint when all of a sudden the pipe down at the other end starts to spout. It's a challenge."

Like that of the old-fashioned stand-up stars of the 1950's, Brenner's life story was one of hardship. He grew up in a changing neighborhood in South Philadelphia. Talking about this period, he sounds a bit like an older comic describing the tears and laughter of New York's Lower East Side: "I had to run a gauntlet of snarling kids after school who wanted to remove my head or at least a leg every day. But when I made it home there was always a laugh. My father used to be a vaudevillian. He taught me what humor is."

Brenner attended Temple University and went on to write scripts and produce television documentaries. He was making money, but he was restless. He gambled with his life savings, taking a stab at stand-up comedy. Again, the story sounds like something out of an old showbiz legend:

"I was listening to the news on the radio. It was so depressing. All the reports about everything that was wrong in the world. I thought to myself, 'Why don't people laugh? If you don't laugh, you'll never get through the day with that news.' So then I thought . . . let me be a comedian. . . . I gave myself a time limit of one year and then extended the deadline six months in order to get on television."

Confident that he would always have a future in writing or producing, the relaxed young comic scored at such New York clubs as The Improvisation and Catch a Rising Star, ignoring the fear of failure.

A gawky 6'2", 150 pounder, Brenner looked comic enough. He was all nose and teeth, a long Pontiac schnozz sitting on top of blazing grillwork. Brenner did nose jokes: "At first I thought it was going to be an extra arm. I kept waiting for the hands to appear. . . . I always admired people who used only one Kleenex."

Influenced by Rodney Dangerfield's rhythms, he worked up amusing bits based on the reality of his tough beginnings: "It was a tough neighborhood. The gang from Third Street would always fight the gang from Fifth Street. They'd throw things at them. And what they used to throw at them were the kids from Fourth Street."

Brenner, carrying a tape recorder with him constantly, developed skills in ad-libbing and started to create more and more original routines. One of his best jokes is a true story, the result of what happens when you're constantly looking for material and "thinking funny." As he tells it:

"I sat down on a newspaper on the subway and a guy asked if I was reading it. I said yes, stood up, turned the page, and sat down again."

A favorite Brenner device is to question the logic of things people take for granted: "Have you seen that Evangelist who cures people on television? And he wears a toupee? I don't get it! He can fix a guy's legs and he can't put some hairs on his own head?"

Brenner questions putting "seeing eye dogs only" signs up for blind people to read. Hearing on the radio that the air in New York was unacceptable, he says, "What do we do, suck in air from Colorado?" And he questions the simple habit of giving money to panhandlers asking for "spare change": "Oh, am I glad I ran into you. I was about to throw all these quarters into the street."

Brenner uses clean material only, pleasant to all. He does the kind of

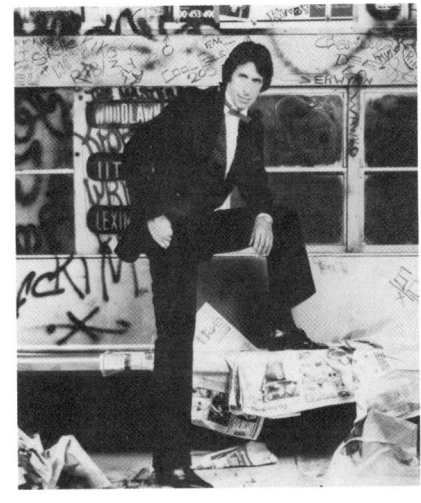

b. February 4, 1945, Philadelphia, Pennsylvania

Record:
"Excuse Me, Are You Reading That Paper?" (MCA Records 5457).

Video:
Casino Gambling (Karl Video), Catch a Rising Star 10th Anniversary (RCA Video).

Books:
Soft Pretzels with Mustard, Revenge Is the Best Exercise.

jokes old-timers used to do, but now there are few old-timers around to do it. He talks about his next door neighbors: "They were the toughest family in New York. Nine brothers—they were three months apart. And one sister . . . every day she had to brush her hair a hundred times. Then she'd do the other leg. . . ."

Slick, polished, the kind of nice, well-mannered boy America would like to see more of, Brenner went to an open audition for "The Tonight Show" just before Christmas, 1970.

On January 8, 1971, David Brenner was standing before 15 million TV viewers, doing his act. 20, 40, 60, 80 appearances would follow, rolling like the "billions served" sign at McDonald's. He told jokes on himself, on the old neighborhood, jokes like: "I went into a bar once and said, 'What do you have on ice?' The bartender said, 'You wouldn't know him.'"

"I have the premise that an entertainer's job is to entertain," says Brenner. "If one person walks out of the audience upset, then I haven't really done my job. . . . It's no challenge to shock the audience into a laugh with a dirty word. I look out and I see 10 year olds there. Now, they probably wouldn't be upset by an off-color remark, but their parents might. Working clean I know that the whole family can come and no one will be embarrassed. . . ."

In Vegas, Brenner easily pulled down $50,000 a week. "My mother had one good dress, my father had one good suit. You know what this business means to me? Money. It means to me that no one in my family has to worry."

The *Chicago Tribune* gave him a compliment, of sorts, describing him as "the comedic equivalent to Barry Manilow. A gifted synthesizer of styles who is able to please a broad public by giving almost everyone something to identify with." He was the young old-timer, the guy who could look nice in gold chains and Tuxedo, but never forgot his roots. He was a success doing a commercial for a Philadelphia beer company, Schmidt's. They were relatively unknown. How could they compete with famous name labels? They hired Brenner, who good naturedly held up the brew and then chided his audience. Labels? Why wear a designer label, Brenner asked. Do designers wear *your* name on *their* clothes? And here he had an unpretentious, good beer, sans "fancy label."

Patrons bought. And they bought Brenner's act all over the country, the lone toe-stub being "Snip," an attempted TV sitcom that didn't make it.

Brenner produced a solid-selling anecdote-filled autobiography, the title based on an appalling Philadelphia specialty, *Soft Pretzels with Mustard*. He also created a concept album that went beyond the traditional "live show transcript" record.

"The unfortunate thing about the album is MCA never distributed it. That's a good joke. A horrible truth. You go into some stores and they don't have it." It was particularly annoying when Brenner promoted it in local interviews, but local shops hadn't got a shipment. "I did dramatizations from my book and tied it in with live performances. My mother and father played themselves."

Brenner remains a popular favorite, especially in the casinos, and when he's teamed up with his friend (and one-time rival for "Tonight Show" guest-hosting) Joan Rivers, they smash box office records. While many frantic new comics are hot for one year, only to be replaced by a new fad entertainer, Brenner's conservative style, professionalism and slick ability to put together an entertaining show guarantee his continued success. Brenner is destined to become as durable as the "traditionals" have been over the decades, the Alan Kings, Myron Cohens and Jack Carters.

LENNY BRUCE

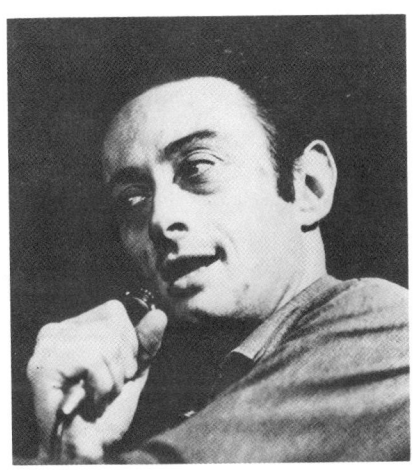

b. Leonard Alfred Schneider, Mineola, New York, October 13, 1925; d. August 3, 1966

Of all the stand-up comedians, only Lenny Bruce transcended the genre. "I am not a comedian," he once said, "I'm Lenny Bruce." Since his death, Bruce has been declared a martyr, a genius, a folk hero, a philosopher, a social satirist, an iconoclast and a moralist. Now and then, he's also been described as a very funny comic.

Says Lenny Bruce's daughter, Kitty, "My father had so much effect on so many that it is difficult to put him in perspective when thinking about him. His efforts to fight for his own beliefs, or maybe just against the quizzical idea of being told 'No'—I can't be sure which—caused a restless fire to burn within the man's very soul."

Lenny grew up in Freeport, Long Island, an area that was lazy and rural in the Depression era. His father was a reasonably affluent and educated businessman. Mr. Schneider married a happy-go-lucky local girl, Sadie, for one reason: she lied to him and claimed to be pregnant.

By the time she was really pregnant, the two opposites were no longer attracting. When they separated, Lenny was shunted back and forth between them. His father was serious, conservative but loving, and the boy was indulged with gifts including a real Wurlitzer jukebox. His mother showed him a good time and even took him to burlesque theaters, and when she was busy he fended for himself. It was a childhood that made a bewildering mix of love and loneliness.

"I volunteered for the Navy in 1942," he wrote. "I was 5'2" weighed 120 pounds, and had a heavy beard that needed removing about once every six months." After the war and service aboard the USS *Brooklyn*, he joined a drama workshop and studied acting. He won a contest doing a comic drunk parody of "To Be or Not to Be," and on April 18, 1949, tied for first place on "Arthur Godfrey's Talent Scouts," encouraged by his mother, who herself occasionally worked as an emcee and comic.

He was a raw talent back then, doing silly jokes and impressions of Maurice Chevalier and Frankie Laine. The evolution from amateur shtick comic to professional sick comic was a long, slow grind over a decade. Along the way he emceed strip shows, married stripper Honey Harlowe and pulled a few unusual stunts demonstrating his abilities as a suave and irresistible conman and showman. In 1951 he was arrested in Miami Beach for, according to the police, being "dressed as a priest, soliciting funds for some non-sectarian organization that had sponsored a leper colony."

Like every comedian, Bruce was influenced by those ahead of him and around him, from life-of-the-party friends (Joe Ancis), pioneering sick-niks (Will Jordan), bawdy bad boys (Buddy Hackett), TV satirists (Sid Caesar) and free-association hip leaders (Mort Sahl). Lenny played clubs so small there was "no pressure, I could try anything. Every night doing it, doing it, getting bored and doing it different ways. And up until 1957 I had never gotten any write-ups."

Out in California, Lenny finally made a stir, first at the Crescendo and then at Ann's 440 in San Francisco. It was there in 1958 that Fantasy Records first put his bits on wax, including his movie satires, gags on high fidelity and his joke about a genie in a candy store who can do anything with his magical powers. "You can do anything?" the suspicious store owner asks, having rubbed him out of an old bottle. "Then make me a malted." The genie gestures and roars, "You're a malted!"

Lenny's bits got wilder and hipper. His prison movie bit, "Father Flotski's Triumph," was a shock: jokes about vibrators, homosexuality and religion. Lenny was after laughs, and laughter comes from surprise.

Records:
Interviews of Our Time (Fantasy 7001), Sick Humor (Fantasy 7003), I'm Not a Nut—Elect Me (Fantasy 7007), Lenny Bruce, American (Fantasy 7011), Best of Lenny Bruce (Fantasy 7012), Lenny Bruce Is Out Again (Philles 4010), The Midnight Concert (UAS 6794, later rereleased in an expanded, 3-record set as "Carnegie Hall Concert," UAS 9800), Thank You Masked Man (Fantasy 7017), At the Curran Theater (Fantasy 34201; also available on Murray Hill Records), The Berkeley Concert (Reprise 6329), Politics (Douglas SD 788), To Is a Preposition Come Is a Verb (rereleased as "What I Was Arrested For," Douglas KZ 30872), Law, Language and Lenny Bruce (Warner SP 9101).

Compilation:
Arthur Godfrey Talent Scouts (Radiola MR 1084).

Films:
Lenny Bruce Without Tears, Lenny Bruce Performance Film.

Book:
How to Talk Dirty and Influence People.

Bios:
The Essential Lenny Bruce (John Cohen), Honey (Honey Bruce), Lenny Bruce (Frank Kofsky), Ladies and Gentlemen, Lenny Bruce (Goldman and Schiller), The Unpublished Lenny Bruce (Kitty Bruce).

Lenny made it come from shocking surprise. At first it was bad boy sniping: "Smokey the Bear eats boy scouts for their hats." Soon it became more focused.

From baring his backside while introducing strippers, or giving the finger to dull-witted customers, he shocked with words. "Sitting ringside," he said, opening a Chicago show, "are two boys who got their start right here in the Windy City—the wonderful Leopold and Loeb!" Smashing through the traditional type of "wife and mother-in-law" joke, he mentioned, "My mother-in-law broke up my marriage. My wife came home and found us in bed together."

He gained notoriety as a sick comic, and this encouraged him to become the sickest of them all. The more he was opposed, the more outrageous he became. *Time* magazine reported on the sick humor phenomenon and wrote that he "whines, uses four letter words almost as often as conjunctions, talks about rape and amputees, and deserves distinction for delivering the sickest single line on record. Taking a minority view of the Leopold-Loeb case, he said 'Bobby Franks was snotty.'"

The New York Times disagreed, noting in 1959 that Lenny was "scarifyingly funny . . . a sort of abstract-expressionist stand-up comedian paid $1750 a week to vent his outrage." His 1959 "Sick Humor" album was nominated for a Grammy. But Lenny had just begun to swing. He would go beyond the shock of going on the Steve Allen show to ask, "Will Elizabeth Taylor be bar-mitzvahed?"

He was fueled by bad boy impudence, hostility, morality, self-destructive impulses and the need for laughter and applause. He was fired up with the joy of creativity, of making sense of all the guilt, confusion and hypocrisy, "the shit running through my head" about hurt, pain, marriage, hookers, Vegas comics, law, language, sex, drugs, politics, love and life. If such old-timers as Milton Berle urged him not to be dirty or blasphemous, he would combine the two:

"To a Jew, fuck and shit have the same value on the dirty word graph. A Jew has no concept that fuck is worth 90 points and shit ten. The reason is that both priests and rabbis shit, but only one fucks."

He said, "The truth is what is, not what should be. What should be is a dirty lie." And the truth was in all his bits, the ones attacking organized religion, comparing Adolf Eichmann's death to the bombs dropped on Hiroshima, reflecting his own guilt at making $60,000 a year when teachers got $7,000, dissecting his feelings of love, lust, distrust and bitterness toward women, his disgust at drunks, bigots and politicians, and his almost childlike questioning of why something is declared right or wrong, legal or illegal:

"Obscenity has only one meaning—to appeal to the prurient interest. Well, I want to know what's wrong with appealing to prurient interest. I really want the Supreme Court to stand up and tell me that fucking is dirty and no good."

"All my humor is based on destruction and despair," he once said. Much of it describes the vulnerable and pathetic: the husband begging his wife, "Touch it, just once"; the frantic riff "To Come"; a brief blue note on "people who come to a nightclub on New Year's Eve at 8:30— they sit there with a hat and a horn, waiting." There was the dark, achingly accurate reportage on dead time in a sad town, "Lima, Ohio," with a woman who had "a vaccination mark as big as a basketball, a mole with hair in it," and where there was depression in a friendly old couple: "the most I can say to people over 50 or 55 is, thank you, I've had enough to eat."

Lenny's vulnerability was as important as his rage. He was the first comic to break the barrier between artist and audience. He talked intimately, as though to his peers, or his therapist. It was always from the gut. When he was sick, that sick humor reflected everyone's occasionally sick or selfish thoughts. When he blazed about having sex with white Kate Smith vs. black Lena Horne, or saving patriotic secrets at the expense of a hot lead enema, he shared his own human thoughts on morality with his audience—an audience also doubtful and confused. He was embarrassing, outrageous but always touchingly vulnerable in his bits on divorce, toilet jokes, Christians, Jews, or something like removing snot from suede. Other comics weren't doing this—the self put-downs were not about themselves, the wife jokes not about their wives.

Many couldn't stand having such intimacy aired. They wanted to ignore their moral problems, their excrescence, their own twisted sense of what's sick. Here was a guy who once held up a fake newspaper headline: "Six Million Jews Found Alive in Argentina." This was the man who questioned whether Jackie Kennedy was trying to get help or just get away when the bullets flew in Dallas.

"Satire is tragedy plus time," Lenny once said. Time was running out. As quickly as he became the famous "Dirty Lenny," he was set upon. A one-two punch: Bruce was busted for narcotics on September 29, 1961, and a week later for obscenity. Next year, a repeat: narcotics arrest October 6, obscenity bust October 24. The effect on Bruce could be seen immediately.

At Carnegie Hall on February 3, 1961, he was at the height of his powers, mixing hysterical older bits with free-form raps. At the Curran Theater in November of that year, he was speaking largely about his harassment, rambling and missing. At first he could laugh at the court procedures. But soon he was studying law night and day, trying to meet the establishment on its own terms. He believed in the system.

In October of 1965 he was declared bankrupt. And one day, with "Conspiracy to interfere with the fourth amendment const" in his typewriter and a needle in his arm, he was found dead. It was a suspicious-looking death scene. It might have been an overdose of drugs, or, as Phil Spector said at the time, "an overdose of police."

"I learned the truth from Lenny Bruce," sang Paul Simon, who included the announcement of Bruce's death in one of his song lyrics. 1967's "Lenny Bruce Without Tears" documented his legacy. A young generation became fascinated with his charisma, his raps on censorship, prejudice and hypocrisy, and the martyred comic became one of their icons. More records came out after his death than in his lifetime, and he was nominated posthumously for Grammy Awards in 1967 and 1969.

In 1971 Julian Barry's play *Lenny* premiered on Broadway, at the peak of Bruce's new-found fame. Cliff Gorman gave an awesome but inaccurate performance in the title role, turning Lenny into a zealous evangelist speaking the truth in blazing sermons delivered with more rage than humor. Bob Fosse's 1974 movie with Dustin Hoffman offered Lenny's routines performed with more of his own sense of irony and comedy. But by then there was no need to convince anyone of Lenny Bruce's greatness. The culmination was the publication of the kind of exhaustively researched biography usually reserved for a president: *Ladies and Gentlemen, Lenny Bruce*.

Those interested in Lenny's drugs and sex got vivid titillation. Those concerned with his self-destruction and guilt could read a letter Lenny wrote to his father, a parable about a self-sacrificing man and his ungrateful son who "ate the father's desserts and took the only pillow." It ended, "I'm going to jail tomorrow because you spoiled me. I love you, Lenny." Those looking for anecdotes of his zaniness and outrages found dozens, and there was ample room for discussions of his social, political and comic relevance.

That just about ended the craze. The public went on to the next dead star, and in comedy, George Carlin and Richard Pryor updated Lenny's drug, sex and social raps, and smoothed over the roughness, the harshness and the Jewishness.

In 1983, Bob Dylan suddenly wrote a song about Lenny: "Lenny Bruce is dead, but his ghost lives on and on." His place as a martyr, outlaw, social critic, trailblazer and cultural figure was assured. But Dylan added, simply, "He sure was funny and he sure told the truth," and that is his story.

"Dig," Lenny said, "the only honest art form is laughter, comedy. You can't fake it."

LORD BUCKLEY

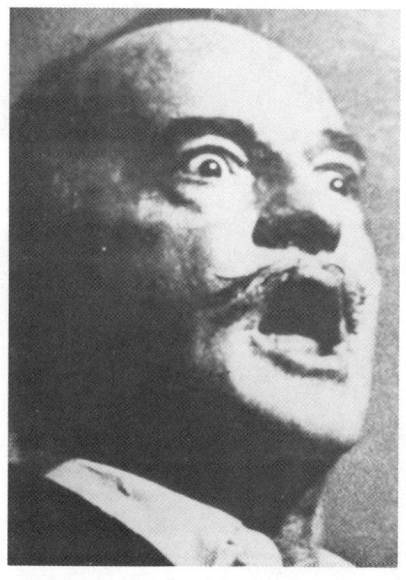

b. Richard Buckley, April 5, 1906, Tuolumme, California; d. November 13, 1960

Records:
Lord Buckley (Vaya 101 & 107), Blowing His Mind (World Pacific 1849), In Concert (World Pacific 1815), Way Out Humor (World Pacific 1279), Bad Rapping of the Marquis de Sade (World Pacific WPS 21889), Buckley's Best (World Pacific WPS 21879), A Most Immaculately Hip Aristocrat (Straight/Reprise STS 1054), The Best of Lord Buckley (Elektra/Crestview CRV 801, reissues of the Vaya recordings).

"The immaculately hip aristocrat," Lord Buckley was a unique figure on the comic stage in the 1950's. A tall, straight-backed eccentric, he looked like dignified royalty but spoke in jazz and black dialects, offering bop rambles, hipster fables and beat lectures on figures from history, from Jesus Christ to the Marquis de Sade.

"Negroes spoke a language of such power, purity and beauty I found it irresistible," the Lord said. "I could not resist this magical way of speaking, nor the great power it had for good in its purity and sweetness." At their best, Buckley's jazz monologues are a joy to listen to. Like Lenny Bruce, Buckley was not always hysterically funny, but he was an engrossing talker who enjoyed the rhythm of words and created jazz-like riffs of sweet sound and truth.

Typical of the Lord's monologues was "Jonah and the Whale," a rich retelling in "hipsomatic" of the old bible story. The humor, like that of folk tales and tall tales, is largely in the telling. As Buckley describes it, God comes upon a happy Jonah to say, "I dig you, Jonah! I dig you, Jonah, I dig you, Jonah, 'cause Jonah is the Lord's sweeeet boy! Put the message on the Israelites—they squarin' up over there."

Jonah takes some marijuana with him for courage, and vows to do what God has told him. But he meets a blustery whale who gobbles him up, throwing Jonah inside, onto his "blubbery rugs . . . fear and terror was in his heart, he couldn't go out the front end and he was scared to go out the back. He said 'Lord! Lord! Can you dig me in this here fish?' God answers, 'Jonah, I got you covered.' Jonah chuckles ironically: 'Maybe that's the reason I dig the cat so much, sayin' he got me covered. He got me sooo-rounded!' "

Jonah lights up some pot. "Jonah," the whale mumbles, "what is you smokin' in there?" Before long the whale's "engine room" is smoked up and his controls are warped. The whale sneezes, blowing Jonah "out on the cool, groovy sands of serenity."

For his audience, there was the joy of watching Buckley work, putting all the ethnic inflection into the story. And, at the small jazz clubs in the 50's that hired Buckley, most knew they were watching an offbeat original. Many loved Buckley's hipness—and their own for hanging out listening to him in some offbeat club.

Buckley's bits mixed philosophy with the riffs. In his version of "The

Raven," he says: "Poe didn't want the bird, he didn't need the bird, he didn't dig the bird . . . if they knocked the bird on him postpaid he wouldn't have dug it. 'Cause he was hung for a chick named Lee-nore who already swooped the satellite. But that didn't bug Eddy, he still knockin' that torch. . . ." It was like this: "When you don't want the bird, when you don't need the bird, when you don't have no possible use for the bird—(razz) that's when ya get it!"

At his worst, Buckley is as dated as a beatnik's bongo. Bits such as "Gettysburg Address" or "Marc Antony's Oration" are simple translations into the hip lingo, very much a one-joke idea:

"I came here to lay Caesar out, not to hip you to him. The bad jazz a cat blows wails long after he's cut out. The groovy is often stashed with their frames. So don't put Caesar down."

There were many sides to Buckley as a performer. He started in the tough, gangster-run Chicago clubs of the 1920's, where he developed his art at adroitly handling all kinds of people. Offstage he was a charmer. On stage he conned the audience, using put-on humor, turning the patrons into puppets—stooges for switched hats, switched drinks and other routines.

For the hip clubs, he did his hip lectures and such extraordinary "pure sound" bits as "Governor Slugwell" and "The Train," which orally duplicated, building to a tense finale, marching bands, crowds and hurried conversation. His train bit frantically duplicates the shriek of a whistle, the clatter along the track ("bibbity-bibbity-huppity-huppity") and all the excitement of the machine's approach.

In private, Buckley lived an eccentric lifestyle, charismatically attracting a small group of sycophants and an even larger group of acquaintances willing to lend him the money or audience needed to perpetrate the latest wild scheme. Loaned money was rarely repaid, but few objected. Most were happy just to be in The Lord's presence.

Reportedly he could reach his hand under a girl's dress with such a complimentary, "Oh, I say! This is wonderful!" that the lady would even allow others to share The Lord's joy. He would stave off the landlady when she demanded rent by dressing up everyone in the house (including guests) in ballet tights and inviting her to join "the class." He organized 16 naked people to parade through the lobby of the Royal Hawaiian Hotel. Again, as with Lenny Bruce, Buckley stories are legion. Here was a caring, crazy, cool leader of his own cult.

Sometimes he would simply come out on stage and say, with a twinkle in his eye, "What a great thing it is to be alive. Milords and Miladies, would it embarrass you very much if I were to tell you . . . that I love you? It embarrasses you, doesn't it? Mmmm."

Listening to Buckley's routines, it's amazing to realize that he performed them in 1950. They sound more in tune with the flowering hippie movement of the late 1960's and early 70's. At that time there was a mild resurgence of interest in Lord Buckley, including the rerelease of many of his old records. These consist mostly of studio recordings from 1950, live recordings made just before his death in 1960 and some home recordings that show with what ease Buckley could "put on" his black accent and then take it off when conversing with the recording engineer.

"It's all so very alive and jumpin'," Henry Miller said of Buckley, "and in the pauses one can hear the atoms exploding out there in the milky way where the grass comes up one in ten billion years and there are no moth balls or Frigidaires, no box office receipts, no railroads, no crucifixions, rosy or otherwise . . . it is very far out, your Lordship."

Buckley encountered problems during his performing career, largely

Compilation:
Golden Age of Comedy (RCA Victor LPV 580; includes "Friends, Romans").

due to his drinking, his erratic choice of materials and occasionally his championing of marijuana from the stage. At the time of his death, from a stroke, Buckley had had his performing license suspended by New York police. They cited "falsified information" on it as a reason for prohibiting a gig at the Jazz Gallery.

Survived by his wife and three children, Buckley remains one of the most unusual figures in stand-up comedy for his innovative approach to monology and his ability, at least in the noncommercial clubs he played, to move away from the standard pattern of jokes to an exciting and so far unduplicated form of humor.

Buckley ended his monologues with a kind of benediction that was very much ahead of its time. He would pause and say, "The flowers, the gorgeous, mystic multicolored flowers are not the flowers of life, but people yes people are the true flowers of life . . . and it has been a most precious pleasure to have temporarily strolled in your garden."

BURNS AND SCHREIBER

It was supposed to be Burns and Carlin. Jack Burns, a Boston radio station newsman, got acquainted with disc jockey George Carlin and the two were going to repeat the history of Bob and Ray all the way to stardom. But after a morning radio show, getting bookings through the help of Lenny Bruce and spending two years in nightclubs, it was just not working. The duo split amicably in 1962.

After Burns met native Chicagoan Avery Schreiber at the city's improvisational club Second City, a new team evolved. Burns and Schreiber found themselves working well in improv together. They honed some of the routines they developed and eventually sought club bookings.

One of their classic routines was a 13-minute dialogue between "The Cab Driver and the Conventioneer." The thin, slick-haired Burns played a brash and boorish bigot to Schreiber's affable, chubby Jewish cabbie.

At first the humor is in Burns's trademarked routines of annoying repetition and relentless jabbering. Never paying attention, even to what he's saying, Burns drives the cabbie crazy by demanding acknowledgment. "I guess there's still some life in the old trooper, huh?" "Yeah," Schreiber acknowledges politely. "Huh?" Burns barks again. "Yeah." "Huh?" "Yeah." "Huh?"

This is only the beginning of it. As the bit escalates, Burns becomes infuriating with his insistence on a response even when one isn't necessary. In fact, as unlikely as it seems, this "huh/yeah/huh/yeah/huh/yeah" bit became a kind of catch-phrase, cheerfully parroted by the team's fans.

Gradually Schreiber manages to dryly play along with the conventioneer's nervous excitability: "I met this blonde girl, good lookin' blonde, blonde, a good lookin' blonde," Burns babbles. "Blonde girl," Schreiber acknowledges. "Huh?" Burns grunts. "Good lookin' blonde," Schreiber says. "Ya know her?" Burns demands in confusion.

Handled with the same slippery smoothness as Abbott & Costello's "Who's on First," the routine progresses, and the bigot emerges. The talkative Burns begins to fill the cabbie in on his friends. One of them has a real cross to bear: "His son is an albino," Burns whispers. "But I told Dave—you can never be *too* white . . . but I'm not prejudicial. Don't get me wrong. Know what I hate?" "I got a good idea," Schreiber answers.

JACK BURNS b. November 15, 1933, Boston Massachusetts
AVERY SCHREIBER b. April 9, 1935, Chicago, Illinois

Records:
The Second City Writhes Again (Mercury SR 61224), In One Head and Out the Other (Columbia C 32442), Pure B.S. (Little David LD 1006), The Watergate Comedy Hour (Capitol ST 11202).

TV:
The Burns and Schreiber Comedy Hour (ABC 1973).

Gradually Burns makes a fool of himself with the kind of ignorant-but-outrageously-funny ethnic remarks that, years later, would bring fame to Carroll O'Connor in "All in the Family."

"I don't care about the color of a man's skin. I was the first guy to scream when they took 'Amos and Andy' off the air . . . by the way, your name on the nameplate there. You're of the Judeo-Hebraic tradition?"
"You mean I'm a Jew," Schreiber says.
"Hey," Burns backs up, "I don't go in for name calling! But lemme tell ya, pound for pound Hank Greenberg was one of the greatest ballplayers who ever lived."
"What about Sandy Koufax?"
"Don't tell me he's one of them too!"

Burns and Schreiber had a hit with this, and over the years used variations on it to successfully tackle controversial issues such as the war in Vietnam and drugs, with Burns on one side, Schreiber the other. Unfortunately, the team found themselves on opposite sides offstage. After their first brush with fame, they broke up.

As actors, the two men immediately found work. They were both "types." Burns was the annoying type, and turned up on "The Andy Griffith Show" replacing Don Knotts. Here his thick-headedness and his delusions of being a well-oiled and faultless machine had the good-natured Griffith going in "huh/yeah/huh/yeah/huh/yeah" circles. Schreiber, the big bear with the rubbery features and woolly hair, played a comical villain on "My Mother the Car."

Both shows took a turn for the worse. "Deep down inside, you say to yourself, gee, I really depend on him for my income," Burns once said, describing some of the chafing a partnership causes. Both men proved they could go it alone, but they had a better shot at success together. They reunited, after a three-year split, and by 1973 had their own television show.

"The block-jawed Burns is still largely doing variations on his boorish conventioneer," *Newsweek* reported, "but his rotund, mustached spar-mate, who manages to look like all four Marx brothers at once, has unveiled a Jonathan Winters talent for all manner of extravagant characterizations."

The show offered some of the experimentation the team enjoyed from the Second City days, and while it lasted, audiences were treated to inventive sketches that went beyond the standard "straight man/stooge" routines. The "Cab Driver" bit was a favorite (and even then they weren't working side by side: they sat in chairs, Schreiber in front, Burns in back, imitating on the sparse stage the inside of a cab) and they added Burns's already developed and perfected "Faith Healer" and sketches that saw Schreiber imitating a machine that, for a quarter, would say friendly things to lonely customer Burns.

The duo did a Watergate album and then, along with Richard Nixon, disappeared. Since 1974, Schreiber has been seen on a variety of shows and has become a popular character in commercials as well. Burns became head writer for a number of shows from "The Glen Campbell Show" to "Hee Haw" to "Fridays," and wrote for The Muppets and *The Muppet Movie*.

GEORGE BURNS

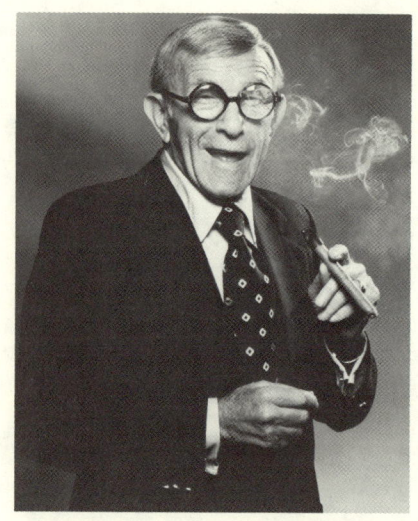

b. Nathan Birnbaum, January 20, 1896, New York, New York

Records:
Kings of Comedy (Longines Symphonette SYS 5282, as narrator), Golden Age of Comedy (Evolution 3013; Burns and Allen), My Favorite Story (20th Century-Fox TFM 3106), The Burns and Allen Show (Memorabilia M 722), The Burns and Allen Show (Mark 56), Jest Like Old Times (Radiola 1; Burns and Allen), Show Business (Epic; Burns and Allen), George Burns Sings (Buddah BDS 5127).

TV:
The George Burns and Gracie Allen Show (CBS 1950–58), The George Burns Show (CBS 1959), Wendy and Me (ABC 1964–65); George Burns Comedy Week (CBS 1985).

Films:
The Sunshine Boys, Oh God, Going in Style, Oh God You Devil.

Video:
Burns and Allen Show 1951 (Video Yesteryear), George Burns Show 1959 (Video Yesteryear), The Big Time Variety Show (Video Yesteryear), George Burns in Concert (Vestron).

Books:
I Love Her, That's Why; Living It Up, Third Time Around, How to Live to Be 100—Or More, Dr. Burns' Prescription for Happiness.

"Thanks for the standing ovation. I'm at the point now where I get a standing ovation just for standing.... They're talking about making a movie of my life. I hope they do it quick—I'd like to see it.

"There isn't a thing I can do now that I couldn't do at 18. You can imagine how pathetic my love life was. I never was a great lover. When I was young the only thing I wanted to get into, was show business ... even today, when I put my cigar into the holder I close my eyes."

George Burns at 80, performing stand-up comedy. With his sly wry delivery and tangy rasp, he's been rediscovered as a monologist in the same league as Jack Benny. And, in films, he can hold his own with the likes of Walter Matthau or Lee Strasberg. Into the 80's, Burns has demonstrated more than endurance. He's that rarity, an "entertainer," who can amuse and satisfy with songs, reminiscences and jokes. He makes it look easy. As he says, "I walk out on the stage, smoke a cigar, sing a few songs, tell some jokes—and wear the same color lipstick Bo Derek uses." But it takes someone special to stay on top so long, and to remain comfortably predictable yet fresh and modern.

"I'd rather be a failure at something I'm in love with than be successful at something I hate," says George Burns. "I'm very fortunate because I'm doing well in a business I've always loved. I've always been in love with show business and I still am. I love it today as much as I did for the 20 years I flopped at it." His enthusiasm for show business is evident every time he takes to the stage.

When his father died, leaving behind a family of 12 children, 7-year-old George scurried about, shining shoes and selling newspapers. He busked for coins on the street as a singer with the "Peewee Quartet."

In show business since he quit the fourth grade, by the age of 14 he was a seasoned veteran as a singer, dancer, joke-teller and even novelty rollerskater. His string of odd vaudeville jobs has become a monologue in itself. Burns continues to tell anecdotes about the years he put in under obscure names, performing equally unlikely routines.

It was in 1923 that he met 17-year-old Gracie Allen: "We were introduced by a mutual friend (a girl living with Gracie at the time) who knew that I was looking for a new partner. Gracie and I got along just fine. It's true that originally I had the laugh lines and Gracie played straight to me. She got the laughs, and I changed the routine around and forever after that I played straight to her." They were married in Cleveland on January 7, 1926.

Burns and Allen moved from vaudeville to the movies, utilizing one of their stand-up routines in *Burns and Allen in Lamb Chops*, made in 1929. They made 14 shorts and had supporting roles in more than a dozen features.

Pleasantly dizzy Gracie and her tolerant husband, George, turned up on radio often, doing routines like this, with Gracie starting it off:

"... Willie broke his back."
"Broke his back. How'd he do that?"
"Well, on account of he's left-handed."
"He broke his back because he's left-handed."
"Yes. Well, you see what happened was he had a doughnut in his right-hand pocket and when he went to take it out with his left hand he—"

"He broke his back?"

"Yeah."

"Well, you tell Willie that if he's got a doughnut in his right-hand pocket to try and take it out with his right hand."

"Well, that's hard to do when you have your pants on backwards."

"He had his pants on backwards?"

"Yes. You see what happened was he had a suit of clothes with two pairs of pants and he put one pair on frontwards and one pair on backwards."

"So that he could go either way?"

"That's when the truck hit him."

"The truck? What truck?"

"The truck that didn't have its lights lit."

"Why didn't the truck have its lights lit?"

"He didn't have to, it was daytime."

"Didn't the fellow in the truck see Willie coming?"

"He didn't know it was Willie. He saw two pairs of pants coming toward him and he drove in between them!"

In 1932 they began their long-running radio show, bringing it to television in 1950. Essentially Burns played the unflappable, dryly cynical husband enduring with good-natured stoicism the inane non sequiturs of wife Gracie. Today Burns still trades on his unflappable, seasoned attitude toward life.

Gracie was a winsome performer whose innate grace and charm elevated a potentially deadly style of comedy to an enduring tradition. The formula for Gracie Allen jokes is such that listeners today can usually spot the trouble several lines away, knowing exactly what Allen will misunderstand. By the time the team came to television, George was staring at the audience, sharing the inevitable:

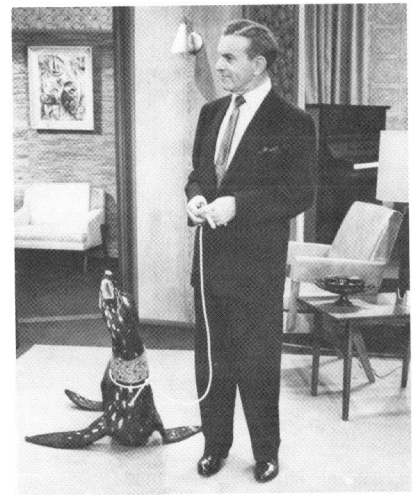

"A woman came to ask the doctor if a woman should have children after 35," says Gracie.

"What did you say?"

"What any sensible person would. I said 35 children is enough for any woman."

The TV show often included Burns and Allen monologues, and solos from George who would step out of the action to confide in the viewer. With a squint that could pass for a conspiratorial wink, he would flatten out his mouth in exasperation, tug a puff or two from his cigar and rasp out an intimate, sly gag or two. "The George Burns and Gracie Allen Show" began to slip in the late 1950's, and the later episodes with adopted son Ronnie Burns were tiresome sit-coms. When Gracie retired in 1959, the program was renamed "The George Burns Show" and the same regulars appeared. But George couldn't start up a show that had already run out of steam.

Many wondered what George would do next. "For every five people who don't like George," Gracie said on one program, "there are 50 who don't even know him, so put that in your hat and smoke it!"

Burns proved that the critics' thinking was as muddled as Gracie's. If some had forgotten George's subtle talents with a phrase and comedy timing, eclipsed as they were by Gracie's spotlight, they soon learned all over again how funny the man could be. He went out on the road, touring on a bill with Carol Channing in 1962. While he foundered with his TV show "Wendy and Me" (co-starring Connie Stevens) he developed a first-rate act of songs and monologues that took him across the country. When his wife died in 1964, Burns stepped up his schedule of performances and tried to keep as busy as possible.

Burns may have developed the character of the "old vaudevillian" with a trunk full of show biz anecdotes, but he never talked about the past at the expense of the future. His jokes were often topical, wry and acerbic. Like Groucho Marx, George Burns embraced the new generation and conquered it. Groucho did a Carnegie Hall one-man show, and so did Burns. And Burns made albums like "George Burns Sings," with his own hip version of "I Can't Get No Satisfaction" as well as the touching "Mr. Bojangles." Randy Newman produced a two-record "Evening with George Burns" which was released in England by DJM Records.

The comedian became a ubiquitous variety show guest, and made the talk show rounds as well. In 1975 he made his first movie since *Honolulu* in 1939. His involvement had come about by a tragic turn of fate.

The Sunshine Boys was supposed to star Jack Benny, but a few months before the start of production, he suddenly passed away. The Burns and Benny friendship was a long and deep one. It was probably with mixed emotions and some strain that Burns filled the empty space in his life by filling the empty part in that movie.

Burns won an Oscar for his performance, and in 1977 played the title role in *Oh God*. Burns was never more in demand. He starred in the 1980 triumph *Going in Style*. He made hit records ("I Wish I Was 18 Again"), came up with several books and made more movies. At 85 he was honored by the building of the George Burns Medical Center at the University of Israel.

In 1983 he continued to prove his box office powers by selling out eight performances at the Sahara Hotel in Las Vegas. In 1984 the unstoppable comic celebrated his 88th birthday by playing Atlantic City. "I'm celebrating by working and getting paid," he said. In 1985 he was paid $500,000 to do ads for LA beer.

He promoted his book *How to Live to Be 100—Or More* as living proof that long life could be achieved in grand style. Burns evolved from vaudevillian, straight man and song-and-dance comic to become a symbol for all America, the embodiment of a dream: a full life and a robust old age. Burns amazes and delights his fans by flaunting his continued love of a good cigar and his wry appreciation of beautiful showgirls. His comedy monologues are often sharper than those of comics one-fourth his age.

Asked endless questions about diets, death and absent friends, well aware that he is perceived as the ultimate success—fame, fortune, with no hint of retirement and no slowing in his zest for life—Burns wrote yet another book, *Dr. Burns' Prescription for Happiness*. To interviewers he always remains up-beat: "The way to live longer is to fall in love with what you're doing, then you've got it made. Then you can't wait to get out of bed in the morning and get to work. Unless . . . unless you got someone in bed with you."

RED BUTTONS

The golden age of television? "World War II was a skirmish compared to what I went through," Red Buttons recalls. "I was picked clean and left to die."

In 1952, Red Buttons was one of TV's hottest stars. His show business career had begun when he was 7, performing songs on street corners, and on the sabbath singing in the famous Coopermans Choir of Cantor Joseph Rosenblatt. At 11 he was a vaudeville singer known as "Little Skippie," then at 16 a singing waiter at Dinty Moore's City Island Tavern. Buttons switched to comedy, cracking jokes after his voice cracked.

He was a comic/singer in the Catskills (sometimes with straight man Robert Alda) known as "The Singing Bellboy." His red hair and 48-button uniform got him his stage name. At 18 he was one of the youngest entertainers in burlesque, "The Only Burlesque Comedian with All His Own Teeth."

When Red had the chance to do a Broadway show, he was willing to swap his $300 a week salary for the $50 rate. The show, The Admiral Takes a Wife, was scheduled to open December 8, 1941, but before the show bombed, the Japanese did, at Pearl Harbor. In 1942 he got his chance in Vickie, starring José Ferrer. The same year Red starred in burlesque for Minsky—and was on stage when the show was raided. Burlesque was finished, but Red had just begun.

After the war Buttons returned to Broadway, and also played the top clubs in the country. Then he got his own television show. Of the Red Buttons style, Jack Gould wrote in the New York Times in 1952, "He does not try to overpower his audience nor is he a believer in frantic antics as a substitute for humor. In appearance he looks like a young man that anyone might know . . . he's easy to like."

Buttons created many likable characters, like the Kupke Kid, and tough little Mugsy. But soon the humble, sensitive comic abandoned Mugsy. The tough guy character had come naturally to him ("I was shorter than most of the kids on my block, so I had to put on a tough guy act to prevent them from picking on me"), but after reading about the upsurge in juvenile delinquency, he felt it was his duty to take a stand. "The last thing I wanted was for any child to mimic Mugsy."

Buttons's self-awareness and sense of duty to his audience led to a great deal of strain. "Don't you realize I have a responsibility to 30 million viewers?" he would demand of his staff. When his ratings began to slip, insecurity turned to panic. Good scripts were hard to get, and Buttons fought with the writers over what was funny and what wasn't. One show was cancelled when the comic fainted from overwork. Haunted by strife and exhaustion, in 1955 he said, "I never took a sleeping pill in my life until this year. This year I ate them by the bushel. It's a back-breaking tension-packed grind."

In hindsight, Buttons recalled, "For 15 years I used the same material in nightclubs and I always got laughs. On TV I use a gag once and it's ready for the glue factory." Buttons used to joke about growing up in the Bronx: "either you grew up to be a judge or you went to the electric chair." In TV, either you killed 'em with your jokes, or they killed you. By 1955, the comic's career was dead.

On his way up, he'd said, "I love people, and I am a mighty grateful little guy. . . . I hope I'll never be too busy or so big a show business attraction as to forget that the crowds put me where I am. I was lucky, I guess." But now, he wasn't so sure of his luck.

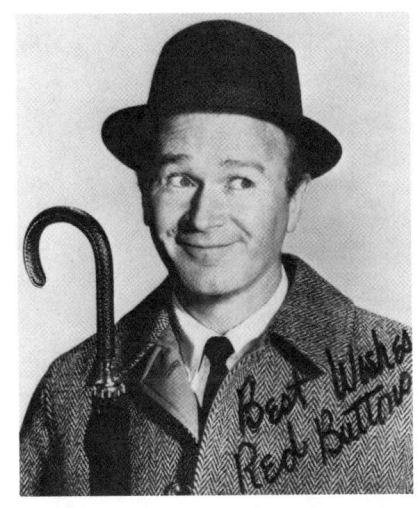

b. Aaron Chwatt, February 5, 1919, New York, New York

TV:
The Red Buttons Show (CBS 1952–54; NBC 1954–55), The Secret Life of Henry Phyffe (ABC 1966).

Broadway:
Vickie, Winged Victory, Barefoot Boy with Cheek, Hold It.

Films:
Sayonara, Imitation General, Hatari, Harlow, They Shoot Horses Don't They, Movie Movie, Off Your Rocker, Pete's Dragon, When Time Ran Out, Reunion at Fairborough.

With his show cancelled, Buttons recalled, "The baptism of firing made a man of me." He made a movie, *Sayonara*. "I'm awfully young to be having a comeback," he quipped. "I have the best part of my career ahead of me. This is a straight dramatic part, not one gag. Of course, some of my comedy shows turned out that way."

The 1957 film was a smash, and he won an Academy Award. Buttons had taken acting lessons to hone his craft and made many films before and after *Sayonara*, accidentally becoming one of the highest paid actors in Hollywood at $1,000 a word: en route to film *13 Rue Madeleine* he was detained. The film continued without him, so he ended up collecting a grand for saying one word: "Go."

Through the 1960's Buttons made more movies and became a leading nightclub attraction in stand-up comedy. In 1966 he even had his own TV show again, a comedy-spy spoof. For his club dates into the 70's, the graying Red did some blue material: "Kirk Douglas doesn't have a dimple. He's had his face lifted so often it's his navel. If he has his face lifted one more time he'll be wearing the strangest necktie you've ever seen!" He also offered fun one-liners: "With prices the way they are, I can't afford wheat germ anymore. Now I eat diseased wheat. . . . I took an economy flight. There wasn't any movie, but they flew low over drive-ins."

A tireless contributor to charity, sometimes Red could be fiery. In 1977 he led 1,000 members of a Beverly Hills synagogue to protest outside the French Tourist Office, pouring 500 bottles of French wine into the sewer, to call attention to the release of Abu Daoud, a French terrorist involved in the 1972 Munich massacre of Israeli Olympic athletes.

On stage, Buttons still performed "Strange Things Are Happening," although young audiences couldn't understand why their elders clapped the moment he sang "Ho ho ho" and cupped his ear. Buttons developed a new trademark in the 70's: his bit about all the famous people in history who "never got a dinner." On the dais of the "Dean Martin Roasts" TV specials on NBC, the veteran comic brought down the house when he upbraided the dubiously famous guest of honor who was being feted while "the greats" never got a dinner.

Opening with bits like "Our guest of honor made a special trip to be here tonight. He got up off the floor," Buttons would segue into lines like:

"George Washington—who said to his father, 'If I never tell a lie, how can I get to be President?'—never got a dinner. Richard the Third—who said to Richard the 2nd, 'Your number is up'—never got a dinner. Michelangelo's girlfriend—who said to Angelo, 'Forget about paint, let's put a mirror on the ceiling'—never got a dinner. Captain Hook's brother—who said to Little Hook, 'For God's sake don't scratch it'—never got a dinner. And Uncle Ben—who was a credit to his rice—never got a dinner. . . ."

He topped himself with every line, getting more choked up with comic anguish with each famous name. In November of 1982, Red finally got his own dinner. At a Friar's Club roast in his honor, he said he was proud and thrilled because "Jesus never had a dinner . . . all he got was supper."

Reflecting on his careers as a fine dramatic actor and outstanding comedian, he once said, "It's much harder to be funny than it is to be serious. There's really no contest." Of his many decades as a comic, he added, "Down deep, basically, I love to clown."

GODFREY CAMBRIDGE

There were three pioneering black comedians of the early 1960's. Dick Gregory broke through with barbed wit. Bill Cosby was the opposite, proving his equality by matching any comic laugh for laugh. And then came Godfrey Cambridge, combining both.

Relaxed and good-natured, he did straight jokes on girls, movies, Vegas gambling and the aggravations of modern life. Using the same broad style, he also did racial jokes. But instead of a Gregory-type lecture, Cambridge used lampooning monologues and frank, "inside" insight. While Gregory tended to keep his audience on the outside of his jabs, and Cosby ignored the racial question, it was Cambridge who made a name for himself by telling it "like it is," on a more personal basis.

Cambridge coaxed his audiences with little human anecdotes all could understand, like the irony of trying to find a "flesh" colored band-aid. Then he built on these with more examples of indignities, indignities everyone suffers, and then indignities only some suffer. He told about the time he was nearly knocked down by a car. The driver got out with an apologetic, "I didn't see you." Cambridge, in disbelief: "Didn't see me? Big and black as I am he didn't see me?"

Cambridge let his audience in on the silliness of white liberal cocktail parties (he considered starting a "Rent-a-Negro" agency so each gathering could have a token black to agree "Joe Louis *is* a heck of a fighter"). And he told simple, sympathetic stories that crossed racial barriers.

He told of a little black boy innocently playing at his mother's dressing table. Smearing white face cream on, he was suddenly yelled at by his furious parents. Crying, the kid mutters, "See that? I don't blame white people. I ain't been white but a few minutes and I hate two colored people!"

Long before Richard Pryor and Eddie Murphy, Cambridge rejoiced in the humor of black slang and custom. He insisted Worcestershire sauce was named when a black man went into a restaurant, tasted it, and asked the waiter, "Wuss dis here sauce?" He had a bit about how Yuma, Arizona, got its name. A black cowboy was shot by a white sheriff. As the black man lay dying, the remorseful sheriff insisted, "I didn't mean it. It's terrible, you dying in this town without a name. Maybe—before you die—you can have the honor of naming this town." The black man looked up and with his last breath said, "You mu. . . ."

At the time, some blacks were a bit embarrassed by these antics, the way Jews were alarmed at Jackie Mason's acting "too Jewish." But it was Cambridge's style to stand up and let it all hang out, to be himself, to use the time-honored comic technique of "look what the little man has to suffer with," and add "hey, take a look at what the black man has to suffer with."

"I'm glad to see some of you wearing colorful clothes," he'd tell an audience. "It takes the pressure off me! I wear a red shirt, people say, 'Look, I told you them coloreds like bright colors!' " In his cheerful, chiding way, he got the message home. Sometimes, though, he underlined the pang of pain with more ironic humor. He talked about a swimming pool down South: "The black pool and the white pool are the same—except there's no water in the black pool. And the diving board is higher."

In private life, Cambridge took pride in fighting discrimination. He also took some pleasure in it, pausing to give a kick in the shins to the telephone company (he would send needling letters pointing out any bill discrepancy). He took down license plates of taxi cabs that passed

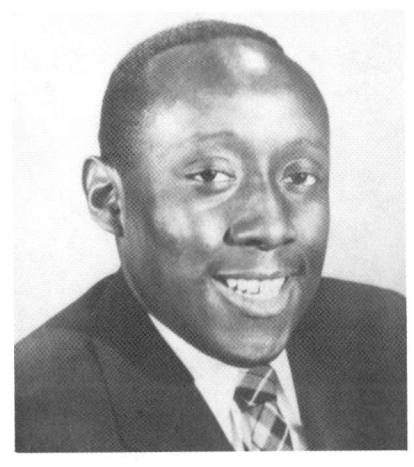

b. February 26, 1933, Harlem, New York; d. November 29, 1976

Records:
Ready or Not (Epic FLM 13101), Them Cotton Pickin' Days Are Over (Epic FLM 13102), Toys with the World (Epic FLS 15108), Godfrey Cambridge Show Live in Las Vegas (Epic FLS 15115).

Films:
The Last Angry Man, Gone Are the Days, The Troublemaker, The President's Analyst, The Biggest Bundle of Them All, Bye Bye Braverman, Watermelon Man, Cotton Comes to Harlem, Come Back Charleston Blue.

Broadway:
Purlie Victorious, How to Be a Jewish Mother.

Book:
Put-Downs and Put Ons.

him by, and complained with letters and with humorous articles in such magazines of the day as *Monocle*.

Cambridge may have taken a different approach to handling racism because he experienced it as an adult first, not in childhood. His parents had come to New York from British Guiana only to discover that despite their skills and education, they could find only menial work. His father worked in the streets as one of Con Edison's "dig we must" men. His mother labored in the garment center. A West Indian of fierce pride, she scraped up the money to send Godfrey to his grandparents' home in Nova Scotia. He attended grade school there, evidently treated as an intriguing foreigner. Attending Flushing High School in Queens, Cambridge found his schoolmates friendly, too.

"Unforgettable Godfrey Wonder Boy Cambridge," was how he was described in the school yearbook, "a laugh, a chat, a gay retort, perhaps sometimes a pun, a friend to all who knew him, a smile for everyone."

He wasn't smiling at Hofstra University where he suddenly ran up against white rage. The white clique on campus ostracized anyone associating with Godfrey, making life miserable for him. He quit school and sought refuge in Harlem. "I had to find out who I was," he said. "I was running away and hiding from a white society which had hurt me."

"I worked as a popcorn bunny maker, airplane wing cleaner, maternity hospital ambulance driver.... I consider these and the other odd jobs I've held as the best source of material and training for me as actor and comic."

He worked in church plays and began to redevelop his self-confidence. "All my life I ignored being colored... it's terrible for someone to reach the age of 21 and realize he's Negro, to spend all that time leading a sheltered life."

In 1956 he made it to Off-Broadway. True, part of his job included sweeping the floor, but at least he was on stage. *Take a Giant Step* ran nine months, leading to New York TV work. In 1961 he won an Obie for his role in Jean Genet's *The Blacks*, then hit Broadway in *Purlie Victorious*. After an improvisational stint in The Living Premise, Jack Paar discovered him and gave him a national audience.

Cambridge became a frequent guest on variety shows, and in 1964 his first comedy album was nominated for a Grammy. He turned up acting on such comedy shows as "The Dick Van Dyke Show" and was earning $33,000 for a month in Las Vegas.

He could tell Vegas-type jokes with the best. He noted that after sex, a "German woman is practical. She'll say, 'Ach, that vas gutt!' A French woman is solicitous: 'Ah, mon cherie, did I please you?' An English woman would say... 'Feeling better?' " And he could do some risque racial material. His wife redecorated the entire bedroom in brown: brown walls, floors, drapes and carpet: "One day she took a bath, came into the room and it took me three hours to find her."

Cambridge mixed comedy and drama when he starred in an episode of Rod Serling's "Night Gallery," playing a nightclub comic who finds himself under a supernatural curse. A fad dieter, Cambridge had trouble slimming down from 360 pounds. When he did, he found himself more in demand for movie roles. He played a white man who turns black in *Watermelon Man*, and later appeared in some of the first big-budget movies intended primarily for black audiences: *Cotton Comes to Harlem* and *Come Back Charleston Blue*. That year, 1972, he was hospitalized for exhaustion.

In 1976, while filming "Victory at Entebbe," he suffered a fatal heart attack. He was playing the role of the mad Ugandan President Idi Amin.

And it was only Amin who could find anything happy about the comedian's early death. "An act of God," Amin claimed. At the time, Cambridge was not married, having divorced his wife some years before.

GEORGE CARLIN

Few comedians can successfully change their image and direction once they've become established. George Carlin did, going from a middle-of-the-road comedian welcomed by TV and Vegas audiences to the country's first successful counter culture comic rapping on everything from long hair and drugs to dirty words and foreign wars.

"The one thing I can remember about my childhood which affects what I do now is having been alone a lot," Carlin has said. "I think that makes one introspective and, oddly enough, it also makes one a critic of the world around him." Carlin's world was a tough, interracial working-class neighborhood in Morningside Heights where taking drugs made more sense than attending parochial school.

His father died when he was two, and for the rebellious youth, the classroom was the place where his hostility and anger erupted: with humor. As Carlin has often said in the many routines about his childhood, he was "class clown," the boy of a million ridiculous faces and dozens of wisecracks.

For a "what I want to be when I grow up" school assignment, he wrote, "I want to be an actor, an impersonator or a trumpet player." He did own a trumpet, but he had another toy, a tape recorder, which he used to create imitation radio shows.

Still a free-thinking discipline problem, Carlin quit high school and worked at odd jobs before joining the Air Force. Several times he was threatened with court-martial proceedings. While stationed in Shreveport, Louisiana, the 17 year old managed to get a job as a disc jockey on a local radio station, and stayed there after his Air Force service was over.

By the time he left Shreveport, at age 20, he was a slick, seasoned pro with a winning one-to-one style that listeners enjoyed. Earning a high school equivalency diploma helped insure better employment prospects.

When he moved to WEZE in Boston, he met Jack Burns. The two became friendly, and when they met again at a Texas radio station (Carlin was fired in Boston for an unauthorized trip in the company car) they decided to become a comedy team. "We had decided not to wash dishes and all that sort of thing people are supposed to do when they get to Hollywood," Carlin recalled. When he and Burns arrived in town, "We went to radio stations. The first one we went to was looking for a comedy team, and we were at work a week later."

Morning disc jockeys Carlin and Burns began to gain a reputation for nightclub work around town. One of the first people to see their potential was Lenny Bruce, who helped get them an agent. In the act Carlin did an accurate impression of his nasal-voiced mentor and often performed, with Bruce's consent, Lenny's old "Genie in the Bottle" bit as an impression/tribute.

Hitting the late night talk shows, they performed safe bits, like the formula-bound routine about punch-drunk boxer "Killer" Carlin:

"Remember your first fight, Killer?"

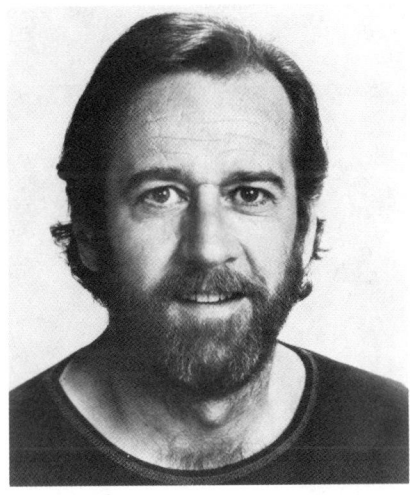

b. May 12, 1938, Bronx, New York

Records:
The Original George Carlin (ERA E-600; formerly titled "At the Playboy Club," ERA EL-103), Take Offs and Put Ons (RCA Victor 3772 and Camden CAS 2566), FM & AM (Little David LD 7214), Class Clown (Little David LD 1004), Occupation Foole (Little David LD 1005), Toledo Window Box (Little David LD 3003), Evening with Wally Londo (Little David LD 1008), Indecent Exposure (Little David LD 1076), On the Road (Little David LD 1075), A Place for My Stuff (Atlantic 19326), Killer Carlin (Laff), George Carlin Collection (Little David 902411), Carlin on Campus (Eardrum ED 100).

Compilations:
Comedy Classics (Era BU 3890), Here's Johnny (Casablanca SPNB 1296).

TV:
Apt. 2-C (HBO, 1985).

Video:
Saturday Night Live 1975 (Warner), Carlin at Carnegie Hall (Vestron), Carlin on Campus (Vestron), Tonight Show 1969 (Video Yesteryear).

Book:
Sometimes a Little Brain Damage. . . .

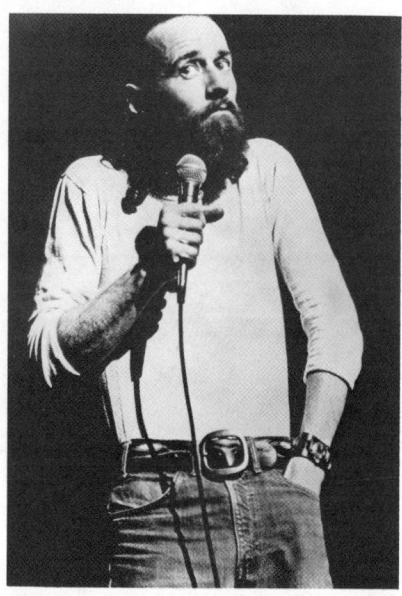

"Sure, that was against Slugger Hogan."
"He had quite an impressive record."
"Yeah, he did have quite a record. Eleven years at Leavenworth! I remember . . . the crowd was yellin', I threw a left and a right and an uppercut and a left and a right—it was great. Then Hogan came out of the dressing room. . . ."

For hipper audiences, Carlin and Burns satirized kiddie shows with commercials like this: "Little girls, send for your Lolita kit! In this kit, you get an autographed picture of Vladimir Nabokov, and a little instruction booklet. If you do the exercises prescribed (that's kind of fun in itself, girls) in just two weeks you'll be walking and talking and acting like girls twice your age. And you can pick up a little cash after school. . . ."

They satirized politics, and a senator (played by Carlin) who announced, "I think bigotry is the coming thing in this country . . . with great leaders like Orville Faubus. . . ."

The team reached a plateau and in 1962 amicably split. For the first time in his career, Carlin had trouble getting gigs. It took a few years to make it as a solo. In 1965 he began turning up regularly on TV variety shows, finding a market for his more inoffensive material.

The newest rubber-faced young comic had an array of funny characters to display, from slack-jawed dizzy quiz show contestant Congolia Breckenridge to lazy-eyed Al Sleet, the "hippy dippy weatherman" who would announce "Tonight's forecast: Dark." There was also sportscaster Biff Burns (later changed to Biff Barf when Carlin realized the name had been subconsciously lifted from Bob and Ray) who would offer fast-paced, pointless information: "Quickly, the basketball scores: 110–102, 125–113, 131–127 and in an overtime duel, 95–94. And here's a partial score: Pittsburgh 37!"

Carlin was adept at both character comedy and straight gags, like his quickie commercial set in a dentist's office: "Say, nurse, what was that good-tasting red mouthwash the dentist gave me?" "That was muscatel, he's a wino." Carlin found work both performing and writing for "The John Davidson Show" and at 29 was named star of "Away We Go," a summer replacement for Jackie Gleason's show.

The turn of the 1970's wasn't exactly a peak period for comics. Young audiences weren't going to nightclubs, sit-coms were stagnating ("All in the Family" didn't catch on until 1972), and the generation gap made it difficult for existing comics to successfully appeal to a wide audience. Carlin's star ascended in 1967 (the year his first solo album was released) but he became restless. He wanted to perform more provocative comedy.

At the Frontier Hotel in Las Vegas in 1970, Carlin reached a turning point. For months he'd been told to cut "dirty words" like "ass" from his show and stick to the straight stuff. That night he began to rap about dirty words. Today it's a joke: "I was fired for saying shit in a town where the big game is crap." Back then, it was serious business. And business was off for George Carlin. Even the Playboy Club gave him the boot.

At the same time, another young comic, Richard Pryor, was experiencing similar dissatisfaction with Vegas safe jokes. He couldn't find a solution. The answer came quicker to Carlin. Carlin, after all, had been experimenting with Lenny Bruce-type humor right along with Lenny himself. The new interest in Bruce was growing at colleges around the country. Carlin dropped out of the clubs and moved on campus. He grew his hair long, embraced the "freak" element and began doing the kind of raps he had toyed with since 1960.

"People change all the time," Carlin said at the time. "Formerly I used to do a lot of characters. Now I'm myself, I just talk as a person, more naturally."

Carlin did audience-recognition bits on all sorts of mildly taboo topics: the folklore of lighting farts, how to make rude noises with a hand in the armpit, the way dogs never urinate all at once in one location, how neighborhood kids he knew turned their eyelids inside out, etc. etc. These were lightweight but immensely funny vignettes, made vivid by Carlin's warmly natural delivery and talents for facial and vocal mimicry.

From childhood riffs, body function humor and audience participation improvisation (hippie audiences were especially delighted when Carlin told them to put finger into cheek and pop—and the whole hall erupted with unearthly pings and pongs for a comic, natural high), Carlin established a bond and vulnerability with the audience. Then he would bring out the heavy ammunition, the political insults ("Nixon looks like he hasn't taken a shit in a month"), interesting studies in semantics ("Please, *please* man, please man—police man") and a favorite tool, the logical conundrum: "Muhammad Ali had an unusual job, beating people up. The government wanted him to change jobs. They wanted him to kill people. He said, 'Nooo, that's where I draw the line. I'll beat 'em up but I don't want to kill 'em.' And the government said, 'If you won't kill 'em . . . we won't let ya beat 'em up!' "

Carlin was viewed as a more accessible, less intense Lenny Bruce. Carlin's raps on dirty words were on target, but were delivered with amused good humor. Using caricatured voices and faces, he put dirty words into the mouths of average people and laughed at how "bad words" were actually common in daily life, from a frumpy housewife blurting "Oh shit! I dropped the broccoli" to a dunce tough's "Ayyy, I don't give a shit 'cause I don't take no shit!" In the midst of these shocking yet good-natured raps, he'd make his points. He talked about the word "fuck . . . it means to make love . . . yet it is a word we use to hurt people, the last word of the argument: ohh, fuck you! Why not substitute the word fuck for the word kill in old movies: Mad fucker still on the loose . . . stop me before I fuck again . . . fuck the Ump!"

If the material was broad, so was the delivery. Carlin was adept at "talking down" to his audience, accentuating his words with popped eyes, comic inflection, body English and funny faces. He knocked the serious edge off with a clowning delivery.

While some resented Carlin for "imitating" Lenny Bruce, he is certainly an original in his own right, and he deserves credit for daring to switch styles, and for continuing to challenge "words you can't say on TV." He paved the way for a new generation of comics by solving the problem of the "rock crowd" audience. His exaggerated delivery got through to even the most stoned-out or uninterested patron. As "All in the Family" suddenly found fame with all generations, Carlin was the stand-up who bridged the gap between the hippies and college kids and adults, even if he had to begin with silly things like his rhyme about long hair ("some really despair of my hair but I don't care . . . they're just square. They see hair down to there say beware and go off on a tear. I say no fair . . ."). From the Grammy-winning 1972 album "FM & AM" on, Carlin sold enough lps to bring comedy records back from limbo, making record companies again take an interest in signing new talent.

Carlin was rolling along with recognition humor ("Be honest. When you first heard of 5-day deodorant pads, how many of you thought you had to wear 'em?") and social commentary ("Eating meat on Friday, man—imagine, are there people in purgatory still doing time for a meat rap?"). But he was pushing himself to be more daring, more Brucian. On stage some bits were not funny and not working. Offstage, his cocaine habit roared out of control. He went for days without sleep, then did nothing but sleep. His mood swings nearly ended the marriage that began in 1961. He suffered his first heart attack.

The mid-70's were not strong ones for Carlin, a problem compounded by the comic's malaise, predictability. Audiences tend to "solve" a comic's style of "trickery" and there's usually a slump before the comic becomes an established star or fades away as a momentary novelty.

A problem for Carlin was new material. He exhausted some of his specialties: dirty words and gross-out bodily functions. For one video concert, he was reduced to simply reciting dirty words cheerleader style, and talking about stomach growling and nausea. Other topics included smoking breakfast cereal, the invention of the flamethrower, raindance techniques and how to get into a car. Offbeat subjects, but aside from a football vs baseball word association routine, the bottom of the barrel.

But today there is still a wide audience for his older bits, and for his new, whimsical observations ("Have you noticed that mice have no shoulders?"). Now with short hair and trimmed beard, Carlin has achieved a balance between his old straight humor and his hippie style, which is in keeping with the changing times: where the straights today were the hippies of yesterday.

JOHNNY CARSON

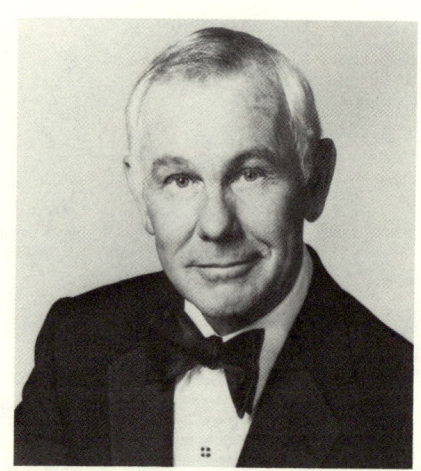

b. October 23, 1925, Corning, Iowa

Records:
Introduction to New York and The World's Fair 1964 (Columbia CS8999), Here's Johnny: Magic Moments from the Tonight Show (Casablanca SPNB 1296).

TV:
Carson's Cellar (KNXT 1954), Earn Your Vacation (CBS 1954), The Johnny Carson Show (CBS 1955-56), Who Do You Trust? (CBS 1956-57; ABC 1957-62), The Tonight Show (NBC 1962-); Carson Classics (syndicated 1985).

For over 20 years, Johnny Carson has delivered a nightly monologue to the American people. Many see more of Carson than they do of their relatives, and enjoy him more. Carson has proved to be an enduring talent, partly because of a very special quality: people are familiar with him, yet they don't know him. Despite his high visibility, viewers can't say that they know much about Johnny Carson, personally or emotionally.

The Carson "cool" has been with him a long time. He doesn't talk about his childhood much, except to indicate that he grew up shy and inhibited. In her book on him, Nora Ephron wrote that his friends "are certain that everything about Carson—his withdrawn nature, his fear of being used, his apparent hostility—can be traced to events in his childhood, though few of them are certain as to exactly what those events were."

Carson's father worked as a lineman for a utility company. The family did some moving about before settling in Norfolk when Johnny was 8. He's remembered as a boy who enjoyed getting into mild, prankish trouble. At 12 he found a new way to call attention to himself: he bought a magic set and developed an all-consuming passion for trickery. He practiced incessantly as "The Great Carsoni" and conquered classmates, audiences at church affairs and later the Norfolk Rotary Club. He learned ventriloquism too, and eventually owned his own dummy, named Eddie.

By the time he reached high school, Carson was writing comedy for the school paper. "I, John Carson, being of sound mind and body (this statement is likely to be challenged by my draft board and the high school faculty) deem it advisable to give you the lowlights of 1942 and 1943 . . .," he wrote for the school yearbook. He warmly described a highlight of September: "Football season opened this month and I went out to make the team. I would have, too, if they hadn't found where I hid my brass knuckles."

Carson joined the Navy in 1943, and before his hitch was over had even managed to get the Secretary of the Navy to play stooge for some of his card tricks. He majored in English at the University of Nebraska and the subject of his thesis was "How to Write Comedy Jokes," a dissection of the techniques for creating stories and snappy punchlines.

He also received some TV exposure back in 1949, playing a milkman in a closed-circuit student epic, "The Story of Undulant Fever." The same year he married for the first time. The marriage produced three children, Chris, Ricky and Cory. He worked first as a radio announcer, and then as a TV personality on WOW-TV in Omaha. In 1951 he moved to California.

"Carson's Cellar" was the comic's first major effort, a low-budget KNXT-TV show loaded with the kind of hip humor, throw-away lines and free-form skit comedy that thrived in the "who's watching anyway" environment of 1950's local TV. Carson opened with a monologue, using a style remarkably similar to today's pattern. He would initiate the jokes with mildly nervous gestures, ask rhetorical questions to get the audience involved ("Anybody bet on the football game yesterday? You know when people bet they do funny things . . .") and employ a deliberately paced delivery that looked restrained.

Carson's improvisational sketches and fresh wit amused many comedians, and such stars as Red Skelton and Fred Allen made good-natured visits to the cellar. Carson began writing for Skelton, and when Red hurt himself during rehearsal in 1954, Carson filled in for a week, earning excellent reviews and national exposure. He briefly had his own prime time show, but it was beset with problems. Some quiz shows followed, and one, "Who Do You Trust," was a hit, and a perfect vehicle for Carson's ad-libs and easy rapport with contestants. His work made him a likely choice to replace Jack Paar on "The Tonight Show" in 1962.

Carson was a change from the emotional Jack Paar, a return to a strong emphasis on monologue, sketch comedy and light-hearted guests. He resurrected some Steve Allen devices, like "The Question Man" (now called "Karnak"). Carson's influences were obvious to the critics.

"He's got a Jack Paar smile, a Jack Benny stare, a Stan Laurel fluster," *Time* reported. "If a joke dies, he waits a second and then yawns a fine Ed Sullivan 'ho-o-okay.' A sudden thought will launch him into an imitation of Jonathan Winters." And there were also helpings of Oliver Hardy, Jackie Gleason and Fred Allen. Yet for all that, Carson *is* an original, a synthesis of many styles distilled into perhaps the ultimate "average American comedian," who appeals to both rural and urban audiences.

"I'm strictly a product of TV," Carson says. "I think you steal a little from everybody, particularly when you are starting. You pick it up here and there, and ultimately you have your own style and people start stealing from you." He has indeed influenced an entire generation of comics. Each night they watch him steer his way through new jokes, trying them out for the first time on an audience. They see him blend the styles of gag-smart Bob Hope, pleasant and vulnerable Jack Benny and topical Will Rogers.

Although professional and controlled, Carson has made great use of "sharing" his role as comic with his audience. After a long day, folks can come home and watch *Carson* work. And they become co-conspirators in putting over the gags, joining the world of show biz. They wink at Johnny's attempts to segue jokes, they're in on the laughter of a muffed line or an attempt to rescue a bomb. The lowliest clod and smuggest intellect are "in" on Carson's attempt to sell the monologue.

They laugh at the predicament of rolling from topic to topic ("Why am I doing Henny Youngman now?" Carson might ask rhetorically, or he'll give a sarcastic "I'm the Prince of Blends"). They appreciate it when

Video:
Carson's Cellar (Video Dimensions), Timex All Star Comedy Show 1962 (Video Yesteryear).

Books:
Happiness Is a Dry Martini, Misery Is a Blind Date.

Bios:
The Tonight Show (Robert Metz), Johnny Carson (Thomas Lorence), Here's Johnny (Nora Ephron), Johnny Tonight (Craig Tennis).

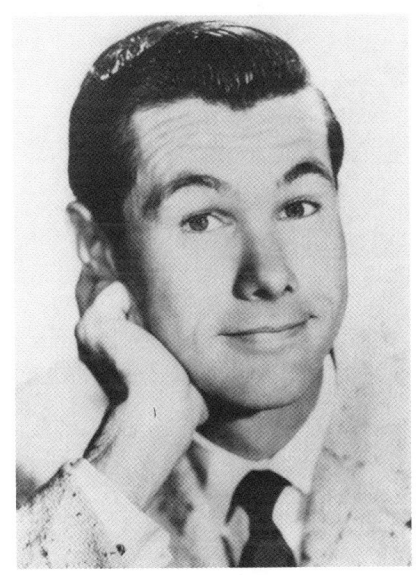

he covers a bomb with a topper, or even nothing (a mock chagrined, "And I don't have anything!" is always good, as is a more frank "I knew that joke would go right down the toilet"). And they applaud Carson's running gag of the ultimate solution to a bad monologue: performing a weary soft-shoe to "Tea for Two."

Perhaps the most famous example of Carson and audience sharing the hip con of putting over a gag is the parody of the set-up. "It was really wet today," Carson begins. The entire audience shouts, "How . . . wet . . . was it?" "All I know is twice on my way to work I was photographed by Jacques Cousteau."

Over 20 years, one could fill a book with Carson's running gags, which include references to: Bombastic Bushkin the accountant, "crack meteorologist" Frank Field, Ed McMahon's drinking, the NBC commissary, the NBC tour, birds and their worms, the San Andreas fault, the Slauson cut-off, or such bomb-savers as the plaintive, "You folks didn't boo when I was raising the flag on Iwo Jima."

Like many comics, Carson has a core of hostility. It shows in the ad-libs bounced off brainless starlets or other comics. And it shows in Carson's sophisticated put-downs of mundane, unexciting things with a sardonic "Whoopee," a cynical "Ya ha," or a sarcastic "that's a real *biggie.*" Many new comics have picked up on Carson's hostility and made it a prime tool: worldly wiseguys like Bill Murray, Chevy Chase and the ultimate Carson imitator, David Letterman.

Because Carson is seen almost nightly (it still seems that way despite his growing vacation time) one would expect to hear criticism from those who have contempt for the familiar. Yet in Carson's case, the complaints are largely directed at the show's format, which is sometimes vapid and glossy, and the guests, who are mostly show biz types with whom Carson feels at ease bantering and whom he makes the target of mild ad-libs. Carson deserves immense credit and respect for pleasing audiences not once a year, as a touring Victor Borge did, or once a month as Bob Hope did with specials, or once a week as Jack Benny did, but almost daily for such an unprecedented length of time. Of course, his eight million dollar a year "Tonight Show" salary goes a long way toward underlining his worth.

Carson is also not given enough credit for keeping the channels open for different styles of humor. He isn't Lenny Bruce, Mort Sahl or Jonathan Winters, but in his way he has helped keep the barriers unclogged for risque humor, jokes about politicians and downright weird gags. In the latter category, perhaps influenced by writer Pat McCormick, Carson has been especially effective.

Over the years he's educated audiences to accept outlandish gags and absurd, sophisticated humor. From the early 60's he began telling jokes like these:

"The weirdos come out on a day like today. A weirdo stopped me on the street and said, 'How about $10 for my grey-haired mother.' I gave him the $10 and he said, 'Now when do you want my grey-haired mother?'"

"We had a little excitement in mid-town New York. It seems that the Jolly Green Giant got ahold of some fermented broccoli, and the next thing anybody knew he was squatting in the middle of Fifth Avenue turning Volkswagens upside down trying to find their sex."

Carson pushed audiences into tolerating odd gags, from "Due to today's earthquake, the 'God is Dead' rally has been cancelled" to visual punchline oddities: "I love to walk to work on a cold, rainy Monday. That's my second favorite thing in the world. My first, my favorite, is taking off my shoes and socks and punting a porcupine." Into 1984, he had the audience with him when he described a Fall TV series: "An ordinary housewife owns a 24-hour instant teller machine at a sperm bank—and is a foot fetishist for the FBI."

Carson has also had a subtle effect on public opinion. There are 15 million or more people influenced when he picks a Spiro Agnew or James Watt as a joke target, singles out a subject to ridicule, or even chooses a name to make fun of. "Bruce" as a name for a homosexual achieved such widespread usage that he received complaining letters about it from various Bruces and dropped the references. Likewise, he stopped making gags about "the heartbreak of psoriasis," when his calling attention to an inane TV commercial called attention to a very real ailment.

Carson will continue to be a popular paradox, known by probably 200 million Americans, yet prone to solitary hobbies like astronomy or drumming in his home studio. He'll be the subject of endless tabloid articles, and books like the "inside" volume by former staffer Craig Tennis, who wrote, "This is a man, after all, who sleeps with his baby pillow—who, in fact, won't travel without it and carries it everywhere in his suitcase."

Says his third ex-wife, in answer to the perennial "what is he really like" question, "Johnny's a survivor. He is probably one of the greatest talents this country has ever had. But he doesn't enjoy the lifestyle, the pressure, the demands that go along with his celebrity. He desperately needs his privacy . . . he's a man who enjoys his work, who loves to read a lot, who enjoys his home and tennis in Malibu and who loves to walk alone on the beach. I find it amazing. Here's a man who's been on TV for 22 years—and yet nobody knows what he's really like."

JACK CARTER

The personification of the "Top Banana" type of comic ("the loud hardsell mode" as *Variety* described him), Jack Carter's style is slick, fast and furious. A simple gag is boosted by mimicry and emphasized with one of a dozen facial or physical takes like "triple skull, the fadeaway, the slow burn, the turnaround, the walking freeze," etc. The style came from burlesque and marched to Vegas to a rimshot drum beat.

The jokes? They're almost secondary to the delivery. Here's a gag from his 1950's TV show. Carter mugs and mimes, playing both Truman and MacArthur. As Truman: "Ok Mac, you're through. Pack up your pipe and get lost!" Now as MacArthur: "You can't do this, Harry. You'll ruin my Korea!"

In Carter's stand-up career, he is more joke salesman than comic. The aim is to get the gags sold at any cost and then get the commission: laughter. If he has to embellish the merchandise with gaudy bravado, he'll do it. The 1955 model joke: "80% of the money is spent by women. The other 20% is spent by men—on women!"

From the mid-60's: A guy sees a fat lady carrying a duck: "The guy says, 'What are you doing with that pig?' The fat lady snorts, 'That's not a pig, it's a duck.' The guy says, 'I'm not talking to you, I'm talking to the duck.'"

Jack Carter, 1970: "If you like to spend your vacation in out-of-the-way places where few people go, let your wife read the map."

And into the 80's: "Canada ran out of silicone and the girls up there are using hamburger helper."

No matter what the joke, Carter can sell it with all the skill and savvy

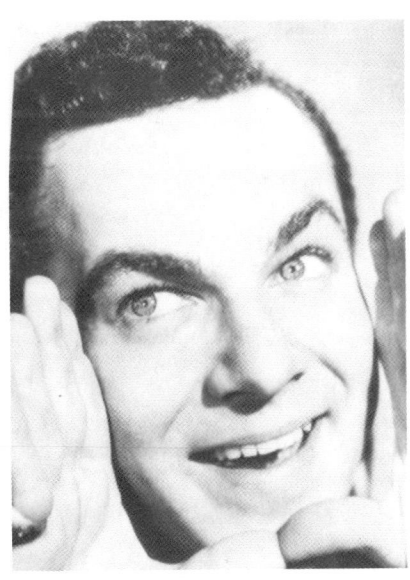

b. Jack Chakrin, June 24, 1923, New York, New York

Record:
Broadway ala Carter (AAMCO).

TV:
Jack Carter and Company (ABC 1949), The All Star Revue (NBC 1951-53), Pick and Pat (ABC 1949), Stage Show (CBS 1956).

of a pro boxer making the most of every jab. He's always been an excellent performer, in fact an extremely versatile one.

He got a taste of show business when he was at New Utrecht High School in Brooklyn, playing Cyrano de Bergerac. An eager student, he worked for Christopher Morley and appeared in Morley's play *Trojan Horse*. He also managed to persuade the team of Pick and Pat to let him take a shot at their blackface minstrel show when it came to town.

After performing in Army shows, he worked on radio and got a break in the show *Call Me Mister*, as the replacement for Jules Munshin. At the time Carter was known mostly as an impressionist, doing Fred Allen, Sidney Greenstreet and Nat King Cole, among others.

"When I was 14 I realized I had talent as a mimic," he said, "but I didn't stay one, exclusively. A mimic is a bromide. He's always the hit of every show but nobody wants to hire one."

Carter made a name for himself when he took over for Phil Silvers in *Top Banana*. The show was built around Silvers's brash "Gladda See Ya" style, but Carter proved he could be "Fun-neee, Fun-neee" not only doing the Silvers shtick but also bringing in his own snappy impressions and personality.

At 26, the young kid impressed Milton Berle and won himself guest spots on "Star Theater." He quickly became known as among the best of the brash bananas. Naturally enough, this glib facade hid a man of tremendous nervous energy, deep insecurity and mournful self-doubt. Fretful over his looks, over his jokes, over his health, his worries drove those around him crazy, but as Red Buttons once said, "he drives everybody nuts but everybody loves him." In another age, Carter might've taken his protective parents, neuroticism and shyness with women to the stage with him and done Woody Allen bits. But in the 50's, audiences were there to laugh, not necessarily to listen. And in the early days of TV, Carter said, "I have to crush an audience or I'm not happy. I swarm all over them, give them 40 jokes instead of four...."

Carter had his own show, "Jack Carter and Company," in 1949 and from 1951 to 1953 was on "The All-Star Revue." "That was like putting on a Broadway review every week," Carter recalled. "Well, that's ancient history. There's nothing like it on television anymore... TV was exciting then. But now it has lost its bigness. It fell into the mediocre class. Live entertainment died. They cut the throats of Durante, Berle, Ed Wynn and the rest of the performers who knew how to belt the public."

The show fell apart for an unusual reason. It preceded "Your Show of Shows," and NBC insisted that Carter not duplicate any topics that might appear on their later blockbuster. When Carter complained about the second-class treatment, his sponsors became disenchanted over the negativity the network seemed to feel toward the program.

Carter headlined in nightclubs across the country and continued to do guest spots on television, especially "The Ed Sullivan Show," where, in the tight five or eight minutes allotted, he could do what not many other comics could: hand-grenade and strafe the audience with gags and mimicry until they were helpless: instant comic annihilation.

About the only problem that Carter saw in himself that had any truth to it was his assertion that "For a performer, I'm very untheatrical. Milton Berle steals gags, Joe E. Lewis drinks, Buddy Hackett talks out of the side of his mouth in that beautiful nasal voice. What have I got going for me? Somebody up there doesn't like me and I think it's me."

Indeed, while almost every comedian has a trademark or a distinctive face or figure, Carter's most distinguishing characteristic is invisible: frantic nervous energy.

To keep himself before TV audiences, in the 70's Carter appeared on game shows: "When you're on a game show your pants are down. On some you're an idiot if you don't know the answers. You take your chances . . . the amazing thing is that the game shows give you more recognition than anything else." Enough recognition to do plays, TV acting and club dates.

On the stage his act consists of songs and impressions as well as fast-paced gags. He still enjoys the challenge of straight drama, but he says, "If you don't go over big in a play, for example, you can kid yourself that the author didn't know his business. But a comedian doing a solo routine is selling himself—personality, style, attitude. I'm offering you me when I try to make you laugh, and if you don't laugh it's like a stab right in the heart because that is personal rejection. That hurts and that's why clowns must be the saddest people on earth."

DICK CAVETT

In 1964, nightclub audiences were treated to the sight of a short, shy, sophisticated comedian who offered up wit, lunatic humor and cerebral one-liners.

It wasn't Dick Cavett.

But Dick Cavett was watching as Woody Allen took the stage. Dick Cavett was, like Allen, a comedy writer. Now he wanted to be like Allen: a stand-up comic.

"I thought being a comic was the route that might take me to acting," Cavett recalled. It was yearning to be an actor more than anything else that characterized his early years growing up in Gibbon and later Lincoln, Nebraska.

Cavett's odd mix of mid-western charm and cool urbanity came naturally enough. His father and stepmother were both schoolteachers (his natural mother died when he was ten). Early on, Cavett developed an interest in literature and the arts. But then as now, he was far from the studious egghead type. He was also an expert gymnast and won several state championships specializing in side-horse competition.

Short and shy, Cavett compensated by learning magic tricks which he performed for school functions, and at 14 appeared in the title role of a production of The Winslow Boy. He earned a scholarship to Yale, majoring in English literature, but switched to drama in his senior year.

He likes to recall with nostalgia and irony the greatest triumph of his young acting career. In 1957 he appeared in a production of The Merchant of Venice with Katharine Hepburn. He had one line, which he can still quote: "Gentlemen, my master, Antonio, is at his house and desires to speak with you both."

In 1958 Cavett came to New York, but found he couldn't get as much stage work as his more successful girlfriend (now wife), Carrie Nye. He took on the usual odd jobs for actors, from typist to store detective. In his case, he wasn't a store detective spying on potential shoplifters. He was to pose as a customer and check up on the manners and efficiency of the department store's own personnel.

Cavett also led the colorful life of a struggling, depressed, miserable, anxious, out-of-work actor. This included the highs of getting small parts in plays and meeting famous stars, and the lows of living cheaply in a run-down walk-up apartment.

He witnessed, firsthand, all the bleakness of a squalid, noisy, crime-filled tenement. At times it drove him to Neil Simonesque extremes. In

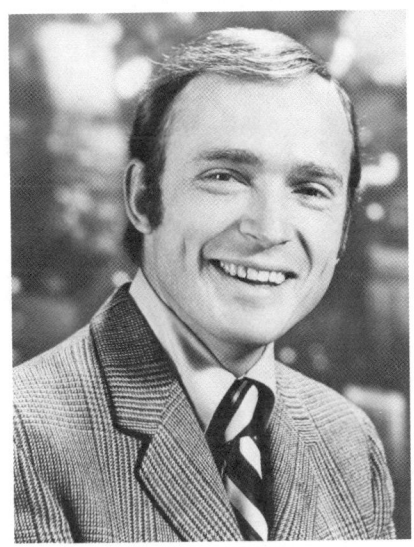

b. November 19, 1936, Kearney, Nebraska

TV:
The Dick Cavett Show (ABC 1968–69, 1969–75; CBS 1975; PBS 1978–81).

Books:
Cavett, Eye on Cavett.

his book, *Cavett*, he describes how irritation turned to exasperation and then mania as he found himself up against Puerto Rican neighbors who couldn't understand why anyone would rather sleep than listen to loud music blasting till 2am. Cavett ended up on his own roof, tossing a Seven-Up bottle through the offender's front window. The next night, he managed to get on the roof of the adjacent building and smash the back window. Of course, in Oliver Hardy fashion, both times Cavett returned only to find, in mute exasperation, his own window broken.

Cavett's big break came when, as a copyboy for *Time*, he managed to use an official-looking *Time* envelope to get past the NBC guards and drop in on talk show host Jack Paar.

"*Time* is planning on doing a story on you," he told Paar. A moment later, Cavett handed the comedian two pages of jokes. The gutsy move paid off. Paar used a few of the gags, Cavett came back a week later with more, and eventually he got a job on Paar's show. From there, Cavett wrote for various "Tonight Show" guest hosts, Merv Griffin, Jerry Lewis and Johnny Carson.

Cavett was not only a good writer but an impressive student of comedy. His dissection of a joke, and how it would be told by various comics (including questions of emphasis, phrasing and timing) makes for fascinating reading in *Cavett*.

When Cavett saw Woody Allen work, he went backstage to express his admiration. Before long, the two were firm friends, and with encouragement from Allen, Cavett took a shot at stand-up comedy. Allen even persuaded his manager to get Cavett bookings.

Dick had one problem: being himself. It was hard to write jokes for himself. There wasn't much to work with. About the most distinctive premise he could find was the thin concept of being a Nebraska farm type who, in witty fashion, could now comment on his new, sophisticated surroundings.

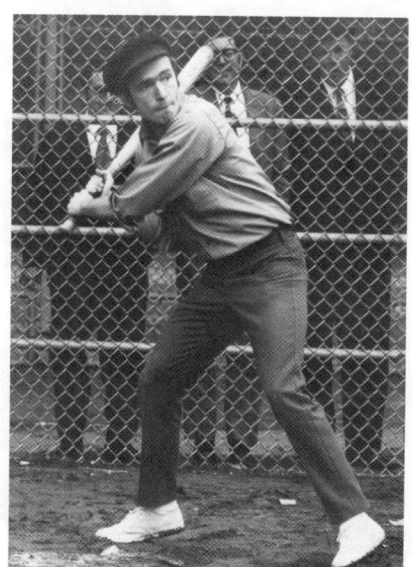

"My whole freshman year I wore brown and white shoes," Cavett told his audience. "Actually they were impractical, because the white one kept getting dirty."

Cavett had some problems with this kind of material, which was far from the truth and more contrived than cute. But worse, in 1964 when he started at the Bitter End, he had deeper doubts about his audience: "I always had a lurking suspicion that the sort of person who would voluntarily pay money for overpriced booze and the possibility of being entertained, and whose idea of fun was to sit in a noisy, crowded room full of foul air and drunks, was not the sort of person I would like to stand up in front of unarmed."

Cavett was at his best with neutral jokes, the kind he could write for any talk show host's opening monologue, only with a thinking man's edge:

"I eat at this German-Chinese restaurant and the food is delicious. The only problem is that an hour later you're hungry for power."

As the laughs slowly filtered up, Cavett's mouth would slip into an ironic half-smile. It might have been a lack of experience, or the wise guy in him, but more likely, this habit, which persisted for years, was more a reaction of pleasure and amazement. He was biting his tongue or sticking it deep in his cheek to prevent himself from giving a full, Cheshire cat grin: "Standing up there getting laughs and having things go well, with people falling over themselves" was amazing. The laughter made him smile a little, with self-satisfaction. Here, in the center of the roaring storm, was a calm, 5'7", 130 pounder with the power to produce laughter.

"That part is great," Cavett says. "If you're one of those people who achieve ecstasy of some sort in a performance, then you love it." At times, he did. Other times he was depressed by the sleaze and the isolation of touring on the nightclub circuit.

In November of 1965 the *San Francisco Examiner* praised the "bright and ingratiating" performer and his "understated lines and hilarious situations." Some of the comedians Cavett had written for, Merv Griffin and Johnny Carson, gave him national exposure on their shows. The sophisticated comedian proved to be naturally witty as a talk show guest. He soon found himself a talk show host, premiering in 1968 on daytime TV.

The following year he replaced Joey Bishop as ABC's rival to Johnny Carson. Samples of his monologues from back then show him still uncomfortable with the odd concept of standing up and throwing off gags. He preferred to insert ad-libs, or at least temper the jokes with "natural" patter between them.

Cavett's wit was an instant hit with the critics, and he won two Emmy awards, although he modestly noted, "You're influenced by everyone who's influenced you. You know, there are things I never would have said if Groucho Marx hadn't existed." While many could easily see the influences on Johnny Carson, fewer seemed aware of the equally shy Dick Cavett's tendency to slip behind a faintly disguised Fred Allen impression or Groucho Marx delivery in order to dare come up with a sly quip to a famous guest.

As Cavett became a household word, both his virtues and flaws were magnified. At times he was self-conscious in the artificiality of the talk show setting, still shy with famous guests. He compensated by being cocky and cute. But Cavett's intelligent discussions and wit intrigued guests who had long refused talk shows in the past.

Like Paar and Carson, Cavett had an intriguing personality. He had Paar's unpredictability and Carson's cool. One never knew if he would be stymied by a guest (he admittedly froze when William F. Buckley, Jr. interrupted a complex discussion to say, "You don't seem too familiar with any of these things") or the hero of the hour, telling Timothy Leary, "I really think you're full of crap." When Norman Mailer made fun of Cavett's use of a question sheet, Cavett told him to "fold it five ways and put it where the sun don't shine."

The rigors of the show produced periods of depression, a sense of being on "a tremendous long treadmill," as Fred Allen might've said, a "treadmill to oblivion." Psychiatric help put him back in control. Although there were downs, there were also ups, times when he felt "it was the best job in the world."

In 1977 Cavett finally made it to Broadway, appearing in *Otherwise Engaged*. It was one of the highlights of his career. Of course, sometimes the unexpected happened. A noisy drunk was at one performance. The fiery Cavett stopped the show: "All right, let's turn on the lights and see who this bastard is," he shouted. "I mean it. Get the house lights on." When the heckler was removed, he said, "Why did it take so long? He was drunk but what's your excuse?" The audience applauded and the show continued.

Over the years Cavett has hosted many TV shows, including a few series for HBO. He's never considered a return to stand-up comedy: "I had an offer to play Vegas once . . . I never did. It just never occurred to me to keep doing it once it seemed to serve its purpose, whatever that was. . . ."

CHEECH AND CHONG

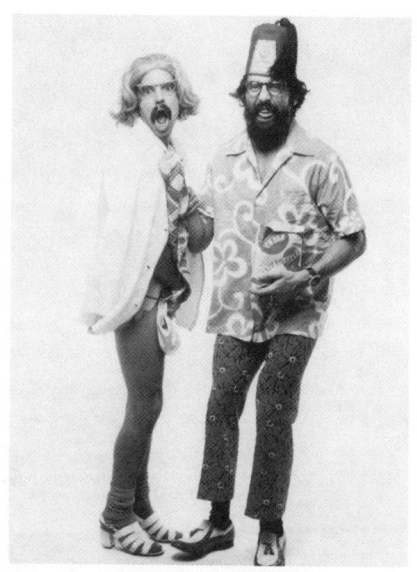

CHEECH MARIN   b. Richard Marin, July 13, 1946, Watts, California
TOMMY CHONG   b. May 24, 1938, Edmonton, Alberta, Canada

Records:
Cheech and Chong (Ode 77010 and Warner 3250), Big Bambu (Ode 77014 and Warner 3251), Los Cochinos (Ode 77019 and Warner W3252), Wedding Album (Ode 77025 and Warner 3253), Let's Make a New Dope Deal (Warner HS-3391), Sleeping Beauty (Warner 3254), Cheech & Chong's Greatest Hit (Warner BSK 3614).

Films on Video:
Cheech & Chong's Next Movie (MCA), Up in Smoke (Paramount), Nice Dreams (Columbia), Still Smokin' (Paramount).

Probably no comedy team in history has been as critically panned and financially successful as the Chinese-Chicano combo of Cheech and Chong. Their first album sold a million copies. The next three sold a million and a half each, and "Los Cochinos" won a 1973 Grammy. Their first movie, made for less than three million dollars, has grossed over one hundred million dollars worldwide, and the others have been box office successes too. Yet for all that, few critics have a kind word for the duo.

The reason is simple. Most critics, and most middle Americans, could care less about the characters Cheech and Chong satirize. Most have had no experience with these people and haven't the faintest idea what is so funny about the team's sketches, which are almost jokeless and based on character comedy. Non-Cheech and Chong fans simply see scruffy hippies and street people engaged in gross, brainless and unappealing action.

"The reason any humor works," says Tommy Chong, "is because you've touched a nerve of truth somewhere. It's like taking a virgin to a sex movie. They say, 'Oh God, that's ugly' because they can't relate to it. Our humor relates to you only if you've done it before. Then you can say, 'Oh yeah, man, I get it.'"

A classic routine of theirs is "Cruisin' with Pedro"—that is, classic for anyone who has experienced drug paranoia. A hippie hitchhiker gets a lift from a gabby, friendly Chicano who offers him marijuana. But when the driver thinks he sees a squad car approaching, he frantically makes his passenger down pot, pills, acid and the rest of the stash. The squad car turns out to be just an ambulance.

Lenny Bruce did drug paranoia humor a decade earlier, a quick 30 seconds on dropping pot down the toilet and later, after the crisis has passed, deciding to do the only logical thing: smoke the toilet. "Lenny Bruce had a great influence on us," Chong says. "We would listen to his records over and over until we had worn out the grooves." But what Cheech and Chong added was recognition comedy. The extended paranoia routine is loaded with typical remarks from the "oh, wow" hippie and excitable Chicano.

Another routine laughs *at* drug users as well as with them. A stoned hippie blows his defense in court by woozily coming up to the stand and telling the judge, "I don't need acid, man, I don't need marijuana," the substances he was busted for. "'Cuz I'm hooked on downers." In the background other courtroom criminals snicker. And the audience laughs too, at the recognition of a typical dumb remark they've probably heard an air-headed druggie acquaintance make.

Some have incorrectly labelled the team the "Abbott & Costello of the 80's." Actually, Cheech and Chong say their main influence has been Bob and Ray. Indeed, Bob and Ray don't do jokes, they do character and situation comedy. The same holds true for Cheech and Chong.

One of the most inexplicably funny routines they do is "Dave," which, like most of their material, has no jokes and no apparent humor to it. A drug dealer, whispering frantically, tries to get into an apartment. "It's Dave," the dealer hisses, "let me in, man!" Chong answers dumbly, "Dave? Dave's not here." "No, man, *I'm* Dave! Dave!" "Dave?" "Yeah man, it's DAVE! Dave!" "Dave's not here." And so it goes for five minutes.

To the average critic, this is a brainless exercise, a typical example of "pot humor" where something ridiculous seems funny because the audience is stoned. Actually, the bit is similar to Bob and Ray sketches where a frantic interviewer must deal with a guest from "Slow Talkers of America," or a guest who can only repeat, with numb regularity, that "The Komodo Dragon is the world's largest living lizard," while the equally opaque interviewer repeats this fact.

The duo's fans get similarly hysterical over the routine where school-teaching nun Sister Mary Elephant constantly lets out blood-curdling screams of "SHUT UP!" before demurely telling her rowdy class, "thank you." And then there's "Basketball Jones" where the team satirize a barely literate street kid's homage to his basketball and such tepidly funky allusions as "I'm bad, I got more moves than Ex-Lax."

The team met in Canada, where Chong owned a topless club, and draft-dodging Cheech (the term is short for "Cheecherone," which is a barrio delicacy, deep-fried pork skins) stopped by and got himself hired. "I got five dollars more for hanging out with naked chicks than I did delivering carpets," says Cheech. "It wasn't much of a choice I had to make."

Chong was more impressed by the blonde Cheech was with. "I always judge a man by his woman. So if you see a little creep with a tall beautiful blonde . . . I hired him on the spot." Ironically, that blonde left Cheech the next day.

Chong was once a member of "Bobby Taylor and the Vancouvers" and he wrote a small Motown hit, "Does Your Mama Know About Me." At the club, he and Cheech did comedy relief and improvisation in between nude sets from the girls. The hippies managed to out-shout the hecklers and the tough truckers who came in for tits'n'ass only, and they unashamedly stole dirty jokes and even used material from other improv groups like The Committee.

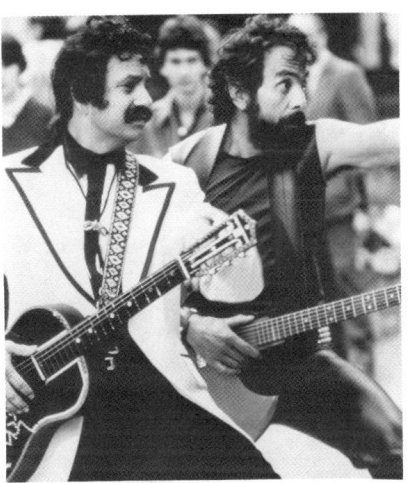

Cheech and Chong's topless dancers and "City Lights" improv group traveled around, landing in Los Angeles. With their tough, earthy humor, they were booked steadily in "trouble clubs" and opened for a lot of black groups and rock acts that normally brought with them impatient crowds that didn't like to sit still for comedy. They gained a certain measure of fame, and some money, which was especially useful to Chong, who had three children, two from an earlier marriage to a young black woman.

The duo prided themselves on their tough stance on stage: "Robert Klein had security guards in the audience to keep would-be hecklers quiet. And he still got heckled. When we were on, our audience—primarily young drunk kids—had to shut up to hear what we were doing. We weren't going to shut up."

The same way Foster Brooks or Woody Woodbury did drunk jokes for their often boozed-out older audiences, Cheech and Chong developed their drug routines. Cheech admitted, "We use dope the way Jackie Gleason and Dean Martin use booze. It's the basis for many comedy situations that can be developed on different levels. But we're essentially dealing in characters."

Goofing around, doing drug and bathroom humor, the team would often throw in old, stolen wheezes ("The Pope at the Vatican") that seemed new to their young, inexperienced fans. Still, they were the only comics around doing real satire and recognition comedy about hippies and "freaks."

"If you're honest in your approach to real life you will always find something funny to share with your audience," says Cheech. Adds Chong, "We're not trying to be good, we're trying to be funny . . . but you know, being vulgar is an art, and to be vulgar and still be accepted you have to be authentically vulgar. That's the power of Cheech and Chong."

After their switch to films, the team decided to change their dope image. The result was the movie *The Corsican Brothers*, but the film was as subtle as the newspaper advertisements for it: "They saw England, they saw France, they saw the Queen in her underpants."

Today Cheech and Chong insist that drugs are part of the past, professionally and personally: "We're not heavy drug users," says Cheech. "We've done it all. I smoke grass. I'm done on cocaine. I did it for a year and never knew why I kept getting sick and was miserable and fighting with everyone."

Director Tommy Chong says, "I'll never be of the caliber of Carl Reiner or Woody Allen," but he's intimated that some day he'd like to try his hand at an *Annie Hall*-type film. Such ambition for a Cheech and Chong movie? Fans and critics are waiting for that one.

MYRON COHEN

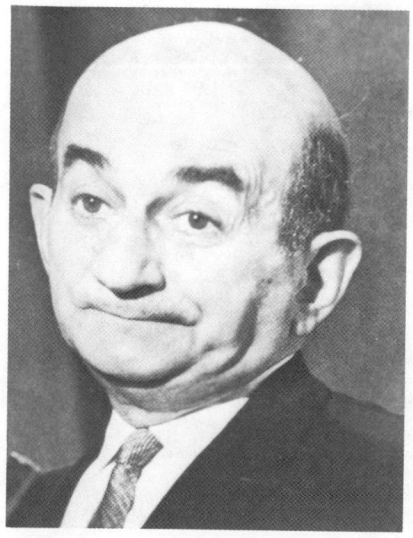

b. July 1, 1902, Grodna, Poland

Records:
Myron Cohen (Audio Fidelity 701), Everybody Gotta Be Someplace (RCA Victor 3534), It's Not a Question (RCA Victor 3791; rereleased on the double set: This Is Myron Cohen [RCA Victor VPS 6052]).

Compilations:
20th Century Yiddish Humor (Banner Records BAS 1004), Variety Yiddish Humor (Banner BAS 1011), Golden Age of Comedy (RCA Victor LPV 580), Fun Time (Coral CRL 57072), Comedy Classics (Era BU 3890).

Books:
Laughing Out Loud, More Laughing Out Loud, Myron Cohen's Big Joke Book.

Myron Cohen was a silk salesman with a smooth line: he amused his customers with a steady stream of jokes. He told definitions: "A shoulder strap is a little piece of ribbon designed to keep an attraction from becoming a sensation." He offered quickies: "I know a salesman who has 100 suits—and they're all pending." And he spread gags he'd heard along his route: "Al Rosenstein of Roseweb Frocks had a model who once told him, 'The nicest thing about money is that it never clashes with anything you're wearing.'" Customers enjoyed the little man who would come around saying, "Piece goods on earth, good wool to men." But as Cohen found out, "They liked my jokes but they didn't always buy my material."

In 1948, Cohen became an overnight sensation in show business. As was his custom, he was entertaining friends at Leon and Eddie's Cafe when owner Eddie Davis insisted he get up and tell the jokes on stage. Not only were the jokes funny and in good taste, the likable Cohen delivered them perfectly, with just the right timing and good-natured flair.

One day Cohen approached his boss, the owner of Wullscheger and Co., and said he was quitting, leaving the garment industry for a show business career. Mr. Wullscheger was astonished.

"I'll be making $1,500 a week," Cohen explained.

"$1,500 a week? For that junk you tell? Go," the boss said, "I'll keep your job open."

The mild-mannered storyteller went down to Miami and delighted audiences with his classics:

"An undertaker called up and says to a young man, 'About your mother-in-law, should we embalm her, cremate her or bury her?' He says, 'Do all three, don't take chances!'"

"Here's one about the small businessman who after six months of valiantly trying to make ends meet decided to call it quits. He posted the following sign in his window: 'Opened by mistake.'"

"A salesman took a girl driving along a lonely country road. They came to a quiet spot and the car stopped. 'I guess we're out of gas,' the salesman leered. With this announcement, the girl carefully opened her purse and pulled out a bottle. 'Wow,' exclaimed the salesman, 'You've got a whole fifth! What kind is it?' She answered, 'Esso regular.'"

When Cohen was booked into the Copacabana in 1952, his old boss, Mr. Wullscheger, came to the show to share Cohen's triumph. For Myron Cohen, "My 25 years in textiles brought me a great many wonderful friends. For me the experience and education couldn't have been bought for a million dollars. It was perfect for me." He could jokingly add, "I'm glad to be out of the business though. My former associates are still jumping out of windows, but they aren't killing themselves because they're falling on their returns."

While some comics had problems with acceptance, or with hecklers, Cohen had a built-in audience: his peers. They were nice people who came to hear nice jokes from a nice man, and he didn't disappoint them. In Miami Beach, in the Catskills and in nightclubs, he developed a following that remained strong.

"You've got to like people and you've got to like what you're doing," says Cohen. "Then it isn't hard to be a nice guy. You've really got to go out of your way to be a louse."

Writer Saul Bellow waxed poetic about Cohen: "In his eyes there is a considerable residue of dark-brown deep down sadness," he wrote. But Cohen calls himself "a nice, pleasant little guy with nothing to prove." Often he begins a story with a humble preamble in which he hopes he will amuse and not offend. He might mention, with a heartfelt word, the person who first told him the joke. If the person is deceased, a phrase like "God love his soul" is not uncommon to hear. It comes without "show biz" sentimentality, from his own sense of what is proper.

He feels he has security in his work because he is not a comic but a storyteller: "I paint a picture when I tell a story. I build a story. This, by the way, is good insurance against robbery. If you just tell jokes thieves grab them."

Cohen's a master of the long, anecdotal story, and like Jack Benny he gently milks each one for maximum enjoyment. He'll introduce the story, revel in the facial mannerisms and accent of the characters (Jewish usually, but Cohen can do many more equally well) and, with a twinkle in his eye and the shared fun of capturing humorously a particular type the audience is familiar with, work his way to the punchline.

For a long time, Cohen turned down TV work because he was afraid he would run out of material. In 1960 he was turning down record offers, too: "Let's say for argument's sake that I make $50,000 from a record of my nightclub show. It'll still bury me . . . the first thing you know everybody knows your stuff."

Later Cohen came to realize that a classic joke *is* classic. Told well, it can even survive a retelling. In fact, many members of his audience requested that he tell a particular favorite story over again. In 1966 Cohen made the first of two albums for RCA Victor, each filled with classics, warm anecdotes and jokes firmly based in laughter at human nature. He put many of his stories into books as well.

Cohen did become predictable: he could always be depended on to be amusing. He took pride in sustaining that level of quality. "Some of my contemporaries," he said in 1979, "I won't mention names, they start to change. They begin to use rough-type words. That's nothing new. I was everybody's stag party mc when I was in the textile business . . . I know the words and how to say them. But in public. . . ."

Cohen remained a popular attraction though he cut back his schedule in the late 70's. He told some modern jokes, on subjects ranging from race relations to infidelity, but they always had that gentle, good natured twist.

He told one about a private detective who says to his client, "I have the proof. Your wife is definitely cheating on you. What do I do now?" The man says resolutely, "Follow my wife and that bum! Keep on their trail night and day, even if you have to track them around the world. And then I want a complete report on what he sees in her!"

On black-Jewish relationships, he described a black man in the diamond district, bewildered at the sight of Orthodox Jews. "What the hell are they?" he asks. "Hassidim," a friend answers. "I see dem too, but what the hell are they?" In another vignette, an angry black man accuses a Jew of bigotry: "I asked him directions, and he called me a black bastard!" The Jew rushes forward and says, in his thick accent, "No! You asked where the drug store vas, and I said—you're a block passed it!"

To a reporter, Cohen insisted, "Today the theater seems to specialize in sex, usually off-beat sex, plays about homosexuals and sadism. If I used that kind of material in a night club, my audience would walk away." The following for Cohen's classic standards and good clean fun never faltered. It was Cohen who, in 1985, retired.

An unintentional little tribute was paid him on an October 1984 "Tonight Show." Tony Randall was a guest, and he told an old fashioned joke, with beginning, middle and punch-line. When it got a surprisingly low ration of laughs from the audience, Randall asked host Johnny Carson if anybody else's delivery could have improved it. Carson thought for a minute and said "No." Then he thought again: "Maybe Myron Cohen could, in a dialect. . . ." Only Myron Cohen.

COOK AND MOORE

Irreverence, cheeky wit and a dash of good old smut characterized the work of Cook and Moore, who, in the manner of most modern comedy teams, have consistently worked individually as well as together.

As Peter Cook has described Dudley Moore: "He was educated (and I use the word in the loosest possible sense) at a local grammar school. Having failed in his attempt to become a pole vaulting champion he turned his attention to music; by diligent study, or possibly bribery, he won an Organ Scholarship to Magdalen College, Oxford."

As Dudley Moore has described Peter Cook: "Educated at Radley College, and Pembroke College, Cambridge, here ostensibly he read French and German, but already driven relentlessly by a lust for power, he concentrated obsessively on seizing the Presidency of the Cambridge Footlights Club in 1959. Revues gushed from his rancid pen. While still at Cambridge he wrote two London shows—*Pieces of 8* and *One over the 8*. Peter was thus the only real professional in the four-man cast of *Beyond the Fringe*."

It was in that satirical show in 1959 that the duo, plus Jonathan Miller and Alan Bennett, won worldwide fame, finally coming to Broadway in 1962. Sketches included a parody of Shakespeare ("So That's the Way You Like It") that became a classic of its kind, and "Aftermyth of War," a mocking bit on England's initial passivity toward Hitler.

Cook performed his own monologues and Moore had his solos too. Still more the musician than the comic, he appeared at the piano to do the popular "Colonel Bogey" theme in an overblown classical concerto, and sing opera in an inane falsetto.

A 1964 *Fringe* followed, including comments on civil rights in the U.S.A. ("What's all this black muslin I hear they're wearing?") and class

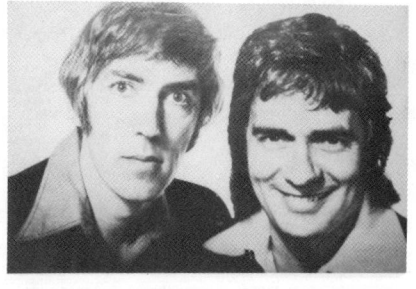

PETER COOK b. Torquay, England, November 17, 1937
DUDLEY MOORE b. Dagenham, England, April 19, 1935

Records:
Beyond the Fringe (Capitol SW 1792), Beyond the Fringe '64 (Capitol W 2072), Not Only Peter Cook But Also Dudley Moore (Decca LKA 4703), Derek and Clive Ad Nauseum (Virgin V2112), Derek and Clive Come Again (Virgin V2094), Derek and Clive Live (Island ILPS 9434), Good Evening (Island ILPS 9298).

Video:
Bedazzled (CBS/Fox), Derek & Clive Get the Horn (Pacific Arts Video), Saturday Night Live 1975 (Warner).

problems in Britain ("I don't want to see lust, rape, incest and sodomy," cries stuffy Lord Cobbold the Duke, "I can get all that at home").

Talented amateurs Bennett and Miller went on to other careers. The team of Cook and Moore appeared in "Not Only, But Also" for British television, had hit records (1967's "LS Bumblebee," with a little help from John Lennon) and movies (*Bedazzled*, which became a cult classic after its initial cool response at the box office).

"I make him laugh a great deal and he makes me," said Moore. "When we work together, you can see the enjoyment in our eyes . . . we listen to each other and react to each other. It's a total involvement in what we are doing . . . and enthusiasm that makes it happen." He later added, "We enjoyed each other, filling in the parts that each didn't have. He always played the know-all, slightly bullying type, and I used to play the compliant sort of twit."

Their first album as a team appeared in 1965, in England, and contained the uproarious "Father and Son" routine. Cook plays the educated, effete son to Moore's raucous, lower-class sewer-worker father:

"What's wrong with the drains then? Ay? I've been down the drains all my life, and my father before me and my grandfather before that. The whole family's been down the drains for centuries. I suppose you're too big to go down the drains! You're too good for the drains! I've seen better things than you floating down the drains! Did I fight in the war for a son like you? Look at this, what's this then?"

"That's your navel, father."

"Get out of my house!"

"It's *my* house, father."

"Oh, pardon me for living! Well get out of your house then, and never darken your doorstep again!"

Through the years, both men took solo movie work as well as team work, with Moore successful as a jazz pianist as well. In 1970 they once again starred on TV in "Not Only, But Two," and then a new stage production, *Good Evening*, which in England was known as *Behind the Fridge*. The original cast lp won a 1974 Grammy.

Though basically stand-up routines, Cook and Moore's material went to Broadway, not nightclubs. The hit of the show was "One Leg Too Few," which was actually one of their older routines, a cruel bit about a one-legged man trying out for the role of Tarzan.

Moore, bobbing up and down on one leg (the other concealed in the folds of his long trench coat) sports a happy, optimistic grin as he confidently meets the casting director. It's up to icy, efficient Peter Cook to damp Dudley's enthusiasm.

"You, Mr. Spiggot," he says with just a tad of condescension, "are a unidexter. . . . You, a unidexter, are applying for the role, a role for which two legs would seem to be the minimum requirement. Need I point out, that it is in the leg division that you are deficient? You are deficient in the leg division to the tune of one."

The smiling, irrepressible Moore keeps on bouncing while Cook admits, "Your right leg I like. It's a lovely leg. I've got nothing against your right leg. . . . Neither have you." Cook finally allows that Moore does "score over a man with no legs at all," and insists that if he can't find a two-legged man, he just might get back to Moore—"in several months time."

It was up to Moore to decide on the taste of such a sketch. The 5'2" comic was born with a club foot: "It was a source of enormous shame for me. It reminds you of Sherlock Holmes films where the villain had a club foot, or The Hunchback of Notre Dame . . . you imagine you are this twisted, undesirable unattractive piece of rubbish. This feeling is very hard to lose. A lot of the projection of charm in the beginning was desperation, I think. . . . I'll never get over the stain of that pain. Of course the actual handicap is very minor."

The most outrageous sketch of the evening was an interview of a shepherd who had happened to witness the birth of Jesus. Part of the dialogue went like this:

"Was the Holy Ghost there?"
"Hard to say, he's an elusive little bugger and I didn't see him. He should've been there, in his capacity as the godfather."
"Three wise men arrived?"
"Three bloody idiots. In they come and call themselves Maggie."

The shepherd, while watching various obscene acts being performed on sheep, wonders about the presents the Magi brought: "What's a kid gonna do with Frankincense and Myrrh? Myrrh is that stuff poofs put behind their ear." Of course, Jesus did appreciate the thought: "He said 'Thank you for your lovely presents, I hope you have a safe trip back. . . . Merry Christmas!'"

Cook and Moore, still favorites among elders with a taste for biting satire, developed a huge cult with young fans. They didn't disappoint them. Their next three albums were done as the characters "Derek and Clive," and they were free-form, ad-libbed and absolutely filthy, "the most obscene thing you've ever heard in your life," Moore said gleefully. "I enjoy a dirty joke, or a pun of scatological nature, 'cause it's all fun."

Sort of like getting a bootleg recording of two very drunk comics trying to be as outrageous and uninhibited as possible, this material was banned by the BBC and by many British record shops. So, naturally, it became their biggest hit. The first "Derek and Clive" record sold a quick 50,000 copies within months of its appearance.

Typical of the rambling is this segment from "Come Again," with Peter Cook describing an encounter with a famous Hollywood star:

"Joan Crawford, J.C. as she's known . . . a tropical storm invaded the bedroom and I was swept away by this huge gust o' wind, straight up her fuckin' cunt . . . tore through the diaphragm she was wearing . . . the biggest fucking disaster area I've ever fucking seen . . . you've heard of the Bermuda Triangle? This was worse . . . fucking fleets of ships, light aircraft . . . they got a pool in there, and there's no water up Joan Crawford at all, so they filled it full of shit."

Dudley admits that he, too, had a terrible experience with Joan Crawford. "I was appalled."
"By the state of her cunt?" Cook asks.

"The people wandering about, lost. I got a bit lost myself. Her asshole was completely blocked with Spanish Revolutionaries . . . I started makin' my way north."
"Did you make your way to her tits? They're frozen over."
"I went into the gall bladder. I fucking fell. Her fucking gall bladder wasn't there . . . I got in her stomach, by osmosis . . . I stuck a pencil up her epiglotis and I came flying out with all this Chinese food . . . I landed straight over the toilet 'cause she was leaning over."

"Fucking Hollywood, isn't it?"

Cook and Moore performed some of their "Derek and Clive" material at public functions. "We are not amused," was the reaction among the elite who had, a decade earlier, taken to satire not quite so beyond the fringe.

Dudley Moore, who was something of a sex symbol in England for years, and who had starred in the English stage version of Woody Allen's *Play It Again, Sam*, took a small part in the movie *Foul Play* as an eccentric sex maniac out after Goldie Hawn. Soon he was out after even bigger things: Bo Derek in *10*. And he became a tremendous star.

"I suppose I've been successful since my early 20's," he says, "but never a star of this magnitude. I've had to learn humility and I've had to get along with other people. Also, being in a partnership with another man, I couldn't let my ego go wild . . . so now here I am, making the most of the movie offers, the work and the ogling. Now I'm cuddly and powerful."

The future for Cook and Moore, sublime satirists, is uncertain. Each has unlimited solo potential in a variety of areas.

IRWIN COREY

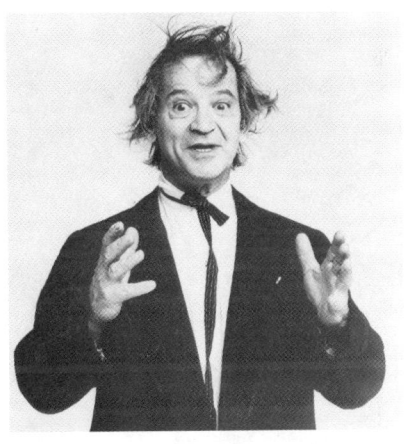

Dressed in an absurdly overlarge frock coat, his hair flying out in all directions, puckish "Professor" Corey delivers wild, free-form lectures that blend ad-libs with prepared gags. In the guise of a windy, befuddled lecturer, he slyly injects social and political satire amid the often-risque audience participation patter.

Lenny Bruce called him "one of the most brilliant comedians of all time." Once a popular raconteur on late night TV talk shows, he found himself persona non grata after doing some controversial lines. "Is there life after birth?" the Professor would ask, eyes wildly aglow. "Yes! Nixon is a great example of afterbirth!"

"When you go along with the policies of Reagan and Nixon, then it's okay, you work. But if you try to discredit or expose their shortcomings you're immediately put on a non-persona list," says Corey. "It's still going on."

Possessing a fierce sense of morality and a complex personality, Corey, like Bruce, has sometimes gone out of his way to be iconoclastic. Sometimes the results cost him, sometimes he made his point, and other times the whole thing could be considered colorfully eccentric. In 1980 he made headlines when he deliberately blocked off his wealthy, bigwig neighbors by parking his car across the alley of a busy private street. The ritzy tenants (the place was actually named Sniffen Court) had to go to court to deal with the feisty little Professor. A short time later he put his house up for sale, choosing to tilt at other windmills.

Nearly 40 years earlier, Corey was just another funmaker, an up-and-coming New York comic. In 1943 he opened at the Village Vanguard, and later became a fixture at Le Ruban Bleu. He displayed his talents in stand-up, summer stock, on radio with Edgar Bergen and on Broadway.

In 1956, he described his Professor character in warm, amiable terms: "He just grew over the years. Sometimes I'm not sure what the Professor is going to say or do until I go on the floor and the character takes over. I'm not sure why, but everybody seems to love the poor-soul absent-minded professor. Just by looking at him you know he's lost in the clouds

b. January 29, 1912, New York, New York

Records:
At the Ruban Bleu (Jubilee 2018), Win with Irwin: Campaigning at the Playboy Club (Atlantic 1236), The World's Foremost Authority (Viva 6009), I Feel More Like I Do Now (Gateway Records).

Broadway:
Flahooley, Mrs. McThing, Happy as Heaven.

Films:
Thieves, Car Wash, How to Commit Marriage, Stuck on You, Crackers.

Video:
The Hungry i Reunion Concert (Pacific Arts).

and doesn't know it. He wouldn't hurt a fly and he loves people. Even children laugh at him."

There was nothing controversial about a typical gag like this one: "Sir Isaac Newton and the law of gravity; there he was, walking through his apple orchard, and he saw an apple falling down from a tree, which amazed him. Because . . . up until that time . . . until the law of gravity was passed . . . all apples fell up."

The Professor would ad-lib, using memory and a skeleton of gags to keep sure-fire material available as he needed it. If his stream-of-consciousness and audience participation bits weren't working, he could go to one of his standard lines, windily weaving his way up to: "Life is memory. So if you don't do anything when you're 13, when you're 51 you got nothing to remember." And when spying some empty seats, "It's impossible to capture the mind of a heterogeneous mass when they ain't even here!"

Once an amateur 112-pound boxing champ, Corey began to add real punch to his act, satirizing the stuffy politicians and professors, able in the 1960's to liberate his humor. "I'm not a comedian," he said, echoing the late Lenny Bruce, "I'm an iconoclast. I'm everybody who has ever been pompous and arrogant, pretending to know all the answers but full of shit. . . . I'm taking off on all those pompous asses. What I do is deflate the coat of righteousness that people wrap themselves in."

Blacklisted from television, Corey's attacks became even angrier, more opinionated, and at times directed even toward those who admired him. "I don't give a damn if I *am* self-destructive," Corey has said, "I just don't want to be associated with scum." The scum include a vast array of show business cliques, politicians, neo-Nazis and fellow comedians who play it safe or sell out.

Among the comics who are "traitors to the profession" he includes everyone from George Gobel ("dullsville") to Pat Cooper ("bullshit") to Woody Allen ("a fuckin' sell-out, a fuckin' shallow, phony liar. Did you see *Annie Hall*? It was an anti-Semitic piece of shit."). It genuinely pains him to be associated with a Rodney Dangerfield or a Joan Rivers ("she demeans the female gender and makes money doing it").

Only a few escape his disdain, comic rebels like Richard Pryor, Jackie Mason, Jonathan Winters, Mort Sahl and Lenny Bruce. Like Bruce in his latter years, Corey can still fire from the hip, though at times he sounds consumed by bitter smoke.

Embraced by the free-thinking porn world, Corey found himself declared "The only real choice for President in 1980" by *Screw* publisher Al Goldstein. Twenty years earlier, similar presidential statements had come about Corey from Hugh Hefner. For *Screw*, Corey gave a rare interview attacking a status quo of "anti-Semitism, segregation, discrimination, poverty and war." He told *Screw* that "Comedy is a very interesting weapon in the hands of those who are fighting the injustices of society. Because people will remember a laugh more than they will a direct quote, however profound it is."

And people still remember the Professor. Despite the network TV blacklist, he is justly proud that after all these years, he is instantly recognizable. He has found outlets in clubs and on cable TV to explore his humor. For the videotaped Hungri i reunion concert he dazzled the crowd with whimsical bits of pantomime and question-and-answer bits like "Is Santa Claus dead? Well, he might as well be." Continuing with a pained expression: "I mean, anyone that comes just once a year? And down the chimney at that! And in *my* sock?"

His brief routine in Louis Malle's 1984 film *Crackers* was the movie's only bright spot, and proof of Corey's talents as a charismatic character.

He continues to wrestle with complex moral issues, often being as paradoxical in his viewpoints as in those he protests. The same man who has said, "New York, where the political view blightens the eye . . . more people per capita than any other city of the same size with the same per capita," has also lent his face and humor to New York ads for Off-Track Betting (OTB), promoting legalized betting and gambling, with revenues going to the state.

Perhaps the greatest stability for Corey comes through in one way that counts: love. He has been married for over 40 years and has two grown children, Richard and Margaret.

BILL COSBY

Bill Cosby projects an image of sweet humor in talking about growing up. But his childhood was the opposite.

"I remember my father beating my mother up three times," he says. "I was too small to do anything about it. These things are very, very painful to think about today."

His father was a heavy drinker who eventually deserted the family. One of Bill's brothers left the family, too. He was only six: dead of rheumatic fever.

At nine, Cosby was shining shoes, delivering newspapers and helping to support his mother and younger brothers. His schoolwork suffered. It took him three years to get through the 10th grade. And from all sides of the Philadelphia ghetto there was the temptation of drugs and crime. "The only reason I stayed out of jail all those years was because I'd say to myself, now if I do so-and-so and get caught, and they lock me up, who'll look out for Mom?"

Bill joined the Navy and from there enrolled at Temple University as a physical education major. By night he found work tending bar in a Philadelphia coffee house. He did some pinch-hitting for comedians who failed to show up, at first failing with set routines that were too much in the artificial mold of the traditional comics:

"I started out making six dollars a night in a burlesque house telling Ivy League jokes to six sailors and a junkie, doing a routine about how Shakespearean actors talk. They didn't want some college darkie talking about Hamlet between bumps and grinds so I got fired. I went to a beatnik dive—you know the kind—full of ugly Negro girls and ugly white men—sort of a Lonelyhearts integration. But they laughed. I was getting closer. Finally some cat called and said, 'Aren't you the one who does the funny bit about the guy with St. Vitus' dance trying to light his own cigarette?' I said yes. He said, 'I'll give you sixteen dollars a night.' Big time."

Cosby moved to New York in 1962 with a confident, loose style of laid-back monology, the same kind of smoothness that had helped him out-talk ghetto bullies and sweet talk the girls. Coming after the "sick-nik" 50's acts like Sahl, Gregory, Bruce and Berman, Cosby was a startling breath of fresh air. He told stories of childhood to a nation that had come to believe in the storybook possibilities of a New Frontier. Even his mildly sick routines (rigor mortis and death at sea, the mating of a zoo gorilla) were done with an inoffensive, amusing style.

Gradually all traces of past influences, either standard comics doing routines or sickniks telling odd jokes, faded away. Cosby emerged as a unique comedian. Groucho Marx was a big fan, telling Charlotte

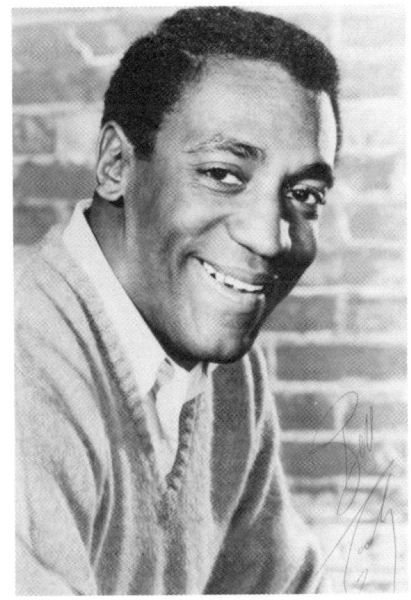

b. William Henry Cosby Jr., July 12, 1937, Philadelphia, Pennsylvania

Records:
Bill Cosby Is a Very Funny Fellow—Right (Warner 1518), I Started Out as a Child (Warner 1567), Why Is There Air (Warner 1606), Wonderfulness (Warner 1634), Revenge (Warner 1691), To Russell My Brother Whom I Slept With (Warner 1734), 200 MPH (Warner 1757), It's True It's True (Warner S1770), Best of Bill Cosby (Warner 1798), More of the Best (Warner 1836), Bill Cosby (MCA 8005), Live at Madison Square Garden (UNI 73082), Fat Albert (MCA 333), Inside the Mind of Bill Cosby (MCA 554), Sports (UNI 73066), When I Was a Kid (MCA 1691 and UNI 73100), For Adults Only (MCA 553 and UNI 73112), 8:15–12:15 (Tetragrammaton TD 5100), Bill's Best Friend (Capitol ST 11731), Disco Bill (Capitol ST 11683), My

Father Confused Me (Capitol ST 115900), Not Himself These Days (Capitol ST 11530), Bill Cosby Himself (Motown ML 6026).

TV:
I Spy (NBC 1965–68), The Bill Cosby Show (NBC 1969–71), Cos (ABC 1976), Fat Albert & the Cosby Kids (cartoon, CBS 1972–), The New Bill Cosby Show (CBS 1972–73), The Bill Cosby Show (NBC 1984–).

Films on Video:
Uptown Saturday Night (Warner Video), Let's Do It Again (Warner Video), Bill Cosby Himself (CBS/Fox Video).

Bio:
Bill Cosby (Smith)

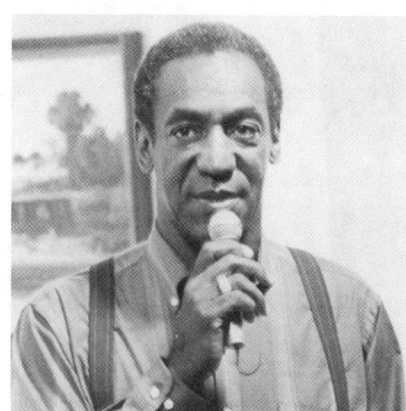

Chandler, "He's fantastic. He doesn't tell any jokes. He does impressions of people. Like how a mother will talk to her child, and how a father will talk to the same child. Things like that. And he'll show you people who take dope. He's brilliant, this man."

Some in the audience were surprised to find a black comedian who didn't do race jokes. But by presenting himself back in 1963 as "a very funny fellow," period, he became one of the most influential of black stars, and a symbol of equality. For many, he removed the last invisible shred of raciality. Sammy Davis Jr. was always the "credit to his race," and Dick Gregory was the "angry black man," but Cosby was really the first to be called "star" without having the word "black" in front of it. He wasn't perceived as a black comedian, or a black star, just a funny comedian, and a superstar. The pressure to take this stance and avoid getting tangled in debate over it must have been intense.

Back in the 60's he told *Playboy Magazine*, "I think there are some people who are disappointed when I don't tell my audience that white people are mistreating black people. White critics will write about Cosby not doing any racial material, because they think that now is the time for me to stand up and tell my audience what color I am and what's going on in America. But I don't see these people knocking the black elevator man in their building just because he isn't doing anything for civil rights by running that elevator. . . . The fact that I'm not trying to win converts on stage bugs some people, but I don't think an entertainer *can* win converts. I've never known any kind of white bigot to pay to see a black man, unless the black man was being hung. So I don't spend my hours worrying how to slip a social message into my act. I just go out and do my thing."

In 1963 Allan Sherman, guest-hosting "The Tonight Show," booked Cosby, and, a few days afterward, persuaded Warner Brothers to sign him. Cosby's first album won a Grammy nomination. In the album notes, Sherman declared one routine, "Noah and the Ark," to be "a masterpiece even though nobody has heard it yet. It's warm, and human, and honest and deeply moving and it's funny. . . . I'm so proud and happy for the chance to introduce you to Bill Cosby. It isn't every day that we come in contact with greatness."

"Noah" did become a classic, a long monologue sketch that plumbed the same fractured history vein as did Bob Newhart. What do you suppose Noah's neighbors thought when he started building this big boat? What did God mean by telling Noah to measure everything in "cubits"? And what do you say when you hear a voice that intones, "This is God"?

Cosby's second lp, "I Started Out as a Child," won a 1964 Grammy with its vivid recollections of childhood, like flapping soles on cheap shoes, getting new sneakers, and drinking from a bottle instead of a glass and leaving breadcrumbs in the family water pitcher. A classic bit described playing 46-man street football: "Arnie, go down ten steps and cut left behind the black Chevy. Philbert, you run down to my house and wait in the living room. Cosby, you go down to Third Street, catch the J bus, have him open the doors at 19th Street—I'll fake it to you."

In 1965 the likable comedian broke the color barrier on TV, co-starring with Robert Culp in the comedy-adventure series "I Spy." The show marked Cosby's emergence as a superstar. He beat out Culp for one Emmy, and racked up two more. But as a stand-up comic he found his row of Emmy Awards rather paltry compared with the six consecutive Grammys his records won, marking him as America's #1 comic from 1964 to 1969.

These early albums are his best, noted not for individual jokes but for funny situations and evocative recollections of childhood. Cosby also displayed a talent for finding humor in such unlikely topics as a pet rhinoceros, groin injuries in football and why men should take Midol tablets. As he shifted to Tetragrammaton and UNI Records, his work became even more relaxed, more keyed to contemporary observations (on golf: "You got the ball. You had it right there. Then . . . you hit it away! And then . . . you go and walk after it again! It's a dumb game!") and filled with ad-libs and light byplay with the audience. One album, he was proud to say, was almost entirely ad-libbed, the result of his rich ability as a raconteur and storyteller. Memorable in this mode was his situation-comedy encounter with an old man who wiped him out playing handball. The humor is almost all in character, in timing and in the comic irritation between fast, athletic Cos and slow, steady nemesis.

In 1969 he started as a teacher in his own situation comedy, which has been more appreciated in rerun than when in its original two-season run. Cosby shifted to movies in the early 70's, making some of the first quality films intended for black audiences. Over the years he peppered the record racks with non-comedy albums of singing and instrumental jazz. None achieved much success, but in the late 70's he finally found the right formula: blending comedy and music for disco-funk parodies.

Cosby quietly opened doors for many blacks, integrating the crews on his TV shows. For such charities as the National Hemophilia Foundation, The Watts Workshop, The American Cancer Society and others, he raised thousands of dollars. Perhaps his deepest concern has been education. He's tried to find new ways to make learning fun for kids, and has lent his talents to various educational film, TV and record projects, including "The Electric Company."

1976 saw him fulfill a lifelong dream, earning his doctorate in education from the University of Massachusetts. He'd built his home in Amherst so he could be close to his studies. It was there that his family grew to include four daughters and a son: Erika (the first, born in 1965), Erinn, Ensa, Evin, and Ennis (the last, born in 1979).

Cosby guards his privacy, and has given few interviews over the years. He resented a *TV Guide* article mentioning the number of cars he owns. Yet, paradoxically, fans know quite a bit about Cosby's personal life. For 20 years he has shared it comedically, describing, with enthusiasm and chagrin, how his children fight with each other, how he and his wife handle discipline problems, and even the time his daughters accidentally saw him using the toilet—and then tried to duplicate the unique masculine ability of standing up while using the facilities.

"As far as my private life is concerned," he once said, "show business is my job. My life at home doesn't differ from any other working man's, other than in dollars and cents. Every man becomes somebody else when he goes to work. You go to New York and get in one of those yellow cabs and sitting up there on the driver's dashboard are color pictures of his kids, smiling back at him. He's your cab driver, but he's their Daddy."

From doing routines predominantly from a child's viewpoint, Cosby evolved bits on a parent's view of children. Cosby had long enjoyed great popularity with children, probably more than any other stand-up comic of his generation. For teens, he was "cool Cos," the man who spun the stories about kids like "Weird Harold" and "Fat Albert." But as Cosby grew older, he gained a more mature following.

It was during this phase that Cosby had his only period of relative stagnance. He didn't produce many albums in the late 70's. It was the era when Richard Pryor reasserted angry racial comedy and Cosby was finding an older Vegas audience sympathetic to his parent-vs.-child routines. It's possible that Cosby's period of mildly low exposure was also tied to his high visibility in television commercials. Advertisers found that Cos was cool and *cute*. Cosby exploited his affable personality by pitching soft drinks, pudding and computers. This may have bothered some fans, suspicious that his "nice guy" stance was really just an act.

Always a top draw in Vegas, a welcome guest on "The Tonight Show," Cosby returned to the spotlight when he made a live concert movie in 1983, and finally accepted an offer to do a new TV sit-com.

The new "Cosby Show" saw the comedian's dream of a realistic family show come true. Powered by his insistence on truth and perfection, the show went through many writers, but emerged as the only hit show of the 1984 season. Gaining even more strength in 1985, it out-rated such strong, if artistically vapid super shows as "Dynasty," "The A-Team" and "Magnum P.I." Only the Super Bowl scored better than Cosby that winter.

"We comedians have a staying power of maybe 20 years," Cosby said in the late 70's. "Unless we come up with something new, we can run out of welcome." With his sit-com, he came up with something new and true, and was greeted with fresh critical praise. With his stand-up act, he continues to explore the human comedy in family relationships. How much of it is based on Cosby's reality, and how much of it translates comedically from his deep childhood pain and his very serious views on a belief in a strong, loving family unit, is still subject for conjecture.

Cosby assesses his comedy:

"What I do with humor is to have three levels hitting all at the same time. There is the middle level which is the total laughter itself, but there is also an overcurrent and an undercurrent. For instance, in my monologues the humor itself goes straight down the middle because of identification. Then the overcurrent is the fact that rather than trying to bring the races of people together by talking about the differences, let's try to bring them together by talking about the similarities. Then there is also the undercurrent that makes an appeal for an understanding of the gap between the ages."

NORM CROSBY

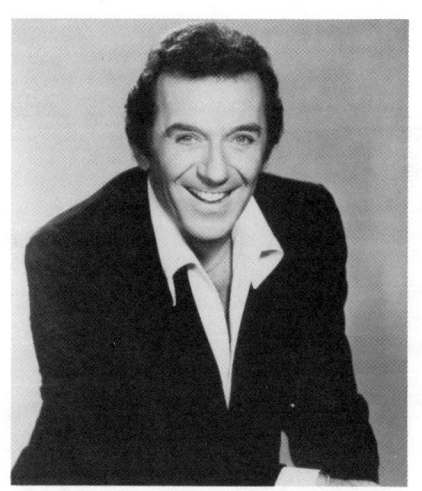

b. September 15, 1927, Boston, Massachusetts

It began with Richard Brinsley Sheridan's character Mrs. Malaprop and was reincarnated with varying twists by Jane Ace, Leo Gorcey, Minerva "Mrs. Nussbaum" Pious and Carroll O'Connor's Archie Bunker. But only Norm Crosby based a stand-up comedy career on malapropism, humor based on punned word abuse. And while most comics used the tool only to make fun of an ignoramus, Crosby smoothed over the limitations by making himself seem lovably befuddled.

While attending the Massachusetts School of Art, Crosby planned a career as a commercial artist. Before completing school he enlisted in the Coast Guard. He was a radar operator during World War II, and when his ship was literally blown out of the water, he suffered a partial hearing loss. He wears a hearing aid and at times has joked on stage about his difficulty making sense of mumbled conversation.

After the war Crosby worked for a Boston shoe store. Although he eventually became the store's manager, he was far from satisfied: "I was the funny kid in school and I loved to do comedy. I didn't want to go through the rest of my life in a job that was not making me happy, so I left the shoe store to take comedy jobs."

He entertained at a party one night and impressed comic Allen Drake, who hired Norm as his assistant for emcee duty at a resort hotel. Crosby made the rounds of nightclubs, charity shows and the grind of entertaining at stag dinners for fraternal organizations. When he finally got a break at New York's Latin Quarter, "It dawned on me that the material I was using was not original, but a combination of a lot of things I had seen on the Ed Sullivan Show. I needed something better for the Latin Quarter."

Crosby had a friend who unintentionally convulsed people with his malapropisms, and Norm developed this character in his act. The Latin Quarter gig was a success, and Crosby perfected his malaprop monologues in other clubs, on TV and in Catskill resorts.

His club act is lecture-oriented, with Crosby urging his audience to accept his "hysterical truths" and understand his interpretations of biblical wisdom, facts of life and advice from great men like "Sigmund Frood who went into a lavatory and friggered out all for himself, on the sperm of the moment, that there was equalness between people."

Crosby may not have gotten a "standing ovulation" from the "masculine men and fennemen ladies" who sat at ringside "meticulously retired," but he did "establish a rappaport" with them that has kept him busy over several decades. For three years he opened for Robert Goulet around the country, and for four years he toured with Tom Jones.

Through the 1970's he shared the bill with such Vegas headliners as Tony Bennett, Olivia Newton-John, Liza Minnelli and Shirley MacLaine. The comic would urge mothers in the audience to guide their impressionable children: "Mothers mold the children's minds. Some of you have done well. There are a lot of moldy-minded kids around." And he would do straight jokes, like this one preaching the real meaning of love:

"Teenagers don't know what love is. They have mixed up ideas. They go for a drive, and the boy runs out of gas, and they smooch a little, and the girl says she loves him. That isn't love. Love is when you're married 25 years, smooching in your living room, and he runs out of gas and she still says she loves him—that's love!"

Enduring for decades as one of the nation's most likable comedians, the gently demented malaprop artist became the spokesman for a light beer company that saw the advantages in having Norm humorously explain the confusing and long name of their product. The same year, 1978, Crosby finally starred in his own TV show, the syndicated "Comedy Shop," which was patterned after the many comedy showcases and workshops on both coasts. He hosted the show, introducing aspiring young comics and old favorites.

Crosby is well known for his charity work, having served as the Honorary Chairman for the Better Hearing Institute in Washington, D.C. He's raised money for the City of Hope by staging annual celebrity golf tournaments. In recognition of his achievements in comedy and his service for charity, Crosby earned a star on the Hollywood Walk of Fame, and was placed, at his request, between the sidewalk stars of his idols Jack Benny and Red Skelton.

He's been married since 1966 to his wife, Joan, and has two sons, Daniel and Andrew. Crosby uses his wife in his monologues, but in a much gentler way than other comics. Talking about the yoga fad on a 1984 "Merv Griffin Show" he remarked, "My wife goes to yogurt class. But lots of people out here in California sit in a chair and medicate. I asked her why she pays somebody so she can sit in one position and go home after an hour, and she said, 'It's better than sitting around the house.'"

Record:
The Funny World of Norm Crosby (aka: She Wouldn't Eat the Mushrooms; Epic FLS 15106/FLM 13106).

TV:
Everything Goes (syndicated 1973); Comedy Shop (syndicated 1978–83).

Crosby maintains a second home in Vegas so the family can stay together: "I have been blessed with the ability to amuse others, make them laugh, help them try to forget their problems," he says. "I consider this a true gift. But, in my personal life, I want to please me, as long as I don't hurt anybody or cause grief to anyone. That's *my* reward."

BILL DANA

In the late 1950's, a Hungarian named William Szathmary appeared on "The Steve Allen Show" under the name Bill Dana and performed as a little Hispanic fellow named Jose Jimenez.

Confusing? Well, confusion was Jose's trademark. The deadpan fellow was a babe in the woods, a dreamer, and no matter what occupations he tried—from astronaut to lion tamer to sidewalk Santa—he met with comical disaster. Shy, unassuming, unable to communicate fluently, Jose would muster all his determination and dignity and proclaim in that little nasal voice, "My name . . . Jose Jimenez"—and audiences would break up laughing. Just introducing himself produced a national catch-phrase. Bill "Jose Jimenez" Dana was an overnight sensation.

Of course, the "overnight sensation" had paid his dues. Bill Szathmary, youngest of six children, grew up in a poor family, attended Emerson College, and at 5'8" and 126 pounds was an Infantryman in World War II. He entered show business with a last name borrowed from his mother, whose first name was Dena.

"I started as a performer," Bill Dana recalled. "I was half of a comedy team with Gene Wood. We played at such night spots as Le Ruban Bleu and The Bon Soir back around 1952–53. Around this time a back injury forced me to give up performing and I turned to writing."

Dana wrote comedy for a young stand-up comic named Don Adams, and in 1956 got a staff job on "The Steve Allen Show," where, as Steve recalls, "For two years he labored in the obscurity of the writer's wing of our offices. Then, amused by his parlor entertainment impression of a Latin-American character, I decided to have him do the voice on-camera. The rest is history."

The first Jose joke was in a "man in the street" vignette, where he appeared as a sidewalk Santa who fractured the language and rang his bell shouting "Jo Jo Jo." Before long, Jose turned up in a number of different jobs. As the terrified (detractors might substitute the term "cowardly") astronaut on his Grammy-nominated first Kapp album, Jose was asked what he planned to do on those long, lonely nights in outer space. "I plan to cry a lot," Jose answered mournfully.

The routine became a favorite at Cape Canaveral, and that particular line was even used by astronaut Wally Schirra for a gag.

Almost from the start, though, Dana had to answer critics who questioned his judgment in making fun of the Hispanic accent. "Jose is anyone in any country with any background who has difficulty in speaking the language," he said in 1961. "I got 7,000 letters when we first did 'Jose' on the Allen Show. I got only one letter saying it was in bad taste—and that came from a non-Latin in Denver."

He amplified on this viewpoint when, his name now synonymous with Jose Jimenez, he was about to star in his own television show for the same network (NBC) where he had once worked as a page for $33 a week: "I speak Spanish, and I'm aware of the Puerto Rican experience. I don't think there's anything about Jose that offends Latins or anyone

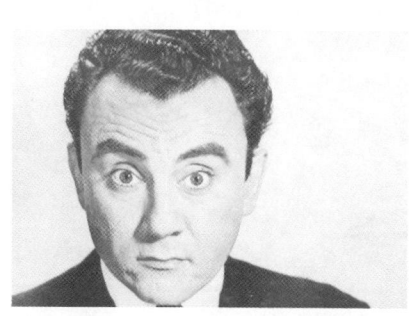

b. William Szathmary, October 5, 1924, Quincy, Massachusetts

Records:
My Name Jose Jimenez (Signature SM 1013), Jose the Astronaut (aka: Bill Dana at the Hungry i; Kapp KL 1238), The Submarine Officer (aka: More Jose; Kapp KL 1215), Jose Jimenez in Orbit (Kapp KL 1457), Jose Jimenez Talks to Teenagers (Kapp KL 1304), In Jollywood (Kapp KS 3332), In Las Vegas (Kapp KL 1415), Hoo Ha (Capitol ST 464), Mashuganah Yogi, with Joey Forman (A&M 4144); The Best of Jose (GNP Crescendo 7001).

TV:
The Bill Dana Show (NBC 1963–65).

Book:
My Name Jose Jimenez.

else. I'm always protective about the character. I was a little worried at first. I didn't want to play this guy in a menial position [as a bell-hop on the show]." Dana once refused to play Jose in a Pontiac commercial because Pontiac wanted to have the little man comically arrested for speeding. "I don't want any cop putting his hand on Jose," Dana insisted. He added, "I don't make fun of him and audiences realize that."

One of his early albums sold 90,000 copies in two months, and Dana saw his salary escalate from $300 a week in 1956 to $35,000 in 1959, until, years later, he could recall that Jose had brought in close to $20 million.

Many wondered how Dana was able to handle the split personality. Actually there were three personalities: "There's Jose Jimenez," he said, "actually the nice side of everybody. There's Bill Dana, who enjoys success to the hilt. And there's Bill Szathmary, who was tremendously insecure and had deep feelings of inferiority . . . but I think Bill Szathmary is just about gone now."

Dana balanced his Jose routines in nightclubs by devoting a portion of his show to straight monologues. Some of these were "man in the street" interviews with himself:

"Excuse me, sir, are you a cigarette smoker?"
"I was. I gave it up. And I was very disappointed."
"Why?"
"I found out my teeth are really brown."

He told dialect stories like the one about the Jewish mother who was visited by her comedian son. The son holds up a color picture of a topless dancer in dark blue leotards. "When I work in nightclubs, Momma, this is the kind of girl I work with." The woman studies the picture and says, "That's the color I want the drapes."

The Jose routines usually involved a straight man (in nightclubs this was often co-writer Don Hinckley) and different professions. But the jokes were usually not based on the Hispanic angle. To Jose the Senator: "Are you a senator? Honest?" "Make up your mind!" To Jose the skin diver: "Would you say skin diving is dangerous?" "All right. Skin diving is dangerous." To Jose the astronaut: "You must have some opinions on the race for space." "OK, I will."

With Steve Allen playing straight, and Dana as a submarine officer, the dialogue went like this:

"Congratulations on your tremendous feat," Allen begins.
"Thank you," Jose answers hesitantly, "but they're only size 8." The bit continues with pure vaudevillian patter:
"You stayed under water for 84 days. How come?"
"They didn't want to come up before the submarine. . . ."
"Under water all that time, did you begin to hate your friends?"
"Just one time. During the third riot."
"As an executive officer you had a specific assignment—"
"No . . . I had the Atlantic assignment."
"In those 84 days that you were submerged, did you have any mechanical trouble?"
"Only with the ballast valve, the one that lets you go up."
"How long did you have that problem?"
"83 days."

In 1967 Bill Dana was the host of a two-hour variety show from Las Vegas on "The United Network," an ambitious attempt to compete with the Big Three networks. When it failed, Dana appeared in "Jose Explores

America" in 1968, a tour of off-beat places around the country. But as the years went on, Jose Jimenez encountered more and more problems. He couldn't get out of the sensitized 60's alive.

On April 4, 1970, Bill Dana appeared at a Congress of Mexican-American Unity gathering and told the throng of 10,000, "after tonight, Jose Jimenez is dead." They cheered.

That year, Dana reflected, "In the first years of Jose, friends of mine like Ricardo Montalban and Anthony Quinn thought he was just silly. But some Latin-Americans thought he was dumb and insulting. I came to realize they were right. I think ethnic humor is fine. What Flip Wilson does is great: a Negro doing Negro humor. But I was doing Latin-American humor, and I'm a Hungarian Jew."

Dana eventually produced an album of Jewish dialect humor, a parody of "Hee-Haw" called "Hoo-Ha," loaded with funny one-liners. It didn't catch on. Meanwhile, the large Kapp collection of Jose Jimenez records went quietly out of print. There has not been a rush from collectors to buy them, either, and they generally sell in the $5–$10 price range.

Listeners rediscovering them will find, especially on "The Submarine Officer" (with straight men Steve Allen and Spike Jones), "Bill Dana in Las Vegas" and "Jose the Astronaut," many first-rate jokes. "Goddamn good jokes," Dana reflected. "I've done Jose Jimenez jokes in Scotch, German, Yiddish dialects. People are laughing at well-constructed jokes" above all else.

It could've been anyone up in that space capsule saying mournfully, "I plan to cry a lot."

Dana has not been a frequent performer over the past decade, but has scored impressively as a television producer and writer. He wrote the famous episode of "All in the Family" that had Sammy Davis, Jr. getting the upper hand on the bigoted Archie Bunker. Recently he's also developed topical humor books with partner Stan Corwin. And, perhaps as a sign that Jose Jimenez was not such a racial insult (especially compared with 1984's "AKA Pablo") re-runs of the old Bill Dana Show have actually been syndicated. Among the stations who bought it is the Christian Broadcasting Network.

RODNEY DANGERFIELD

"My wife's an earth sign, I'm a water sign. Together we make mud. . . . My kid goes to a private school—he won't tell me where it is. . . . I was a very ugly baby. When the doctor cut the cord he hung himself. . . . We were so poor in my neighborhood the rainbow was in black and white. . . . The other day I called up to get the right time. The record hung up on me. . . . Know what my trouble is? I appeal to everyone who can do me absolutely no good. . . . I don't get no respect, no respect at all. I broke up with my psychiatrist. One day I told him I had suicidal tendencies. He told me, from now on, I had to pay in advance."

Indignity heaped on indignity, push to shove to kick, punchlines that boomerang and punch the comic right in the nose. With a sad, pouchy-eyed, basset-hound face, a deep and haunted hollow voice and fidgety mannerisms, Rodney Dangerfield is the personification of the struggling, snake-bit loser.

It's a character he's known well: "People take a look at me and think I

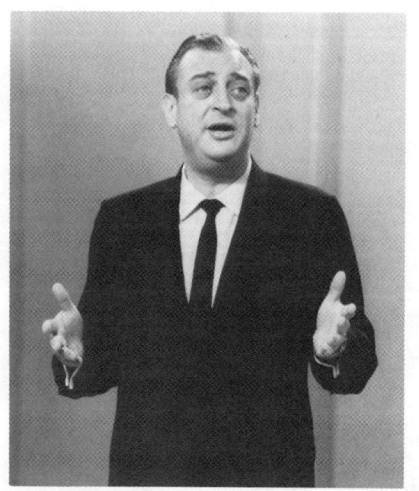

b. Jacob Cohen, November 22, 1921, Babylon, New York

don't have any feelings. There's that joke that underneath this rough exterior is a rough interior, but I'm really a very sensitive person. Peace of mind is what I want, and maybe to love and be loved in return. I believe that's what everyone is seeking."

For Jacob Cohen, growing up in Kew Gardens, Queens, there was a shortage of love. His father was in show business, using the name Phil Roy. He was gone most of the time. Jacob wasn't able to fit in with the kids in the neighborhood. They were opposites: wealthy, attractive, seemingly so poised. "It was pretty high class, but actually it was a place that financially we didn't belong. I found myself going to school with kids, then in the afternoon delivering groceries to their houses. . . . I wanted to date certain of the girls, but I never asked them. I felt I wasn't good enough."

The young man retreated from the misery, from the antipathy and anti-Semitism: "Comedy is a camouflage for depression. Without knowing why, I began to think funny. I went into a fantasy world of my own." He recognized show people as suffering from "a need for love. . . . A lot of people from split homes go into show business because they want applause: tell me I'm wonderful. In my particular case, it was a question of: accept me, tell me I'm okay. Tell me I'm as good as the rest."

The first joke Dangerfield wrote was: "When I played hide-and-seek, they wouldn't even look for me."

At 19, adopting the name Jack Roy, he started out at a salary of $12 a week plus room and board. And as the grinding run of clubs and promises wore on through nine long years, he saw his salary rise slowly, slowly, until he was just about at poverty level. Looking back, he said, "I never earned more than six or eight thousand a year. I got married, and then with a family to support, the future looked bleak. I was disgusted. I decided to give it all up and become a businessman."

In his spare time, the old desires were sublimated by joke selling. Always an outstanding gag man (he writes about 90% of his own material) he sold jokes to many comics, including Jackie Mason and Joey Bishop. A typical Dangerfield joke that turned up on a Jackie Mason album was: "This is a comeback for me. You didn't know this. I was in show business years ago. But do you know—to give you an idea of how bad I was doing, when I quit, I was the only one who knew I quit!"

Other jokes he wrote became public domain. Henny Youngman uses the line about visiting a doctor's office, hearing bad news, and saying, "I want another opinion." The doctor says, "Okay, you're ugly, too."

In his 40's, his children, Brian and Melanie, grown up, Dangerfield decided to give show business one more try. He "went down to the Village and just started telling the truth. I don't get no respect. Everyone has felt that way." It worked. The middle-aged, battered-looking comic looked the part.

The fresh start was accompanied by a fresh name. It was a club owner who dreamt up "Rodney Dangerfield": "I decided I was depressed enough to keep the name. What a handicap. . . . I went to work for nothing with a wife, two kids and a dog to support. I think I even noticed a change in my dog. With no money coming in, it seemed he barked at me more often."

Dangerfield's pressured, pop-eyed, florid face perfectly underscored the jokes about being a dumped-on everyman. Unlike the woeful, introverted Jackie Vernon, Dangerfield portrayed himself as a loser who keeps on trying. Vernon acts born to his baleful condition, but Dangerfield shows a hostility to his fate, a longing for the right break to bring him fame and fortune.

He used quick jokes, fast and punchy one-liners about his rough

Records:
Rodney Dangerfield, the Loser (Decca DS 6009; rereleased as Rhino Records RHLP 012), I Don't Get No Respect (Bell 6040; rereleased as Arista ABM 4281), No Respect (Casablanca 7167), Rappin' Rodney (RCA Victor AFL 14887).

Compilation:
Comedy Classics (Era BU 3890).

Films:
The Projectionist, Caddyshack, Easy Money.

Video:
Easy Money (Vestron).

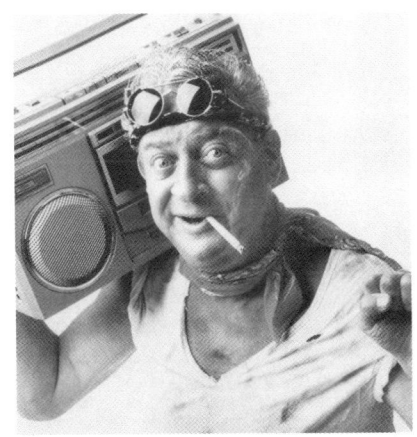

neighborhood, troubles with the wife and kids, conflicts with an outside world where even an elevator operator gets the upper hand on him, giving him the once over and asking, "Basement?" His nervous mannerisms have been captured by impressionists: the twist of his neck, the adjusting of his tie, the shifting of his weight like a man literally caught with his head in a noose.

In the mid-60's, the former paint salesman landed an audition for "The Ed Sullivan Show" and made the most of it. He began to appear more and more frequently on TV, he made a record album in 1967, and within a few years he scraped up enough money to open his own nightclub.

Most figured that Dangerfield's, opened on the East Side of New York in October of 1969, would close by 1970. But the loser's lounge turned out to be a winner. In 1970 he made headlines by turning the tables, banning William Morris agents from the club. Needless to say, Dangerfield had been one of their clients.

A perfect symbol of the dead end to the American dream, Dangerfield developed a strong following among teens and young adults. He's the laughable parent/teacher/establishment man who believes in the system even as it steps on his face. He scored with a song, "Rappin' Rodney," for the youth market, and made a rock video in which, taunted by back-up singers, he appeared in an actual *Death of a Salesman* scene, ending up in prison, walking the last mile.

In reality, Dangerfield is a success who perpetuates the American dream, although he's come through a bit shopworn: "I was 40 when I came back. I was always in love with love, the American dream. There was a need in me to write jokes, to try to perfect something, to create a character that people could identify with. I had to do it, it was like a fix. I'm a writer, writing all the time, like a maniac, you know, I just had to do it."

Into the 80's, Dangerfield has modified his style. He still has plenty of self put-downs, but he also does many more general one-liners. He's also a master at the heckler squelch, fighting back when raucous audiences try to gang up on the guy who gets no respect. "Rodney, how did you get so ugly!" someone shouts. "You're contagious, that's why," Dangerfield yells back.

After stealing the show in *Caddyshack*, Dangerfield starred in *Easy Money*, solidifying his position as a major comedy star, even though that film was strangely ill-conceived and untrue to the character he's perfected over nearly two decades of stand-up comedy.

Dangerfield is respected, he made it the hard way, and now he's gotten a piece of the dream. But, he admits, "I'm basically a down guy. I don't walk around smiling. My most exciting activity is going to the health club. I walk over, take a swim, weigh myself, hate myself, take a steam." Fame and success? "It came late in life," he says. He takes it in stride. "I'm too old to start doing cartwheels."

PHYLLIS DILLER

When she was close to 40, going nowhere, Phyllis Driver's audience was a fleet of bill collectors. Once an amateur pianist and singer, she had enrolled at a music conservatory in Chicago and later attended Bluffton College, but her hopes for a musical career faded. She married Sherwood Diller in 1939 and moved to California in 1941. Her dreams of fame were replaced by marital squabbles and policing her five kids.

At the laundromat she joked with other housewives about how she kept her ironing in the freezer, had minor grease fires—in the sink, and lorded over a spotless kitchen (the dog died). The Food and Drug Administration was investigating one of her puddings. But Diller couldn't laugh her problems away. She wrote them off, instead.

"When I was a housewife I could see no way out of my dilemma other than writing. I was writing from the third grade on, writing, writing, writing. When I was a child I wrote romantic stuff—princes and dragons and things like that. As I got out toward high school, puberty and I became comic together. Whenever I could, I'd hand in a funny assignment for literature or whatever. I remember the little kids were all around the floor, the little rug rats, and the drape apes going up the drapes, and I was writing on the top of a small upright piano so that they couldn't get at my papers."

Diller began writing for a local paper, the San Leandro News Observer, and was encouraged to move from advertising copy and straight articles to humor. At 37, she pieced together her comedy writing and mustered the nerve to try and be funny with it live, on stage.

"I started with involved, chi chi, cerebral material, high brow and very uncommercial. I played certain places, and when I took it out of those places it didn't go at all." As a somewhat arch, deliberately madcap prima donna, she told jokes and performed cabaret-style songs. She was an after-hours comic, a caricature of the sophisticated lady, prone to remarks like, "A boy of nine came in here last night . . . when he left he was 38." Her first album was recorded at this stage in her career.

"It's very painful to become a good stand-up comic," she recalls. "It's extremely painful to get there. Once you're there it's just total joy. But some people don't want to pay the price and go through all that pain."

What pain?

"The pain of being lousy!" she snaps.

Referring to the particular problem of being a female stand-up, she says, "I truly believe that it's terribly difficult to really get up on stage and do it because it's rather unlovely. And I think a lot of women would rather not lose their loveliness." Few male comics are notably handsome, especially when performing. As Steve Martin would say, "Comedy is not pretty."

Although in person she is the soul of good taste, attractive, sophisticated and quietly elegant, Diller's stage costume has always been a compendium of thrift-shop oddities and a garish gown topped with a fright wig. Although her housewife persona doesn't suggest "women's liberation," Diller has often attacked aspects of the male-dominated world. She shucked the fright wig for a different disguise in 1983 when she dressed in male drag to invade a "men only" Friar's Club roast for Sid Caesar. Even after it was over, Buddy Hackett was saying, "There were no women at the roast—they're not allowed," until he was shown shots of Phyllis, as "Phillip Downey," coming out of the men's room.

Of her years spent perfecting her style, she says, "Comedy is not easy. No one can teach it to you. It's something that comes out of your childhood. Something happens to you that makes you a comic . . . all comics are hyper-sensitive or they could never do comedy. Once you're sensitive, you never change. And what's so humiliating about becoming a good comic is that there's no such thing as a good beginning comic. You train in front of the audience and you don't know what's funny yet because the audience hasn't told you. You learn little by little, year after year, what is funny and what they will laugh at."

Diller found that her audience responded to the truth: to the more personal jokes in her repertoire. "I started talking more about what I had lived, what I understood and what I knew about. But in a very comedic

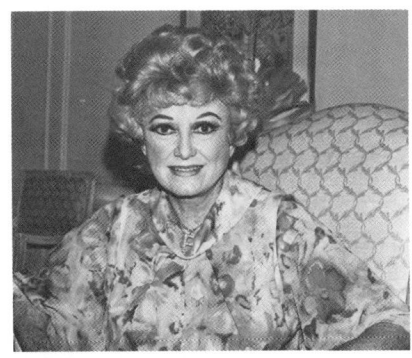

b. Phyllis Driver, July 17, 1917, Lima, Ohio

Records:
Wet Toe in a Hot Socket (Mirrosonic SP 6002), Phyllis Diller Laughs (Verve V 15026), Are You Ready? (Verve V 15031). Reissued and reedited versions: Great Moments (Verve V 15046), What's Left (Verve V-15059), Best of (Verve V-15053), Beautiful Phyllis Diller (Verve), Born to Sing (Columbia; a noncomedy album).

TV:
The Pruitts of Southampton (retitled "The Phyllis Diller Show" during its run; ABC 1966–67), The Beautiful Phyllis Diller Show (NBC 1968).

Broadway:
Hello, Dolly.

Films:
Boy Did I Get a Wrong Number, Eight on the Lam, The Private Navy of Sergeant O'Farrel, Did You Hear the One About the Traveling Saleslady, The Fat Spy, The Adding Machine, The Sunshine Boys.

Video:
Minsky's Follies.

Books:
Housekeeping Hints, Marriage Manual, The Compleat Mother, The Joys of Aging and How to Avoid Them.

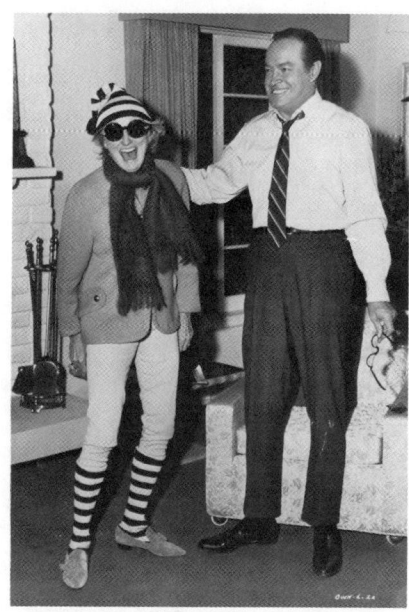

way, in other words, hyperbole. If you're gonna become great, you should write from the gut, from what you've been through."

Gone was the chi-chi sophisticate. The housewife jokes doubled, along with references to her husband, "Fang." "I went through a lot. I went through all those kids which wasn't easy. Taking care of all those kids without any help. In the old days there weren't even washing machines. This was during the war. That was World War II, which you don't remember, do you? No. Of course you don't. 'Cause everyone who remembers that is old.

"In those days you had to color your own margarine. It came white and looked like lard and it was a messy, dreadful job and I hated it. And ironing—I had the greatest ironing jokes in the world and women related to them. It was true, I froze my ironing, buried my ironing, anything not to do it."

She was a smash at the Purple Onion, and appeared often on Jack Paar's show. Her trademark was a cackling laugh that punctuated jokes with a leering "Ah ha HA" or fueled the audience's response with loud, sliding quacks that were infectious. She says she developed the laugh "probably out of desperation and nervousness," trying to cue the crowd.

Influenced strongly by Bob Hope, Diller became his female equivalent, shrewdly, almost scientifically crafting her monologues to get the most gags per minute: "My style is machine-gun; I do it rapidly. A set-up and a payoff and the quicker the better. The gag must reach everyone in the audience. You go for the simplest denominator. Set-up and pay-off with the key word at the end. Like, 'She's so fat that . . . when she takes her girdle off her feet disappear.'"

She developed punch and counterpunch. Punch: a woman "with a mouth so big she accidentally bit off an earring." Counterpunch: "From another woman!" Most of the jokes poked fun at herself: "My Playtex living bra died . . . of starvation! I've turned many a head in my day . . . and a few stomachs. I never made 'Who's Who' but I'm featured in 'What's That!' I once went braless and wore a peek-a-boo blouse. It was embarrassing. First they'd peek, then they'd boo!" Sometimes there was a deeper dig: "The more beautiful the single red rose he brings you, the more gorgeous the tramp he's fooling around with."

Despite her sensitivity, Diller professes to enjoy these self-deflating lines: "If it's funny material, I use it. If it's clean I buy it. Bob Hope has a joke on me, the most beautiful one I ever heard. He said, 'A peeping tom threw up on her window sill.'" She breaks into an infectious laugh: "Isn't that great?"

By 1962 she was averaging $4,000 a week and pushing higher. She became the first superstar stand-up comedienne, and in the 60's starred in a pair of short-lived TV series and some movies, several co-starring Bob Hope. Her first marriage ended in the 60's and another failed as well. She quipped, "The first one lasted 25 years, the other 25 minutes."

Energetic and very much in demand, Diller maintains a heavy concert schedule, and also performs as a classical pianist for fund-raisers. And to the many who have found inspiration in her story (at one time Alex Haley was commissioned to write her biography) she unceasingly recommends the book that helped her get started, *The Magic of Believing* by Claude Bristol.

It taught her to focus on her goals, "and that meant I gave up all activity except the one thing I wanted to do. That's all I thought about, that's all I worked toward, and that's all I did. I focused all my attention and it happened. The book taught me to pay no attention to what other people say or do. A dirty look would deter me from anything, the slightest criticism and I would give it all up. There were people who advised me, early on, to give up that 'stupid' laugh. And if I could tell you how many commercials I've been hired to do with huge money involved just to get my laugh! People said, 'You'll never make it.' Don't listen! I learned to accept nothing negative from other people. Negative people are amazing, you tell them you're gonna do something and they have to tell you why you can't."

She also doesn't believe that you have to be miserable offstage to be funny on stage. "I'm totally happy personally," she says. Her humor comes from remembering hard times, empathizing with the audience, and "inventing unhappiness. You've got to have tragedy. See, comedy is tragedy revisited." Diller has found many ways of making herself happy. She un-wrinkled through plastic surgery (and has produced a video tape on the subject) and in 1985 went to Dallas for a tattoo-like operation that has given her permanent eye liner.

"I'm for mental attitude being up and positive. Don't take things that seriously. Nothing is permanent. When something goes wrong, it isn't going to stay that way." For Phyllis Diller nothing is more fulfilling than making other people laugh. "Nothing. Oh, brain surgery, plastic surgery, outer space engineers who put something on the moon and all that, I think that's fulfilling, but I don't think anything's as gratifying and as pure pleasure as hearing laughs. Having fun is the best medicine, the perfect rejuvenator. The biggest thrill of my life is to hear the laughter."

FLANDERS AND SWANN

Very few comedy teams have appeared on Broadway in their own "two-man" show. Flanders and Swann did it twice, to the delight of audiences seeking a sophisticated mixture of satire and silliness.

The shows, or "after-dinner farragos," consisted of the portly, bearded Flanders in his wheelchair and the slim, mild-mannered Swann at the piano, singing their delightful songs of whimsy, sentiment and literate, civilized humor. The set was an English sitting room: rug on the floor, lamp in the corner and a polite audience out front watching.

Songs like "Wom Pom" and "The Reluctant Cannibal" were frantic gibberish, doubly funny coming from such staid-looking gentlemen. They were especially known for their repertoire of light-hearted animal songs, in which the slants were as unusual as the animals: an armadillo falling in love with an armor-plated tank, a gnu lecturing on the correct pronunciation of its name, a horrible joke-telling boar, a spider lurking in a bathtub, and a hippo delighting in "mud, mud, glorious mud, nothing quite like it for cooling the blood."

Many of these numbers contained warm elements of wit and pathos, and audiences delighted in hearing of the foolish warthog who learns she needn't tint her gums or wear perfume to be attractive (at least to another warthog) and in the tale of two "uncultivated" flowers who, because one twines to the left and the other to the right, are denied the chance at happiness together. A few songs, such as "Slow Train" or "Twenty Tons of T-N-T," were more serious and ironic.

But most of the Flanders and Swann repertoire consisted of cheerful, energetic swipes at everyday life: bus drivers who love to clog traffic, status-seekers, chic interior decorating ("curtains made of straw. We've wall-papered the floor . . . ivy everywhere, you mustn't be surprised to meet a cactus on the stair . . .") and how world problems could be solved if the leaders would "get together, face to face" in a bathtub.

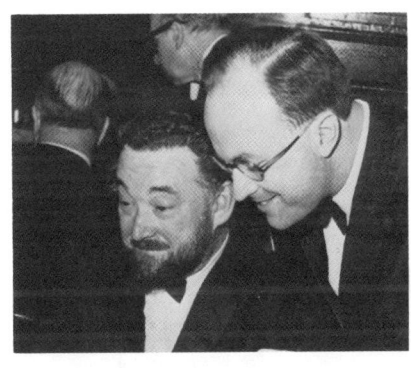

MICHAEL FLANDERS   b. March 1, 1922, London, England; d. April 14, 1975
DONALD SWANN   b. September 30, 1923, Llanelly, Wales

Records:
At the Drop of a Hat (Angel S 35797), The Bestiary (Angel S 36112), At the Drop of Another Hat (Angel S 36388), And Then We Wrote (EMI EMCM 3088), Tried by the Centre Court (EMI TS 116). Flanders alone: Peter and the Wolf (narration; Seraphim). Swann alone: Songs from the Middle Earth (music; Caedmon).

Broadway:
At the Drop of a Hat, At the Drop of Another Hat.

Books:
Swann's Way Out, Between the Bars, The Space Between the Bars.

Between numbers, Flanders would offer introductions laced with subtle humor. He might call a bit of current news "just an idea in the mind of God," or remark on "the things we see around us every day—the sky at night, for example." He tossed off sly literary jests, translating "La Belle Dame Sans Merci" as "The beautiful lady who never says thank you," while admonishing "Always be sincere—whether you mean it or not." He paced the song program with a few intricate monologues, from the delightfully ridiculous (olive stuffing as a ritual comparable to bull fighting) to the brilliantly sublime (an intricately rhymed discourse on the tediousness of tennis). At some points along the way he would delight in lightly twitting his slight partner's dignity.

Swann's contribution, the music, has endured not only as a complement and accent to the humor of the lyrics, but often as legitimately entertaining light music. Without lyrics, the melodies are still memorable. Swann also possessed a Stan Laurel-esque hysteria. Just as the slim, quiet Laurel could explode with helpless laughter, Swann had the giddy habit of letting his eccentric tenor voice slide up with comic histrionics, usually to the muted annoyance of Flanders.

It was Swann who sang, in just four lines, a compact and mannered devastation of astrology: "Jupiter's passed through Orion and come into conjunction with Mars. Saturn's wheeling through infinite space to its pre-ordained place in the stars. And I gaze at the planets in wonder at the trouble and time they expend. All to warn me to be careful . . . in dealings involving a friend."

Flanders and Swann began singing together in 1940 when they wrote revue songs together at the Westminster School. Flanders, whose mother was a violinist and father an actor, had always had an interest in the stage. Swann's father was a doctor, born in Russia of English parents. His mother was a Russian Moslem. At Oxford, he studied Russian and Greek while Flanders was president of the dramatic society.

During World War II, Swann was a conscientious objector, volunteering for work with medical units in Greece and Albania. In World War I, his parents had served in medical units. Flanders joined the Navy, and saw action in far-off Malta and the Gulf of Ob in Siberia. He endured a torpedo attack off the coast of Madeira, and later spent a year on duty guarding the Scottish coast. In 1943 an attack of polio forced him to spend six months in an iron lung.

"I do not look upon my years in hospital as the least valuable in my life," he wrote, noting that being "given time to think and study has its advantages. Nor is life in a wheelchair all a handicap. I drive a hand-controlled car and with my wife's devoted help am rarely debarred from going anywhere I want to go or doing anything I can reasonably do."

After the war the duo wrote songs for such revues as *Fresh Airs, Penny Plain* and *Airs on a Shoestring,* which were very successful through the late 1940's and 50's, performed by such British stars as Max Adrian.

Enjoying their success as songwriters, but feeling their songs were being performed "not nearly enough," they decided to stage a revue of their own, performing their songs in the same casual way they auditioned them for friends. They would perform these songs *At the Drop of a Hat,* but for two years (January 1957 to May 1959) they ended up performing their revue 759 times for audiences who doffed their hats and raised their hands to applaud. The show came to America, and a few years later the sequel, *At the Drop of Another Hat,* appeared.

Through it all, Flanders, awarded an O.B.E., maintained his own career as a lecturer, radio and television program host and actor. He also wrote opera libretti. Swann wrote the music for several operas including

Perelandra and *Requiem for the Living,* as well as carols, lyric songs and pieces based on the poems of J.R.R. Tolkien.

Flanders and Swann fans awaited another show, but other commitments interceded. In 1975, Michael Flanders died. Since his death, several British albums have been released, scraping up remnants from radio shows and live appearances to bring forth the team's 1950's revue songs and previously unreleased numbers, to add to the small but potent and memorable shelf of Flanders and Swann records.

In 1980, Swann teamed with bearded Frank Topping, who superficially resembles Flanders in vocal cadence and temperament. But the songs of Swann and Topping are mild and sentimental, the monologues and lyrics far too ordinary for the extraordinary "Drop of a Hat" revues. *Swann with Topping* played on stage in England, but did not come stateside.

FRANK FONTAINE

Show business was Frank Fontaine's career from start to finish, as it was for his parents (vaudevillians) and paternal grandparents (circus strongman and trapeze star for Ringling Brothers).

By the time he was 16, Fontaine was married, trying to support his family as a singer and an impressionist. As his family grew to include 11 children, he had to work extremely hard at his craft.

He first made his mark as a vocalist. A popular style of the 1940's was the "sweet"-sound featuring a singer with a pure, golden voice. Fontaine's was a very gooey baritone with a low warble many found hard to resist. He crooned with the Vaughn Monroe band after World War II, but found that his abilities as an impressionist and comic could help him get even more work. Under contract to MGM, Fontaine made 12 movies, but at the same time insisted on taking on all the freelance nightclub work he could get.

"When I was a boy," Fontaine once said, "my father was in vaudeville and my mother went with him. Sometimes my brother and I went with them and I went to 53 schools. But sometimes we didn't and we were boarded out. I don't want my kids ever missing going to the ball game, or being without their Dad over any Christmas holidays or birthdays or times like that."

Fontaine continued to push himself to gain the security he desperately wanted. At times he turned down lucrative offers if it meant being separated from his family. He developed a stand-up routine called "The Sweepstakes Ticket Winner: John L.C. Savony," and in 1948 he was a hit with it on "The Ed Sullivan Show." The routine became an enduring favorite when Fontaine became a regular guest on Jack Benny's TV show.

As John L.C. Savony, Fontaine would come center stage to tell, with eyes wide, lips slurred, and many a simple-minded giggle of delight, how he happened to win the prize: "I was jus' hangin' around," he'd begin, amazed to the point of stupefaction, "I wasn't doin' nothin' see. Jus' hangin' around." The more vacant and dim-witted he acted, the more laughs he got. And he matched them with his own inane laugh.

After meandering through the wide-eyed routine, he'd say, "I'm glad I won," and break into an infectious chuckle that built into a gooey giggle and finally to full-blown goose-like quivers of hysteria, ending with a sudden intake of air to "put the brakes" on himself.

Fontaine's idiot laughter, spontaneous and uncontrollable, was the

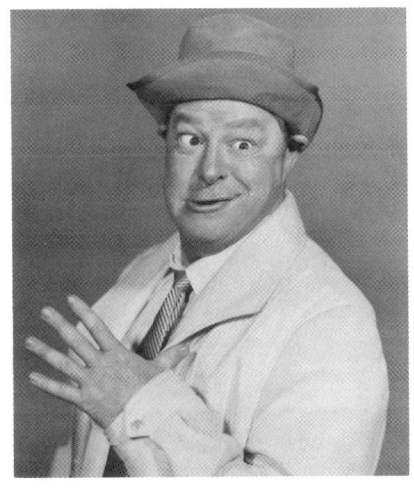

b. April 19, 1920, Haverhill, Massachusetts; d. August 4, 1978

Records:
Idiot's Delight (Guest Star G 1412).

Compilations including "Sweepstakes Winner":
Comedy Hits (Capitol DT 1854), They're Still Laughing (Capitol T 1651).

key to the routine and his gleeful, empty-headed character. There were no real jokes, just extended laughter, meandering, and a constant repetition of the sweepstakes ticket number: "They asked me if I had the right number, and I said it was 6-9-8-4-5-3-4-3-4-3-Oh-Oh-Oh . . ." on and on, each number gasped out as though he were on a pogo stick.

Fontaine's was still a naive age, and merriment could be gotten from the portrayal of a sappy-go-lucky character who was possibly suffering from some form of mental illness at worst, simple-mindedness at best.

With eyes bulging, lips twisted and giggling endlessly, Fontaine did look like some kind of moron. But to his credit, he made the character good-natured and lovable. By 1962 Savony had become "Crazy" Guggenheim. The Guggenheim character was featured in stand-up sketches on "The Jackie Gleason Show," with Gleason as straight man. As "Joe the Bartender," Gleason would call "Craze" from the back of the bar (there must've been a good reason for keeping him shut up out of sight) and the two would do a routine, Gleason warily asking questions, Fontaine blithely giving forth with inane answers. Sometimes Guggenheim would offer jokes like this:

"Two little mice went in swimming. And one of the mice started to drown. The other mouse dragged him out and tried to save him. How did he do it?"

Gleason ponders as Guggenheim giggles delightedly. Gleason doesn't know the answer. Guggenheim says, "He gave him mouse-to-mouse restitution!" And bursts into hysterics.

But Fontaine was also adept at being his own straight man. For his obscure album on Guest Star Records, he plays both subject and interviewer in a shaggy dog story that extends over both sides of the album. The interviewer thinks he's got a man-in-the-street exclusive with a florist, but after the man exhaustively details his knowledge of flowers (replete with non sequiturs, cackles and repetition) he confides, "I don't know anything about flowers . . . I'm an expert on rocks!"

A treatise on rocks follows. Then the man giggles and says, "But . . . I don't know anything about rocks. I'm really a dance instructor!" He then launches into jokes on dancing: "Some of you may not be able to do The Twist—you don't have the background for it. Or, you may have too much background!" After some coughing, gasping giggles, he continues, "I was always a great dancer, I used to do the jitterbug. I could throw a partner straight up in the air and do 22 jitters and a mess of buggin' and still catch her before she hit the floor!" Finally the dance instructor is banished by a gruff-voiced guy who demands that he resume his job. He's a "man in the street," all right: a janitor.

Fontaine was able to make mild routines like this work. Audiences seemed to enjoy indulging in his "Crazy" Guggenheim brand of light-hearted, light-headed humor. And most enjoyed his straight singing. Fontaine made several noncomedy albums for ABC–Paramount.

After the Gleason series ended, Fontaine resumed his performance schedule of stand-up and song. In 1970 his health began to fail. A year later he lost his house to the Internal Revenue Service in a settlement over back taxes. Finding the club scene changing, he joined one of the "vaudeville revues" run by the late Roy Radin. These were family shows of comics, singers, jugglers, magicians, etc., put on in town halls, schools and civic auditoriums.

Appearing in a true vaudevillian's outfit (orange hat, green jacket, plaid pants) he looked older and heavier than before, but he still had that patented laugh that slid up and down his throat, a set of rubber-faced comic expressions and all the warmth an audience could want. He did a traditional monologue updated for the 70's ("I got a 16-year-old boy at home—wears his mother's beads—we're praying he's gonna be a hippie") and ended with a set of songs including an audience sing-along.

"Success? What is it? It's not five million dollars," Fontaine told *Celebrity Register*. "It's your being contented and your family being contented."

He began along the vaudeville trail, and that's where it ended. In 1978 he was the star attraction at a convention of the National Order of Eagles in Spokane, Washington, and suffered a heart attack moments after being given a check for the $25,000 he'd helped raise in that area for charity.

REDD FOXX

To the general public, Redd Foxx was a new face in 1972 when he starred in the TV series "Sanford and Son." But nightclub audiences had known about him for more than 20 years, first in black clubs and then in integrated rooms, where he developed a specialty for "adults only" material.

Record buyers in specialty stores found literally dozens of his albums available, starting with his first releases in 1956. With many on obscure labels and others reissued, reedited or sold to other labels, the total of Redd Foxx albums is now about 50, easily the greatest selection available by any comic. Each album was studded with mild (by today's standards) jokes typical of those to be found on the humor page of one of the saucier men's magazines. He did one-liners like this series of definitions:

"What do you give an elephant with diarrhea? Lotsa room! What's a sardine? A little fish that smells like a finger. What's a brute? A guy who puts a prophylactic on with a tire iron. How does a French girl hold her liquor? By the ears."

Once a musician who played a washtub for The Five Hip Cats, young Foxx knocked around for more than a decade, hooking up with various bands, performing a series of low-paying menial jobs between gigs and getting himself arrested for poor man's crimes like stealing a bottle of milk (for which he was sentenced to 5 days at Riker's Island) and trying to sneak out of a restaurant without paying the check (90 days in The Tombs).

In the late 1940's Foxx was seeking work as a novelty singer and stand-up comic. He was already known by the nickname Red. As he said, "Red's a nickname they used for light-skinned Negroes. I made it 'double d, double cross' so it wouldn't be a color or an animal." The last name was a tribute to his foxiness, with only a slight amount of attention paid to ballplayer Jimmy Foxx, the only celebrity who used the same spelling.

The up-and-down struggles of Redd Foxx continued. He teamed up with Slappy White and they began to make good money, but the team broke up in 1951. More odd jobs followed, mixed in with Foxx's cross-country treks as a stand-up comic.

Years of working in small clubs and struggling in front of indifferent, drunken audiences honed his style, which was marked by a wary hostility. Eyeing the audience, casually smoking a cigarette, Redd would almost grudgingly rasp out the one-liners, showing a certain bitterness and distaste which fortunately registered more as hard, crusty hipness to fans.

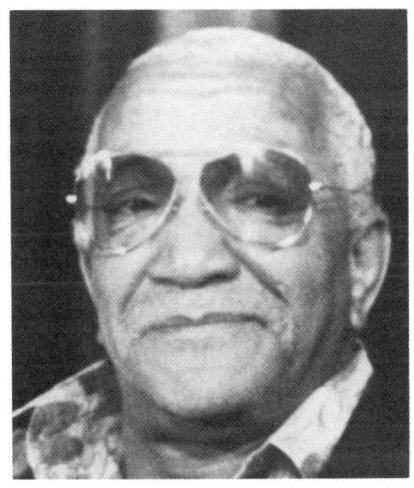

b. John Sanford, December 9, 1922, St. Louis, Missouri

Records:
Both Sides of Redd Foxx (Loma 5901), Redd Foxx at Home (MF Records RF-3), In a Nutshell (King 1074), Pass the Apple, Eve (King 1078), You Gotta Wash Your Ass (Atlantic SD 18157), Laff of the Party (Dooto DTL 214, 219, 220, 227), Burlesque Humor (Dooto DTL 249), Best of Redd Foxx (Dooto DTL 234), Sidesplitter (Dooto DTL 253), Sidesplitter, Vol. 2 (Dooto DTL 270), Have One on Me (Dooto DTL 298), Laffarama (Dooto DTL 801), He's Funny That Way (Dooto DTL 815), This Is Foxx (Dooto DTL 809), Wild Party (Dooto DTL 804), At Jazzville (Dooto DTL 820), Sly Sex (Dooto DTL 295), Foxx Live '85 (Reddy Freddy).

TV:
Sanford and Son (NBC 1972–77), Redd Foxx (ABC 1977–78), Sanford (NBC 1980).

Films:
Cotton Comes to Harlem, Norman, Is That You?

Video:
Dirty Dirty Jokes (host; Vestron), In a Plain Brown Wrapper (Vestron).

"When I first started doing dirty jokes," Foxx recalled, "everybody told me if I cleaned up, I'd be famous. I didn't clean up, but I got famous anyway. Now, everybody's doing it.... Actually, I revolutionized the sex revolution with my party records. Twenty years ago those party records got sneaked around and played, and people got less and less guilt feelings about sex."

Over the years, Foxx developed a following and found a home for his blue material in Las Vegas. After 30 years in the business, he was able to open his own nightclub in Los Angeles. Comfortable at last, the comedian was reluctant to leave his niche even for a chance to do movies or a TV show. Such things were gambles, costing a lot of time and money.

Foxx did accept a role as a junk dealer in Cotton Comes to Harlem, and it was that performance that created interest in this "unknown" when it came time to cast the black version of "Steptoe and Son," an English series about a crusty old man (Wilfrid Brambell) and his adult son (Harry H. Corbett).

Using his own real surname for the main character, Foxx brought himself into the role. He *was* Fred Sanford: temperamental, irascible, hostile, prone to the wisecrack but worldly wise and sympathetic in spite of himself. His Sanford had a set of mannerisms that were not part of the Steptoe original, and audiences loved Foxx's feigned aches and pains, his mock heart attacks, gullibility toward a gamble and ceaseless raunchy or insulting jokes aimed at everyone he met.

Foxx proved these mannerisms were original by making real-life headlines out of them. He used a faked illness to walk off the show (and come back with a better salary). He temperamentally demanded windows in his dressing room (Johnny Carson didn't have one, but after Foxx got one, he demanded one, too) and a golf cart to get around the NBC set. His attitude toward people was crusty at times, to put it mildly, and he saw his name in the scandal sheets often in connection with violent threats to his employees, his problems with mistrusted agents and some messy divorces. He was noted for bewildering highs and lows, and shifts between warmth and coldness.

Like most veteran comics who had been through years of struggle, Foxx was entitled to his suspicions, and to turn the tables to gain the upper hand in salary negotiations with the hated "fat cats" of TV and clubs. Unlike those old-time hard-knock comics, he had the added burdens and bitterness of the arrests, the assaults on his dignity.

Even in doing "Sanford and Son," his new-found stardom seemed to bring only resentment that it had all come too late in life. He gloomily said at the time, "When you get to be 60, material things don't mean so much, you don't have that long left to enjoy them. I'd just like some peace of mind."

Through the "Sanford and Son" years, he made some manic headlines. In 1974 he streaked the stage of The Apollo, clad only in pantyhose. Fans saw a lot more of Redd Foxx than they'd bargained for, including the face tatooed on his breast, the nose being his nipple. In 1976 he allegedly pulled a derringer on the vice-president of a cosmetics company he owned, and, in Three Stooges style, poked the man in the eye. The following year he married for the third time, to Yun Chi Chung, 20 years younger. It didn't last.

For his show, Foxx was able to create the truest portrait of black life yet seen in a sit-com. For himself, he called attention to the discrimination that he felt prevented him from getting Emmy Awards, TV specials or guest-host duties on "The Tonight Show." The comedian bitterly announced, "A lot of things I've lived through are supposed to be life, but it was more like death. You work for a lifetime in a business that you love, and I love it like a woman, so it hurts when it treats you this way."

"Sanford and Son" was NBC's most popular prime-time series during its first four seasons. In fact, it was NBC's *only* show in the Top 20 for the 1975–76 season. But Foxx was not to be soothed. He quit the show. He made a Grammy-nominated record, and in 1977–78 starred in his own series for ABC, a blend of stand-up and variety. It was a disaster that lasted barely half a season.

A movie, Norman, Is That You? was roasted by the critics. In 1980 Foxx returned to NBC for "Sanford," but it was too late. The show didn't have it and viewers lost interest. Foxx returned to Vegas and the nightclub circuit where enthusiastic audiences still wait for his blue humor.

"We were poor," Foxx tells the crowd. "At Christmas time if I wasn't a boy I had nothing to play with. . . . Some folks say Negroes always carry knives. That's a lie! My brother has been carrying an ice-pick for 25 years." And to a heckler in front: "Rest your lips, 'cause you got a busy night ahead of you!" And to a heckler in back: "Hey, Nigger, pay more and get a good seat."

In the clubs Foxx can be as raunchy and insulting as he likes, and when he tours, he fills the clubs with many who have come to hear how legendarily uncensored he can be. A video version of his club act was released in 1983 under the appropriate title "Redd Foxx in a Plain Brown Wrapper." Foxx also often performs for free in prisons around the country, "but people don't want to hear about the good things I do," he says, "only the stuff in the papers."

Most any Foxx album on Dootsie Williams's old Dooto Records label has representative 1950's Foxx. Also recommended is the album he did for Loma (Frank Sinatra wanted him for this division of Reprise Records) and his Atlantic lp, the most uninhibited, although his voice was troubling him during the rigorous tour of club dates and is harsh and worn.

DAVID FROST

Among the "angry young men" in Britain in the early 1960's was this son of a Methodist parson from a rural English village who made two countries stand still and listen—at least for a moment or two.

Young David Frost was an excellent soccer player, with offers to play professionally. He turned them down and accepted a scholarship to Cambridge University instead. It was there that he starred in the traditional student revues loaded with antiestablishment sass and satire.

It was the right time and the right place. There were angry young writers like John Osborne and Alan Sillitoe, and even the beginnings of angry young musicians playing new music in Liverpool. The sharp, satirical angry young monologist found himself, at 23, starring in England's "That Was the Week That Was," a topical TV show gleefully poking fun at morality and the passing parade of politicians.

Frost and his cast lampooned sex, offered a "Consumer's Guide to Religion" and served up political satire, with lines of dialogue like this:

"You don't think that black people are inferior to white people?"
"Of course not. If we did do you think we'd go to all this trouble to suppress them?"
"Aren't there a lot more black people than white ones in South Africa, and so shouldn't they perhaps run the country?"
"That is precisely the point. There are so many more of them they have less need to say as much as the few white people."

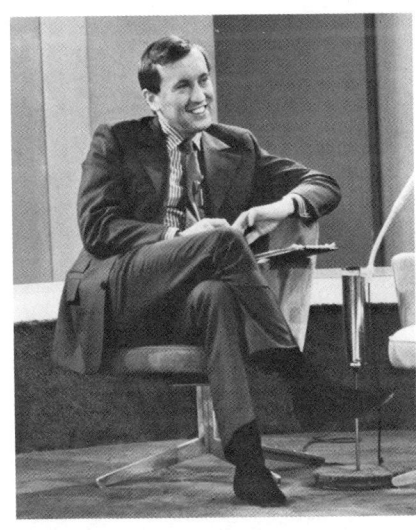

b. April 7, 1939, Tenerdon, England

Records (U.S. only):
The Frost Report (Janus JLS-3005), Live in Las Vegas (United Artists UAS 5555), That Was the Week That Was (Radiola MR 1123).

TV:
That Was the Week That Was (NBC 1964–65), The David Frost Show (syndicated 1969–72), The David Frost Revue (syndicated 1971), Headliners (NBC 1978), That Was the Week That Was (ABC 1985).

Books:
The World's Worst Decisions, David Frost's Book of Millionaires.

Bio:
Will You Welcome Now . . . David Frost (Frischauer).

And two men, talking about the sincerity of world leaders, remark: "Wilson's sincere . . . Jack Kennedy's sincere. So's Khrushchev. Give him his due . . . he's sincere." "True, true. Thank God there aren't any Machiavellis in world politics today." "You knew where you were with Machiavelli."

As was his custom, Frost surrounded himself with good writers. Ned Sherrin, Peter Shaffer, John Braine and Peter Cook contributed to the show, and Tom Lehrer and Buck Henry were among those who worked on the later American version. But in America the show was ahead of its time and lasted only half a season. "The Frost Report," another British series, utilized co-stars Ronnie Barker and Ronnie Corbett, and contained material written by the five Englishmen who would later become part of the Monty Python troupe.

Always more of a monologist than an actor, Frost was prone to do stand-up and then introduce sketches in which others appeared. His monologues were always tart and sly ("Somebody broke into the Kremlin yesterday and stole next year's election results") with cerebral throw-away lines ("He has a wonderful head for money . . . there's this long slit at the top") and thinking-men's gags ("There's a masochist who loves a cold shower every morning . . . so he takes a warm one").

Following in the tradition of Jack Paar and Johnny Carson, from stand-up comic and emcee Frost became a talk-show host, and it was with the Emmy-winning "David Frost Show" that he scored with American audiences. He became known for his ready smile, seeming total absorption in what his guests were saying and attracting controversial guests. Of course, not only people like John Lennon and Phil Ochs felt comfortable with him. So did Richard Nixon, who did a series of special interviews with Frost in 1977.

Frost continued to host a variety of shows and began producing novelty and humor books. In 1981, he married for the first time. It was to Lynne Frederick, who had lost her husband Peter Sellers a few months earlier. For two decades, Frost had been one of the world's most eligible bachelors and was linked at one time with Diahann Carroll.

In 1985 he was ready to give American audiences another look at his stand-up satire. "Irreverent political and social satire hasn't been done in prime time for twenty years," he said, promoting the new version of "That Was the Week That Was." On the show he offered typical Frost quickies: "What is a liberal? A liberal finds it in his heart to forgive Jane Fonda for being in Hanoi but not for being in Barbarella. . . . Statistics in today's Pravda show that 88% of Russian homes have a video camera. But of those, only 5% know about it."

DAVID FRYE

David Frye always seemed to have doubts and worries inside, even as he provoked laughter outside: "We're in such a frightening time," he once said. "I hope I'm giving the country relief, but sometimes it's like making fun of cancer." Frye seemed at times to literally turn himself inside out, letting famous politicians and actors inhabit his body for his mimic routines: "The next step," he said glumly, "would be to become the person—and then I'd end up in the insane asylum."

The comedian/impressionist has often been described as insecure and intense. Backstage he would fret in front of a mirror going through alarming split-personality changes to make sure all the celebrities were still with him. At his peak in 1968–74, David Frye was, after the president himself, the country's foremost Richard Nixon impersonator. He was also as unusual and moody a personality as Nixon.

A key to Frye's inner drive can be found in two lines spoken to a *New York Times* interviewer. The first is typical of any political satirist, the second is not: "Audiences need a way to vent their feelings and fears about these big political figures and they can do it with me. That's why it's so important to me to get not just a few characteristics but the whole presence of the man."

Frye was driven to catch that *whole* presence, the "inner image" or, in other words, the soul. To this end he not only spent the mandatory hours with a tape recorder, matching his voice to the star's and adding the right amount of exaggeration, he also studied photographs meticulously and developed a talent for literally rumpling his face into grotesque caricatures. From Jekyll to Hyde, Frye actually did in some way create gargoyles that showed the souls inside the famous men.

Frye's best impressions were the grotesques. Audiences were shocked by his Lyndon Johnson, eyes benignly half shut, mouth oozing from ear to ear in a parody of a grandfatherly smile. They were convulsed by his political cartoon of William F. Buckley, Jr. with anteater tongue, popping eyes and head cocked like a striking reptile. And he became a star with his grubby version of Nixon, with puffed-out jowls, cruel and predatory open mouth, shrugged shoulders and shifty eyes.

The nervous, tumultuous late 60's saw a nation divided on almost every political issue. It was the perfect time for a tense, tumultuous impressionist like Frye, who would fade when more benign and soporific political leadership, order and reason came in. Frye not only made political impressions a specialty, he was the first impressionist (discounting Vaughn Meader, who did John F. Kennedy and only John F. Kennedy) to come anywhere near a gold record. And he did this thanks to the record-buying habits of his many young fans who were openly rebelling against Johnson and Nixon on college campuses.

He'd come a long way from Cary Grant impressions when he was starting out doing University of Miami amateur shows, from 1959 when he came back from the Army to be a comic by night and work for his father's office cleaning firm every day.

"Life was pretty dismal," Frye recalled of that period. "You live in the images of your parents." But after living in the inner images of movie stars, politicians and even obscure character players like Lloyd Nolan and Zachary Scott, Frye won a shot on "The Tonight Show" in 1962. He didn't click, but it was a step forward. Four years later he displayed a full arsenal of LBJ, Nixon, Hubert Humphrey and Bobby Kennedy on "The Merv Griffin Show."

Frye blistered Nixon with his jokes and caricature, giving the chief executive the catch phrase "I *am* the President" to reinforce the notion that the man was so neurotic and insecure he needed to remind himself. LBJ was not allowed to disappear. Instead, Frye dragged the beaten politician down farther: "My fellow Americans. I come here tonight . . . because I no longer have any place to go."

But Frye's own personality was also in turmoil. Behind the scenes the fretful behavior continued with a wired-up intensity that, after the Lenny Bruces and Shelley Bermans, was almost expected of stand-up satirists. On camera, the nation saw a man uncomfortable being himself, offering no eye-contact to TV interviewers, avoiding personal topics to present nonstop mimicry.

Frye actually longed to do characters as Jonathan Winters did: inventions from within. That was the next step, but he was having trouble

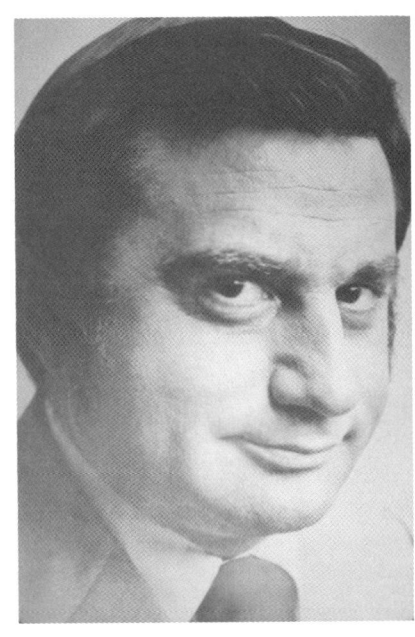

b. David Shapiro, 1934, Brooklyn, New York

Records:
The New First Family 1968 (Verve V 15054), I Am the President (Elektra EKS 75006), Radio Free Nixon (Elektra EKS 74085), Richard Nixon Superstar (Buddah BDS 5097), Richard Nixon, A Fantasy (Buddah 1600), The Great Debate (Frye Productions D-80).

getting there. So he did the famous figures, and to add a further dash of Freud to it, he admitted that "The kinds of impressions I do have very little to do with how I feel about the people." He was a political satirist who was relatively apolitical and uninterested in government beyond the general view that everything is botched at best, corrupt at worst.

Nixon didn't last forever, but while he did Frye made the most of it. Each new album offered a different attack. How about Richard Nixon running his own radio show? How about a Nixon version of "Jesus Christ, Superstar"? And finally, there was the Grammy-nominated Watergate album, bold and biting, which included a fantasy execution of the president: "Esteemed executioner, honored guests . . . I think I can safely say that this is my last press conference. I appreciate this opportunity to make myself perfectly clear . . . as for this great country of ours, ladies and gentlemen, I HATE America . . . try spending 21 years in Whittier, California—try loving America after that!"

Meanwhile, Frye seemed to be becoming as erratic as Nixon. There were incomplete shows. At times Frye would have to take his celebrity photographs on stage with him, and refer to them like cue cards, to trigger the facial caricatures.

Perhaps it was just as well that Jimmy Carter was prone to smiles, not snarls. This gave Frye the opportunity, whether he wanted to or not, to take stock of himself. Looking back, he produced some exceptional, breathtaking work, impressions done with acid-etched accuracy and driven home with absolute fury. Even his impressions of Al Capp, Rod Steiger or Henry Fonda have that distinctive, bold stroke of full, down-to-the-bone authenticity.

The Carter and Reagan years have not lent themselves to the ferocious mimicry of David Frye, but he continues to work nightclubs regularly, amazing patrons with new impressions and the surviving old: Buckley, George C. Scott, Billy Graham and Howard Cosell.

BROTHER DAVE GARDNER

A Southern comic philosopher, Dave Gardner was the hip man's Will Rogers: "Love your enemies and drive 'em nuts!"

Educated at Union University in Jackson, Tennessee, Gardner joined the Navy and later found a career in music, as a drummer in various combos. He gradually blended the two unlikely elements of Southern cracker barrel wit and a jazz musician's sense of cool.

In 1954 he was looking to the headlines for inspiration. When the Supreme Court ruled for integration in that year's *Brown* vs. *Board of Education* case, Brother Dave was ready. "They were callin' it Black Monday," he recalled of his Southern audience, "and when I went onstage I hit a few licks, and then I said, 'Good Lord, beloved, let 'em go to school; we went, and we didn't learn nothin'.' There was dead silence, and then someone laughed, and then they all broke up, stood and applauded. That's when I realized how powerful the topical stuff could be."

If Will Rogers had been around, he might've used Gardner lines like these: "The only reason the Russians are appearing ahead of us is because they want to get out of their country a whole lot worse than us

b. June 11, 1926, Jackson, Tennessee; d. September 22, 1983

. . . probably with our luck in getting to the moon it'll be a half moon and we'll miss it. Wouldn't that be weird?"

"Ain't that weird" was a catch-phrase for the comic, along with "It don't make no difference," which was his Will Rogers way of getting out of a bombed joke or a line that sounded more serious than satiric. It recalled Rogers's "I just don't understand it—well, maybe I'm not supposed to."

Gardner shared another interest believed to be widespread among musicians: pot and pills. His controversial material that swerved from right to left wing was sometimes matched by a controversial personal life. He had best-selling albums out in 1959, 1960 and 1961, but in 1962 he made headlines for a drug bust he insisted was a frame-up. He managed to pull a prescription for the speed and sleeping pills he was carrying and the case fell apart.

While Gardner, like Lord Buckley, was generally perceived as too jazz-hip for a national audience, Jack Paar was one of the few to give him some exposure, making him one of the first Southern comics to hit TV sans stereotype. To Paar, Gardner was "The Wild Man," and of Paar, Gardner characteristically enthused, "Man, that Jack, he's the swingin-est. He's on such a high celestial orb, that I can't hardly believe it. But I rejoice that I move in such swingin' circles."

His audiences rejoiced in his ironic whimsy ("Do you believe the Washington Monument looks anything like George Washington?") and sharp wit ("I believe in love and kindness and charity and goodness, and if a man's down, kick him . . . that'll give him the incentive to become something").

Gardner used to say, "Success is gettin' what you want. Happiness is wanting what you get." He had an interesting philosophy about taxes: don't pay them. From 1967 to 1973 he waged a war with the Internal Revenue Service, and by the time he was indicted he and his wife had spent all the money and there was nothing left to collect.

Fading into a star with only regional appeal, Gardner had his ups and downs, traveling around from Florida to Mississippi to the west coast, managing to offend members of his audience by refusing to confine his viewpoints to stark black and white, liberal or conservative. He encountered the same coolness Mort Sahl had when he attacked John F. Kennedy in the same way he attacked Dwight D. Eisenhower or when he kidded women's groups.

Gardner's wife, Millie, also his manager, died in 1980. The comic was in the midst of a comeback in the 80's, making a movie, *Brother Dave in Concert*, for South Carolina producer Earl Owensby. It was during the making of the sequel, *Chain Gang*, that Gardner suffered a sudden and fatal heart attack.

Records:
Rejoice (RCA Victor LPM 2083), Ain't That Weird (RCA Victor LPM/LSP 2335), Kick Thy Own Self (RCA Victor LPM 2239), Best (RCA Victor 2852), All Seriousness Aside (Capitol T/ST 2628), Did You Ever? (Capitol T/ST 2498), It Don't Make No Difference (Capitol T 1867), Bigger Than Both of Us (Capitol T/ST 2761), How You Look at It (Capitol ST 2055), Hip-Ocracy (Tower Records).

Compilation:
Comedy Hits (Capitol DT-1854).

Films:
Brother Dave in Concert, Chain Gang.

GEORGE GOBEL

A low-key comedian with a bewildered, cock-eyed gaze and a bird-like face, George Gobel was an unlikely star, but in the late 1950's he was one of television's hottest comics. His laid-back approach was something new.

Gobel began his show business career as a singer, appearing on NBC's "National Barn Dance" radio show. He gradually mixed in some unassuming humor, but didn't really decide on stand-up as a career until after his discharge from the Air Force in 1945.

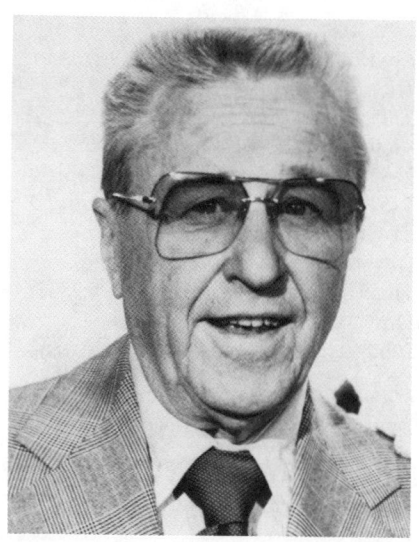

b. May 20, 1920, Chicago, Illinois

Record:
In Person at the Sands (Decca DL 74163).

TV:
The George Gobel Show (NBC 1954–59; CBS 1959–60), The Hollywood Squares (NBC 1966–76), Harper Valley PTA (NBC 1981–82).

Films:
I Married a Woman, Rabbit Test.

He built up a following in the Chicago area, working conventions and nightclubs. "It's interesting how I got to be George Gobel," he would begin, standing in front of the crowd like a kid pushed out from the wings of an amateur production. Pausing, the words coming out with shy wryness, he continued, "See, I come from a very large family. One day Dad calls all 16 of us children into the living room. And he says, 'Now which one of you wants to be George Gobel?' I didn't. I wanted to be Douglas Fairbanks, Jr., but that was already taken."

Actually an only child, Gobel made the most of his folksy style, although at heart he considered himself more of a city slicker. The 5'5" comic and his crew-cut cuteness became a fixture on "The Garry Moore Show" in 1952, and within a few years, he had his own series.

"This show might just keep you from getting sullen," he told the audience. Gobel was a Top 20 attraction for the first two seasons, winning both an Emmy and a Peabody Award. Aside from monologues and comedy songs, his program featured sketch comedy. "Spooky old Alice," the wife of many a monologue joke, was played by an unlikely-named brunette, Jeff Donnell, and later by Phyllis Avery. Alice really did exist: Gobel married Alice Humecki in 1942.

Known as "Lonesome George," the offbeat little comic had a catch-phrase that, in 1954, swept the country. It was an exclamation of bewilderment: "Well, I'll be a dirty bird!" One of his most popular monologues, delivered on a TV special commemorating the 75th anniversary of Thomas Edison's discovery of the lightbulb, described the greatness of electricity. "If it wasn't for electricity," Gobel said in deadpan lecture, "we'd all be watching television by candlelight."

Gradually Gobel developed a set of drinking jokes with which he also became identified. If humor, for Gobel, came from truth (his family, his wife, etc.) so did the drinking: "I've never been drunk," he would say, "but I've often been over-served."

In 1958 Gobel starred with Diana Dors in a mild comedy movie, *I Married a Woman*. It didn't make much of an impression, and gradually Gobel's low-key style allowed viewer attention to fade on television as well. He was finally shot down in the ratings by the Dodge City action of "Gunsmoke."

As the 60's began, Gobel returned to nightclub work, although he had established himself as an amusing character actor through roles in such TV shows as "Wagon Train" (in 1960) and "Daniel Boone" (in 1965). He later became a regular on the comedy game show "The Hollywood Squares," where his brand of sly subtlety and dizzy whimsy made an interesting contrast to the kink of Paul Lynde and the foxiness of Charlie Weaver.

"True or False," host Peter Marshall said, "Christopher Columbus has been buried eight different times."
Gobel: "You certainly have to admire his spunk."
"What do you call a cow that won't give milk?"
"Hamburger."
"Does the Secret Service include any women?"
"Who do you think performs the secret service?"

Following a struggle with alcoholism, Gobel has continued to perform his amusing songs and routines in clubs when he feels so inclined. He also accepts comedy roles on TV shows and in movies, and played the President of the United States in Joan Rivers's *Rabbit Test*, and Mayor Harper in TV's "Harper Valley PTA."

SHECKY GREENE

"He is a gentleman who has done it all," says Jerry Lewis. "But primarily he has made Las Vegas the city that it is. He has performed in every facet of that town and when people come to Las Vegas the first thing they want to know is if he's there. If you see this man perform you're seeing the epitome of comic genius. I remember one night at the Riviera Lounge—I laughed as hard as I've ever laughed in my life. . . ."

The epitome of the "Vegas comic," Greene is at his best in a nightclub setting, working the room with a frenzy of ad-libs, sight gags, ringsider jokes, songs and comedy routines. He's a master at it, and makes a six-figure weekly salary, something he has in common with Buddy Hackett and Don Rickles, the only other comics who rival Greene's ability to destroy a Vegas audience and to be considered "must see" entertainers in that town.

Greene came to Las Vegas when it was first becoming a tourist attraction in the early 1950's. His show business career began in 1949 when, after three years in the Navy, he came back to his home town: "I enrolled at Wright Junior College in Chicago and planned to become a gym teacher. I took a summer job at a resort near Milwaukee called Oakton Manor. They paid me $20 a week and gave me a fancy title, Social Director. We could not afford to bring in acts, so I would get up and tell a few jokes. I certainly was not Red Skelton, but I got a few laughs. I went to college that September and spent a year working toward my degree. In between I kept doing club dates and started to put an act together."

He was booked into a New Orleans club for a two-week engagement—and stayed three years. The only thing that could have put an end to his engagement there was a major disaster. It happened—the club burned down. Greene went back to Chicago, but was soon called down to Miami Beach, at the request of Martha Raye, to play her nightclub.

"They held me over for six weeks . . . I was only 25 years old and I was making $500 a week." In 1953 Greene was the opening act for Ann Sothern at the Chez Paree. "I cannot describe the feeling I experienced when I became a hit in my home town. The Chez was one of the top nightclubs in America in those days."

From there, Greene went out to Vegas, raising his salary to $3,500 a week; by 1959 he was making $5,000 a week. The comic developed a reputation as one of the entertainers to see in town, but found other phases of show business elusive. His style wasn't suited to TV variety shows, where improvisation was frowned upon and ringsider repartee was impossible. Although offered film roles, he turned these down: "I was too busy trying to figure out the daily double and the odds on a hard 10. Besides, I loved to wing it . . . improvise, that's my style and I was making enough in nightclubs so I could turn down the offers. I can truthfully say money has never been that important to me . . . only to my bookies."

He recorded an album in the early 60's, "A Funny Thing Happened on the Way to the Moon." The liner notes stressed that Greene was different from his "contempt-oraries," the sick-nik comics. He was an old-fashioned comedian with a heart, in the show-biz tradition.

Over the next decade he developed a reputation far wilder than that of most sick-niks. One night at Caesar's Palace he knocked down a number of the club's prized Grecian statues. Leaving the wreckage behind, he got into his car and drove into the fountain in front of the casino. "No spray wax, please," he said. His own press bio admits that

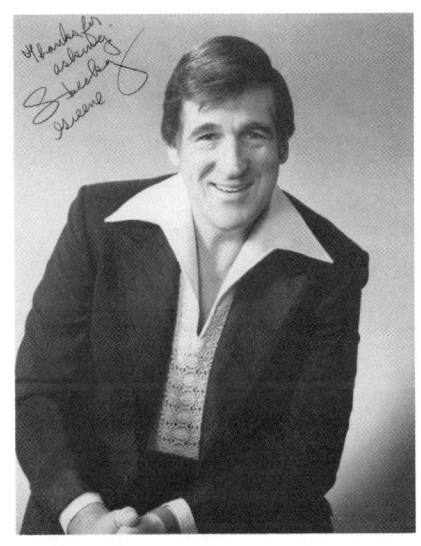

b. Sheldon Greenfield, April 8, 1925, Chicago, Illinois

Records:
A Funny Thing Happened on the Way to the Moon (Majestic T-101), A Day at the Races (Laff A-204).

Video:
NBC Comedy Hour 1956 (Video Yesteryear).

"Tales of his drinking, carousing, gambling, turning over crap tables and busting up entire casinos are legion, and some even have a little truth to them." Often these were just extensions of the antics he'd begun on stage, encouraged by his delirious audience. "However," the bio adds, "Shecky has a different attitude about himself and his career today. He is a new, much better Shecky, who is deeply loved and respected by his audience, peers, friends and family."

In addition to the inevitable mellowing after 15 years in show business, Greene suffered through two sobering traumas in the last few years. Throat surgery devastated him: he lost his voice for a year. Then he had cancer surgery. But Greene has completely recovered from the one-two punch that could have brought an end to his career and his life.

He has acted recently in TV sit-coms and such adventure shows as "The Fall Guy," as well as returning to Vegas. He is, in fact, one of the last of the old school. Few entertainers still do an impression of Maurice Chevalier, for example. He does, for a risque bit: "When I was 76," he says as Chevalier, "I was in the movie 'Fanny.' There was a part in Fanny . . . *naturally* there was a part in Fanny! I said, I love you, Fanny. I want to marry you, Fanny. I want to kiss you, Fanny. . . ."

He'll talk about Vegas shows: "If you've seen one nude girl, you've seen them all. Forgive me, ladies, but I don't believe there's anything sexy about a naked girl. My wife used to walk in front of me at night with a black lace negligee and that was sex! Then I'd wait for her to go to sleep and I would put on that black lace negligee. . . ."

He'd eventually touch on other topics, like his daughter: "I have a daughter who goes to SMU. She could've gone to UCLA here in California, but it's one more letter she'd have to remember. . . . She's an A student. All she knows how to say is 'Ayyyyyy'. . . ."

But the art of Vegas success is not necessarily in the jokes. While Don Rickles works his audience with insults, and Buddy Hackett uses raunch, Greene earns his reputation by putting over standard shtick with slick tricks, facial gestures broad and subtle, throwaway lines and bits of pantomime, all giving him the appearance of a true "life of the party," a master of spontaneity who can make up new comic song lyrics for ringsiders he kids, ad-lib patter and keep a crowd amused.

Greene may indeed be perceived as part of the old comic tradition of tuxedo and corny tales, but that does not take away from his talent, which has made him, at the entertainment center of America, one of the most popular comedians with the people of mid-America.

DICK GREGORY

In January 1961, an all-white audience made up mostly of Southern conventioneers descended on the Playboy Club in Chicago to see the whimsical comic Professor Irwin Corey. But Corey was ill. In his place was a virtual unknown. He was Dick Gregory, and he was black.

"Good evening, ladies and gentlemen," Gregory said, easing the microphone off its stand. "I understand there are a good many Southerners in the room tonight. I know the South very well. I spent 20 years there one night. . . . The last time I was down South," he continued, "I walked into this restaurant and this waitress came up to me and said, 'We don't serve colored people here.' 'That's all right,' I said, 'I don't eat them. Bring me a fried chicken instead.'"

Gregory had his audience laughing. He drifted through straight jokes, political jokes ("Wouldn't it be funny if Khrushchev didn't really hate us—his interpreter does?") and always brought his focus back to the racial problem in some way:

"Cigarettes—I wouldn't let a man give me cancer. I'm damned if I'll go out and buy it! And pay state and local tax on it? When that cigarette report came out and said 'Cigarettes definitely cause cancer,' had that report read 'Smoking cigarettes will make you turn jet black,' the tobacco companies would be out of business."

As with Lenny Bruce rapping on sex and morality, or Mort Sahl on politics, it was the right time for "Brother Greg" to talk about racial problems. This was an age when comedians were the ones calling attention to problems. For whatever reasons, talk show hosts, newspaper critics and magazine editors promoted them and audiences were ready to listen.

Gregory was suddenly signed for records, and the same year, 1961, was written up in *Time* magazine. His overnight success marked the end of a lifelong struggle with poverty. His own poverty, that is. It started a lifelong vow to alleviate the poverty of others.

One of six children, Gregory was out on the streets early, working at a variety of back-breaking jobs to help support the family. His father had walked out on the family before Gregory had gotten to know him. The lean, hungry young man worked his way through high school and, while there, discovered a talent he hoped would get him a brighter future. It wasn't acting, although he appeared in some school plays. It wasn't music, although he was a drummer in the school's band.

Dick Gregory was an excellent athlete, a runner who was the fastest miler in his class. He began to break records at track meets. By the time he was ready for college, a dozen schools were offering him athletic scholarships. He attended Southern Illinois University, where he could run the mile in under four and a half minutes. He became one of the country's top half-milers, completing that route in just two minutes, seven seconds.

It was while in the Army that Gregory began to perform comedy in special services shows. After developing his talents as both a comic and an impressionist, he came back to Chicago to work as an emcee. He injected comedy into his chores, and drifted from club to club barely making a minimum wage.

Gregory was working in mostly black clubs, doing risque comedy. He figured the only way out of the situation was to own his own club and give himself freedom to perform the type of routines he was so anxious to do. He managed to scrape up some money, but his club, The Apex, closed not long after it opened.

In 1959 he tried a different approach. He produced his own show at a Chicago club that he rented. He did his emcee work and his comedy his way, and impressed the club's owner enough to be hired on a steady basis. When the Republican convention hit Chicago the following year, the media came out in force. Gregory made a name for himself when a performance clip ran on an ABC documentary, "Cast the First Stone."

Gregory got more bookings, but even so, he had to supplement his income by working in a local post office. This recalled the dreary days after he left the Army—when he worked in a post office until he was fired for doing comic impressions of his superiors. With a wife and daughter to support, Gregory was still working hard, breaking even. Finally that opportunity came to substitute for Corey at the Playboy Club.

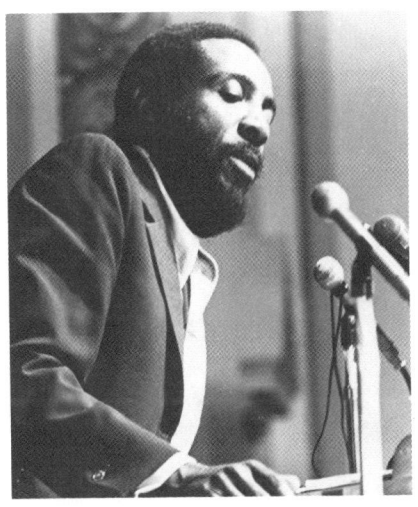

b. October 12, 1932, St. Louis, Missouri

Records:
Two Sides (Vee Jay 4005), Talks Turkey (Vee Jay CJLP 4001), Running for President (Vee Jay 1093), We All Have Problems (Colpix SCP 480), East and West (Colpix SCP 420), Black and White (Colpix SCP 417), At the Village Gate (Poppy 40011), Light Side Dark Side (Poppy PYS 60001), On . . . (Poppy 40008), Kent State (Poppy 60005), Frankenstein (Poppy 60004), Caught in the Act (Poppy 17662), Best of Dick Gregory (Tomato 3-9001).

Books:
From the Back of the Bus, Nigger, Up From Nigger, Write Me In, No More Lies.

The first black comedian to become a success in stand-up, Gregory utilized satire and irony to drive his points home. With dignity, logic and low-key ironic humor, Gregory was a persuasive spokesman who calmly and comically gave white America insights into complex racial issues. But underneath, he was impatient with the slowness of politicians in rectifying the civil rights grievances.

One of his best-known phrases was the gentle, "you see, we all have problems," usually spoken after an ironic joke. Gregory also ironically stated, "In what other country would I have to attend the worst schools, live in the worst neighborhoods, eat in the worst restaurants and average $5,000 a week talking about it?" In 1964 he stepped up his participation in civil rights marches and protests, published a book, *Nigger,* and at year's end made good on his pledge to bring 20,000 turkeys down to Mississippi as Christmas dinners for the poor.

Of the Johnson-Goldwater presidential race, Gregory offered an analogy: "You got two girls and one is a full-time prostitute and the other is a weekend prostitute. If you choose the lesser of two evils and marry the weekend prostitute, you're only fooling yourself if you don't think you're marrying a whore."

By 1966, Gregory announced that he was leaving stand-up behind, and turning to the activities of campus lecturer and social activist. "Entertainment relaxes people enough that they forget about the rent or that deadline for a few minutes. This is all I see myself doing as an entertainer. But when I go and give lectures at colleges and universities I'm not playing games . . . we didn't laugh Hitler out of existence. There will be a cure found for cancer, only it won't be good humor."

In 1967 he made such statements as, "I'm a racist. All my life I've been trying to sit on white folks and now I'm being paid for it." Citing the race riots and ghetto fires, he told a Yale audience a year later:

"How many of you read where Henry Ford hired 6,000 Negroes. Did you also read that they didn't have to take tests when they hired them? Hired 6,000 niggers in two days—because of non-violence? The fire got too close to the Ford plant, baby . . . let me tell you something tonight. We will burn your house to the ground and we mean that—if you think you're going to keep on insulting us."

He ran for president in 1968, although few thought he had much of a chance with lines like this: "If Democracy is as good as we tell you it is, why in the hell are we running all over the world trying to ram it down people's throats with a gun?"

"Much of his humor is inescapably racist," the *New York Times* said in 1969, "but it is a revenge-twist racism in which he drives black paranoia and white prejudice to sublimely ridiculous extremes . . . it is the kind of plain, honest talk that black people have been engaging in for years and white people have been ignoring."

Of Spiro Agnew, Gregory said in 1970, "Agnew reminds me of the kind of guy who would make a crank call to the Russians on the hot line." And with his assertion in 1975 that the CIA killed John F. Kennedy, and lines like "We should love America a little less and respect the constitution a little more," he got his wish—he was considered an activist, no longer a comedian. He released his last comedy album when Richard Nixon resigned.

Over the last decade Gregory has continued to write books, father children (ten) and tour the nation with lectures. At times he's suffered through spells of debt, most recently in 1982 when he was $100,000 in arrears on his Massachusetts home.

His name has appeared in the media most often in connection with protest fasts. "I'm a better person today," he says of these fasts. "I'm more ethical and more honest, more decent and more understanding of a whole lot of people's problems today. You see, once I lay there and got hungry I could relate to that hungry hillbilly in Appalachia and before . . . the only thing I would see was his being a bigot and a racist. But when I lay there I could really relate to this cat just not getting his dinner." Gregory's fasts began in the Vietnam War era when in protest he stopped his intake of solid food and dropped from 170 pounds to 98. He's fasted to protest the death penalty in Georgia, to call attention to the hostage situation in Iran in 1980, and has even fasted for health: he restricted himself to a water diet for two months to help a New Orleans agency gather data on the effects of malnutrition.

BUDDY HACKETT

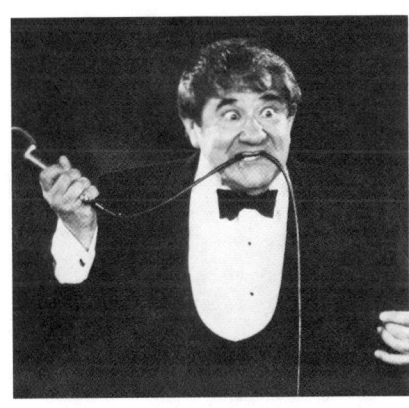

"I'm not a human being. I'm a cartoon," says Buddy Hackett. "And if I say something serious it comes out funny anyway."

He's starred in movies, Broadway shows and his own TV series, but his greatest success has always been in stand-up, ad-libbing and telling raunchy anecdotes for the Las Vegas crowds. Perhaps the last old-time practitioner of the classic risque story in the Belle Barth tradition, Hackett's also a master of spontaneous, free-wheeling party comedy where ringsiders become part of the show, inspiring by-play and encouraging Hackett to be as shocking as he can.

Hackett can get away with many a hardcore remark thanks to his soft, puckish appearance. Back in 1954, *New York Times* critic Brooks Atkinson saw the 5'6", 200 pounder as "large, soft, messy . . . with a glib tongue and a pair of inquiring eyes."

With a streak of little boy mischief, he'll grin and say, "If I wasn't a Jew I would be a Catholic. They got the world by the balls." And just before the audience has gotten over the shock, the kick: "They do whatever they want then they confess they didn't do it!" The impish grin broadens and the laughter starts.

He can do material that would've gotten Lenny Bruce crucified: "As soon as you become a Catholic you're very wealthy. The Vatican has paintings, statues, jewelry . . . I said to a Cardinal, 'Your holiness, if you sold one of these paintings you can feed all the starving Catholics in Rome.' He said 'Get outta here you fat bastard!' Of course, he said it in Latin: 'Absconde, obeseri illegitimo.'"

Coming from the side of his pudgy mouth, spun with reverse English and a Brooklyn accent, it comes out funny. The curious contingent that comes to see this prurient Puck are more than satisfied by the outrages: "I lose half my audience every night," Hackett says, only half in jest.

A graduate of New Utrecht High School in Brooklyn, Hackett learned the ropes in clubs where losing half the audience was not the result of risque jokes, just few good ones. He "tummelled" in the Catskills, tried song and dance patter, and took friend Red Buttons's advice and brought his Chinese waiter shtick to the stage. The routine became so popular Hackett had an unlikely hit album with it. It was broad humor performed with a stereotypical Chinese accent.

Viewed as that rarity, the completely comic character in both voice and physique, he was persuaded by playwright Sidney Kingsley to accept a role in his 1954 Broadway play *Lunatics and Lovers*. This success led

b. Leonard Hacker, August 31, 1924, Brooklyn, New York

Records:
Original Chinese Waiter (Dot 3351), How Do You Do? (Coral [7] 57422).

Compilations:
Do You Wanna Have a Laugh (Coral 57380), Here's Johnny (Casablanca SPNB 1296).

TV:
Stanley.

Broadway:
Lunatics and Lovers, Viva Madison Avenue, I Had a Ball.

Films:
God's Little Acre, Walking My Baby Back Home, The Wonderful World of the Brothers Grimm, It's a Mad, Mad, Mad, Mad World.

Video:
Buddy Hackett in Concert (Family Home Entertainment).

Hackett to TV in 1956 for a show called "Stanley." But already critics were complaining that such vehicles only stunted and slowed his spontaneity.

It was the same in movies. With Abbott and Costello aging, Universal groomed Buddy Hackett and Hugh O'Brien as their new duo, tossing them into *Fireman Save My Child*, a film initially intended for the older comedy team. The reception was cold.

While he continued to experiment with acting roles, appearing to good reviews in *God's Little Acre*, and doing comedy on "The Jackie Gleason Show," a revolution was occurring in stand-up. While ringsider banter was not new (many comics had stock comic answers in such opening wheezes as "You sir—where are you from? Buffalo? Gee, what strange parents!"), performers like Lenny Bruce were reaching audiences with more personal, less formal material. Hackett thrived playing off the crowds, indulging in shockingly personal ad-libs aimed at ringsiders and also at himself. With set jokes in between, he created a euphoric atmosphere where the audience, always off-balance, is constantly giggling and receptive for the next line.

Although he finds Don Rickles "as far from truth as the North Pole," Vegas audiences come to see Hackett for the same reason as Rickles: to be shocked. Bad boy Buddy doesn't disappoint. Shaking hands with a ringsider in a low-cut blouse, he stares down and asks to shake hands again: "Sometimes they jump out when you do that!"

On television, the results are usually mixed. Late at night, on Johnny Carson's show, Hackett does a decent, restrained version of his material that intimates there is much more available in the "privacy" of a nightclub. He's been shunned by game shows like "The Hollywood Squares," where his ad-libbing has been viewed as dangerously undisciplined, too broadly tasteless.

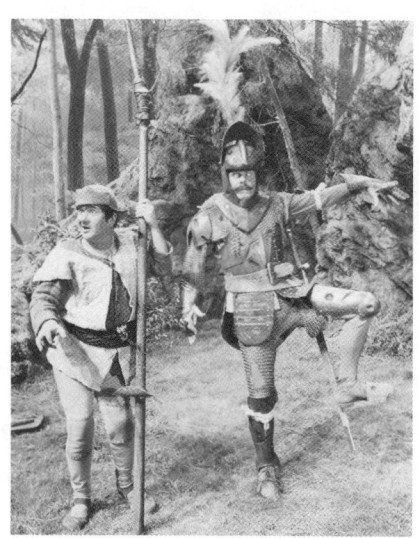

Hackett always considered his comedy influence as "W.C. Fields, W.C. Fields and W.C. Fields. I never cared for Chaplin, wasn't big on Laurel and Hardy. I liked Jimmy Durante, Lou Costello and Harry Ritz." But Hackett never really got hold of a good movie comedy role and managed, solely on the strength of his bright, seemingly spontaneous good humor, to keep afloat a Broadway musical called *I Had a Ball*, which included some modestly amusing numbers such as the Danny Kayesque "Dr. Freud" song.

While it's debatable how cuddly Buddy Hackett is in real life, he was able to show the two sides of a comic's soul effectively in the TV movie biography, "Bud and Lou." It cast him as Lou Costello opposite Harvey Korman's Bud Abbott. Factually, the drama was less than accurate, but Hackett did an effective job capturing the feisty spirit behind a funnyman. Some suggested that the Lou Costello character in the film was akin to Hackett: the little man who needs to prove, via comedy, push or shove, that he is really a big man to be respected.

Hackett remains a Las Vegas fixture, shocking his audience into helpless laughter by doing audience participation twists on Lenny Bruce-George Carlin semantics: "You ever say any of the words I say?" he asks a blushing female ringsider. "You ever say ass? You don't say shit? Then fuck is out of the question! But sometimes ya gotta say it. If you're puttering around the garage and an anvil falls on your foot what are you gonna say? 'Spring is here'? Like a normal person you say, 'Oh shit, I broke my fuckin' foot!'"

With living-room coziness he'll describe the humorous horrors of prostate trouble or taking a barium enema ("the pipe fell out and I left a white line to Pittsburgh . . . I got a big ass but it's not gonna take three gallons of chalk"), and while it's obvious he ad-libs most of his material, he uses vintage jokes and throwaways: "Think what a crowded elevator smells like to a midget."

Couched in Las Vegas sentiment, which means a benediction at the finale or an old-fashioned love song, little of Hackett's performance, no matter how offensive, is unforgivable. And most of it is hysterical because, whether "licensed" by the Vegas atmosphere or not, it's still outrageous, and it comes from a true human cartoon, a man with a naturally funny voice, face and mannerisms.

Hackett's most recent foray into television was as the star of a new syndicated version of "You Bet Your Life." He'd hoped to prove that he was the best ad-libber since Groucho Marx, and figured that this setting would be perfect for his brand of spontaneous fun. Unfortunately it was one of those shows that seemed to have a built-in self-destruct button on it, and it disappeared not long after it premiered.

Recently, something new has been added to Hackett's stand-up show: the appearance of probably the only comedian Buddy would allow to upstage him, his son, Sandy.

HOMER AND JETHRO

"The Thinking Man's Hillbillies," Homer and Jethro were song parodists who brought serious tunes down to earth—if not right into the mud. Loaded (or larded) with puns, the duo's new versions made love ballads sickening ("My poor heart is as heavy as a bucket of liver") and romance ridiculous, as in this line from their "Fascination" parody: "There were nine buttons on her nightgown, but she could only fasten eight."

"Let Me Go, Lover" became "Let Me Go, Blubber": "You're too fat in the first place, you know it's true. You're too fat in the second place too." And "Oh My Papa" became the alcoholic "Oh My Pappy": ". . . sometimes he's good sometimes he's bad. But he can't replace my love for Old Grandad!"

What made the duo endearing was the complete lack of malice in the parodies. The humor usually came from a line-for-line greening of a tune from cosmopolitan to corn, or from turning a tender sentiment into a homely one. Even the legends of country music were not exempt.

Homer recalled, "People used to come to us and say, 'You shouldn't butcher a Hank Williams song because what would Hank think?' Well, Hank, he told us one time, that he didn't think a song was a success until it had been butchered by Homer and Jethro."

Aside from their comic skills, they were both excellent musicians adept at two-part harmony. With short, slim Homer on guitar and his taller, heavier partner clutching what seemed like a junior-sized mandolin in his large hands, they came up with a pleasing sound that often led fans to ask for a few straight tunes mixed with the comedy.

Both men started out as straight musicians. Jethro and his brother were a duo, and Homer was part of a trio. The trio and duo happened to meet at a 1932 amateur show conducted by WNOX in Knoxville. The youngsters were plucking and twanging together offstage when the station's program director came by. He immediately selected four out of five to come to work as staff musicians.

As "The String Dusters," they appeared on WNOX's "Mid-day Merry-Go-Round." Backstage, Homer and Jethro had become fast friends, sharing laughs by slipping new lyrics into hit songs of the day. The program director liked these bits, too, and dubbing the team Homer and Jethro, he allowed them to perform their songs on the air.

"The String Dusters" were blown away by the duo of Homer and Jethro. The team was featured on WNOX from 1936 to 1939. After World

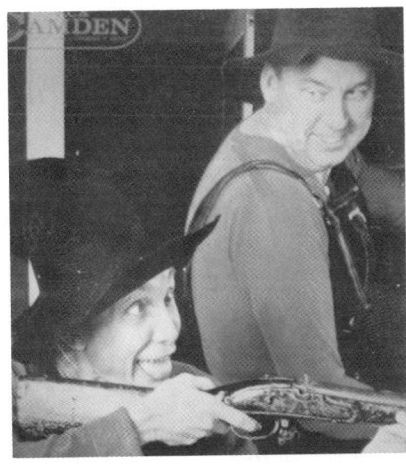

HOMER   b. Henry D. Haynes, July 27, 1920, Knoxville, Tennessee; d. August 7, 1971)
JETHRO   b. Kenneth C. Burns, March 10, 1920, Knoxville, Tennessee

Records:
At the Country Club (RCA Victor 2181), Barefoot Ballads (RCA Victor 1412), Homer and Jethro (King 639), Cornier Than Corn (King 848), Musical Madness (Audio Lab 1513), Songs My Mother Never Sang (RCA Victor 2286), Worst of Homer and Jethro (RCA Victor 1560), Life Can Be Miserable (RCA Victor 1880), At the Convention (RCA Victor 2492), Zany Songs of the 30's (RCA Victor 2455), Playing Straight (RCA Victor 2459), Go West (RCA Victor 2674), Something Stupid (RCA Victor 3877), Wanted for Murder (RCA Victor 3673), Ooh, That's Corny (RCA Victor 2743), Cornfucius Say (RCA

Victor 2928), Nashville Cats (RCA Victor 3822), Any News? (RCA Victor 3538), Homer and Jethro (RCA Victor 3701), Old Crusty Minstrels (RCA Victor 3462), Songs to Tickle Your Funny Bone (RCA Camden 948), Homer & Jethro Strike Back (RCA Camden 707), Humorous Side (RCA Camden 768).

War II, the boys joined a Cincinnati radio station and signed their first record contract. They made five albums for King Records before heading down to Missouri to work on KWTO's "Red Foley Show" with Chet Atkins.

Describing their early years, country comic Archie Campbell wrote, "The first time I recall seeing these two was at the old playhouse in Chattanooga. Jethro started singing 'Sweet Fern' and Homer repeated with 'dad burn.' I know that doesn't sound so funny now, but it tore 'em up that day."

Jethro usually played straight man, although Homer was not conspicuously comic-looking. Predating later comic foils like Dick Martin and Tom Smothers, Homer was only borderline "tetched" in the head. He seemed attractive and almost normal. But that was deceptive. "Boy, it was hot," Homer would say. "How hot was it?" indulged Jethro. "It was so hot I seen a cow layin' on her back giving herself a shower." Homer would grin, Jethro would look mildly chagrined, and then, like George Burns to Gracie Allen, ask a few more straight questions against his better judgment.

In concert they'd do a comic version of "On Top of Old Smokey" with Homer interrupting, saying, "Jethro, give me an E flat." "Now, Homer, you know I can't play an E flat." "Then gimme an E and I'll flatten it out myself!" Later Homer would enthusiastically call out, "Would you folks like to join in and help us sing this song?" After the affirmative applause died down: "Well . . . I wish you wouldn't 'cause we'd like to sing it by ourselves."

The corny comics met up with another king of corn, Spike Jones. They had some hits together including a new "Pagliacci" called "Pal Yatchy" ("When we listen to Pal Yatchy, we get itchy and scratchy"). They left Jones in 1951 for the Chicago-based "National Barn Dance" and stayed there through much of the decade, hitting the charts with a series of novelty tunes. "The Battle of Kookamonga" won a 1959 Grammy award, and their "Country Club" lp was a nominee in 1960.

Like Spike Jones, they were signed to RCA. Through the 1960's Homer and Jethro averaged a pair of discs each year. During this, the era of TV's top-rated "Beverly Hillbillies," the country comics were definitely "in," not only enjoying huge record sales (in 1966 and 1967 eight lps were released) but appearing in a successful TV commercial selling cereal. After cracking some bad jokes, they'd sing: "Ooooh, that's corny, corny as Kellogg's Corn Flakes."

Homer and Jethro didn't do much physical comedy, they simply stood up and sang their songs, adding some routines in between. They could have continued for decades, but after the successful 1960's there was no more. In 1971, Homer, only 51, suffered a sudden heart attack and died. After losing his partner and life-long friend, Jethro resumed his interest in music by taking on occasional session work. Some years later he recorded a solo album for the Chicago record company Flying Fish.

BOB HOPE

America's greatest living comedian was born in England, but moved with his family to Cleveland, Ohio, when he was four. He learned singing from his mother and tap dancing in high school, but the athletic young man's first claim to fame was in sports. As "Packy East" he had a brief fling as a boxer. He also worked as a shoe salesman, and with a girlfriend named Mildred began singing in local clubs.

Hope had limited success with partners. Mildred didn't want to tour. Another, Lloyd Durbin, ate some tainted coconut cream pie and died a few days later. Finally Hope hooked up with George Byrne and as "Two Diamonds in the Rough" they rose to a $300 a week salary for their blackface song and dance routines.

When an emcee failed to appear for a program, Hope was pushed out to take care of the duties. He managed to get a few laughs, and this encouraged him in his dream of being a stand-up comic. Soon he was without Byrne—and without money.

"I couldn't get a job," he recalls. "I was $400 in debt just for coffee and doughnuts. No one came when I was billed as Leslie Hope, song and dance man, so I changed it to Bob and still nobody came. Finally, in 1925, I signed a vaudeville contract." It was then that he learned his craft.

"These young guys today have no way of getting that kind of experience. It was a rare opportunity to master such important things as timing and delivery. Today, aside from the comedy shops, which I feel are very good, there is no such training ground."

After he was told "your face is funny the way it is," Hope dropped the blackface. In 1928, Dallas theater owner Robert J. O'Donnell commented on Hope's rapid delivery: "Where are you going, fancy pants? Why are you working so fast? Let them enjoy you."

"I learned to have enough courage to wait," Hope says. "I'd stand there waiting for them to get it for a long time . . . my idea was to let them know who was running things. I used to defy the audience. I didn't have much talent but I had plenty of guts."

He still remembers one of his first jokes: "I used to go out and say I was eating in the restaurant next door. When I walked up to the cashier I found out I left my money in my other pants. I said, 'Say, I'm very sorry about it but I'll pay you the next time I come in.' She said, 'Don't worry about it, just put your name on the wall and you can pay us the next time you come in.' I said, 'I don't want to have my name on the wall where everyone can see it.' She said, 'Don't worry, your overcoat will be hanging over it. . . .' Then I'd stare at the audience, stare 'em into a laugh."

Hope developed his brash character: "Pseudo-smart, that's the way I describe my stuff," and soon resumed the climb to the top. He was on Broadway in *Ballyhoo* in 1932 and *Roberta* in 1933, and it was during that show's run that he met his future wife, Dolores, a nightclub singer.

Hope was starring in the 1935 version of the Ziegfeld Follies when he made his radio debut. Three years later he had his own show. That year he made his first movie, *The Big Broadcast of 1938*. Typical of his early fame as a song and dance man, the highlight was not his comedy, but his wistful rendition of "Thanks for the Memory" in a duet with Shirley Ross. Hope made five films that year, and in 1939 had a hit with *The Cat and the Canary*.

Hope wrote his first autobiography in 1941, *They've Got Me Covered*, and people wondered how he found the time. He was starring on radio, entertaining the troops overseas and making his "Road" pictures with Bing Crosby. Through the 1940's Hope was one of the "Top Ten" box office attractions in the nation, and in the 50's made the transition to television. "I didn't want to take the plunge. I was still in the Top 10 at the box office. But NBC kept making offers until they made that high stakes one I couldn't refuse."

In 1981 *Variety* wrote, "The specifics of Hope's ratings record tend to stagger the mind. In his 30 years on NBC he has aired 213 specials . . . only nine have scored less than a 30 share, and six of those misses have occurred in the last two seasons."

In the 60's, Hope was still a superstar, but to a growing segment of

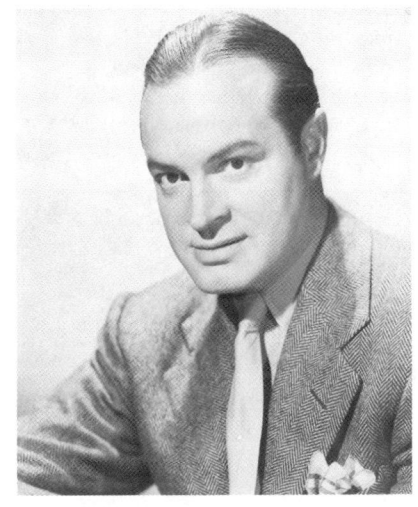

b. Leslie Townes Hope, May 29, 1903, Eltham, England

Records:
Bob Hope in Russia (Decca 74369), Holidays (Spear 4700), America Is 200 Years Old . . . and There's Still Hope (Capitol ST 11538), On the Road to Vietnam (Cadet LPS 4046), Bob Hope & Bing Crosby on Radio (Radiola 1044), Bob Hope Radio Show (Radiola MR 1068), Bob Hope in Hollywood (MCA 906).

TV:
The Bob Hope Show (NBC 1953–56), Bob Hope Chrysler Theater (NBC 1963–67), Bob Hope Specials (NBC).

Films:
Big Broadcast of 1938, Thanks for the Memory, Cat and the Canary, Ghost Breakers, My Favorite Blonde, Monsieur Beaucaire, My Favorite Brunette, Paleface, Son of Paleface, Beau James, Private Navy of Sgt. O'Farrell.

Video:
My Favorite Brunette (Budget Video), Bing Crosby Show 1963 (Video Yesteryear), Masters of Comedy (Video Dimensions), Bob Hope Chevy Show 1956 (Video Yesteryear).

Books:
Have Tux Will Travel, I Never Left Home, So This Is Peace, The Last Christmas Show, The Road to Hollywood, I Owe Russia $1200, Confessions of a Hooker.

Bios:
Amazing Careers of Bob Hope (Morella, Epstein and Clark), Bob Hope (Charles Thompson), Bob Hope (William Robert Faith).

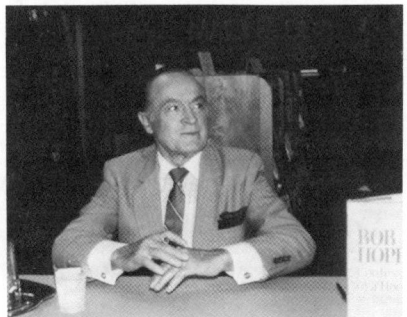

America he wasn't funny at all. The Vietnam War polarized the country, and the comedian's staunchly conservative stance antagonized many. An anti-hippie joke here and there, a pause for some "but seriously, folks" remarks about getting behind the president, and he was perceived as blinded by Old Glory.

Another problem for Hope was a change in the style of comedy. Young fans made heroes out of hip, "human" comics like Bill Cosby and George Carlin, and couldn't warm up to Hope's style or personality. Some may have sensed the fear and contempt that could make a comic plant his hands deep into his pockets and fire one-liners to kill them, each volley followed by an antagonistic stare. Staring down an audience made young fans bridle, and his style, lacking in sincerity, didn't help.

Here was an "Establishment" millionaire (worth $200 million to $300 million, paying his writers a half million a year) who sold his middle name to whatever sponsor he worked for ("Hi, this is Bob 'Pepsodent' Hope"), told safe political jokes and shamelessly plugged NBC stars on his specials. Even such commonsense gimmicks as surrounding himself with appetite-whetting pretty starlets were perceived as crassly commercial, although the technique continues to be used today, even by youth-oriented comics like England's Benny Hill.

It didn't matter that Hope had put in decades of public service, raised millions for charities, helped to cheer thousands in hospitals and hundreds of thousands of GI's in his 30+ years of overseas Christmas tours. Many were likewise unaware of his awards—from the Jean Hersholt Humanitarian Award to a Congressional Medal of Honor given to Hope by John F. Kennedy.

As the Vietnam War became memory, the rift between Hope and Americans under 30 slowly healed, although by that time Hope had competition as "the symbol of American comedy," with the emergence of the equally quick, personable and handsome Johnny Carson, who even replaced Hope for Academy Awards emcee chores.

Into his 70's, Hope maintained his frenzied schedule of 150 charity appearances and concerts a year. His energy baffled even such sports figures as Sugar Ray Leonard: "In 1981, Mr. Hope asked me to be in his 78th birthday special . . . he wanted to do a number sparring with me in the ring. At about 6pm I got in the ring and began to work with Bob. He kept saying, 'We can do this better. Let's try it over again' . . . after about two hours I said I was getting a little tired." Hope, who had been rehearsing for 12 hours, was still going: "That old man wore me out!" For relaxation when out of town, Hope and an aide would often take a long walk after midnight, window shopping in a town's shopping district.

On July 4, 1982, Hope did a concert in St. Louis that must stand as a world's record for a comedian: he played to two million people. "Geez, can you believe it?" he says. "The best I ever did before was 500,000. I must be getting better in my old age." Around the country, Hope's movies featuring his brash, all-American character have become more popular than ever. Woody Allen, a great supporter of Hope's, and an important influence in restoring his reputation among "hip" critics, said of *Road to Morocco*, "I saw this film in 1942 when I was only 7 years old. I knew from that moment on what I wanted to do with my life."

Even at 80, Hope did not slow down. He went overseas once more to entertain the troops. The jokes? Well, they were the typical light and saucy gags everyone expected: "I'm happy to be here for the 181st ceasefire in Lebanon," he said. When a few jokes bombed, he said it would be a good idea to "stuff the bad jokes into the five-inch guns and aim them at the Syrians." He did definition jokes: "Beirut. That's an Arabic word meaning 'Let's get the hell out of here.'" And he did jokes guaranteed to please. A roar from the Marines accompanied this one: "Semper Fidelis. That means 'Mr. T is a sissy.'"

Into the election year of 1984 he trundled out jokes both old and new: "In recent years I've not been going in so much for political jokes because too many of them are getting elected.... How about Walter Mondale's slogan, 'Where's the beef.' If he doesn't know where Tip O'Neill is, why should we?"

Hope reflects, "I don't think my humor has changed much. I talk about golf, flying, my health and other people's health, and politics. But it might be a little more sophisticated because you can do more things these days. People buy sex all the way, but I try to stay away from a lot of it." This joke is about as salty as he gets: "Last night I saw a lot of sailors looking for culture on 42nd Street: The only place you have to be vaccinated to go to the movies."

He doesn't neglect mention of some real problems:

"Almost everything we eat has pesticides in it. That bugs me. The other day I saw a picture of Betty Crocker with a gas mask on. It's always nice to know you can use your birthday cake as a roach motel.... Now they have a new way of killing fruit flies. They poison our food then maybe when you keel over you'll fall on a fly."

Despite recent eye problems, Hope maintains a huge schedule of appearances and looks and acts far younger than his years: "If I look good to you, it's because I laugh a lot. Laughing is the greatest thing for you." On retirement, he adds, "Hell, if I retired I'd have to have an applause machine to wake me up in the morning."

Today, Bob Hope's movies, his old TV and radio performances and his current specials please not only old fans, but also new generations. He is, if not America's greatest comedy attraction, still "Top Ten" at the box office when he chooses to do a concert. And more than that, he is now universally acknowledged as a living legend in American entertainment.

GEORGE JESSEL

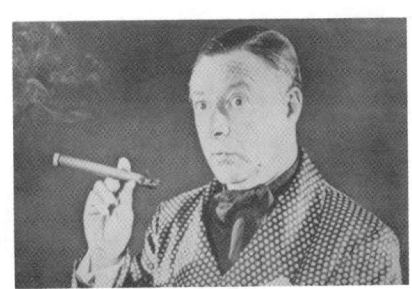

b. April 3, 1898, Harlem, New York; d. May 24, 1981

Records:
Jessel at His Best (Audio Fidelity AFSD 1706), Bedtime Stories for Adults (Riot 304).

TV:
The George Jessel Show (ABC 1953–54).

Dubbed by Harry Truman the "Toastmaster General" of the United States, George Jessel was accustomed to crowds ever since childhood. As the bat boy for the New York Giants, the youngster often entertained after games with songs in the clubhouse—that is, if the Giants won. "If they lost," Jessel recalled, the manager John McGraw "would say, 'Get out of here, you little Jew.' And then I'd go to the visiting club."

With the help of his mother, who worked at Harlem's Imperial Theater, George got bookings with his trio, which included Jack Wiener and a boy named Walter Winchell. By the time he was 19, he was a veteran comic, "The Boy Monologist" of vaudeville. In addition to stand-up, he did songs. His act changed very little over the next 60 years.

His famous "Hello, Momma" routine had its roots in the ancient "Cohen on the Telephone" 78's recorded by Barney Barnard for Victor and Joe Hayman for Columbia. But unlike these routines, which based their humor on the monologist's failure to assimilate or understand American culture, Jessel put the humor not on himself, but his old-fashioned mom:

"Hello, Operator. Fentingtrass 3522. Hello, Momma. This is George.

Video:
The Big Time Variety Show (Video Yesteryear).

Books:
Hello, Momma?; The World I Lived In; So Help Me; This Way, Miss; Jessel Anyone; You Too Can Make a Speech; Elegy in Manhattan; Halo over Hollywood.

Isn't it nice to have your own phone? What? Nobody calls you? Even before you had the phone, nobody called you either?

"Say, Momma, how did you like that bird I sent you for your birthday. You cooked it! But Momma, that was a South American parrot! He spoke five languages. He should have said something?

"How's my sister Anna? Put her on. Hello, Anna, this is Georgie. What's gonna be with that fella—you're engaged now 33 years. You'll get married when his business comes back? What's his business? He milks reindeer? Put your mother back on.

"Mom? Well, the girl is in love so there you are. But you know what Longfellow tells us, 'Tell me not in mournful numbers life is but an empty dream.' I say Longfellow tells us this. I shouldn't go around with him, he's drunk? No, no, Longfellow. He didn't live next door to us at all, that was Lowenstein, the bookmaker!"

Jessel recalled that "it would be a simple matter to romanticize by saying that these phone conversations were inspired by the homey atmosphere of the Bronx, that the gentle humor of my relatives is contained, that my mother used to talk like that. But I cannot tell a lie. At least, not such a big one. My mother did not talk like that ... the business of being inspired has been highly overrated of late, anyway."

Jessel starred in many Broadway shows, singing in 1918's *Shubert Gaieties* before ending up in *George Jessel's Troubles* and finally *The Jazz Singer*. Although it was Al Jolson who starred in the movie version, Jessel never let anyone forget who was the original mammy singer.

A fixture in almost all phases of show business, Jessel started his "toasting" career as an "after-dinner" monologist when he campaigned for New York Mayor Jimmy Walker in 1925. He was a movie producer with dozens of films to his credit, and also wrote songs with such titles as "Oh How I Laugh When I Think How I Cried Over You," "Stop Kicking My Heart Around," "Oooh-La-La Wee-Wee" and his trademark tear-jerker, "My Mother's Eyes."

Jessel did not finish high school, but he was extremely well read and even wrote eight books. He knew every U.S. president from Woodrow Wilson on, and raised over a hundred million dollars for charity. His charity work for Israel was monumental. Yet, over the years, Jessel became a figure of derision.

This was due in part to his weary and ubiquitous presence on the dais, at public functions and, increasingly, at funerals where he would deliver eulogies. Another factor was his act, which didn't change. His comedy could still get laughs, but new generations had difficulty understanding dated references to friends like Eddie Cantor and Jolson and the sometimes maudlin songs Jessel sang. But what truly separated him from other "nostalgia" acts, or other old-time comics, was his virulent, highly unpopular conservatism.

In the 1960's Jessel was as pro-Vietnam War as Bob Hope, but totally humorless about it. He was outspoken and crusty on other topics, too. Wearing quasi-military gear, he launched into a right-wing tirade on a 1971 "Today Show" broadcast, deliberately calling the *New York Times* "Pravda." He became so obnoxious that interviewer Edwin Newman quickly brought the segment to an end. And that ended Jessel's talk show dates. For years he was generally considered persona non grata.

Some of Jessel's friends took it all in stride. George wasn't a conservative in every way. They recalled his affairs with Lupe Velez and Pola Negri, and that two of his three children were born out of wedlock. Jessel was not at all averse to getting his "joint copped" by a convenient show girl or bimbo backstage, on a plane or in a cab, although he was not about to share this information with his more sentimental fans. "When he was a sex machine," Earl Wilson said, "he feared husbands; now that he isn't, he fears Communists."

In 1979 he amazed reporters by proclaiming, "I don't want Richard Nixon sitting up in Watergate stagnating. We deserve him. . . . I was very close to President Nixon. In fact, I was being groomed for an ambassadorship to South Korea. I was the personal public relations officer for Tongsun Park, who was a hero in my opinion and was wrongly accused of any wrongdoing."

Jessel continued to appear in clubs, even at the age of 80, telling mildly risque stories, reminiscing, singing songs. And some began to realize he did have a point when, talking about comedy, he wished more comics took a more universal stance: "A comedian is a fellow who can make my Aunt Tilly laugh . . . these are all very clever people, mind you—Mort Sahl, Jack E. Leonard . . . a few others . . . [but] what would they do at a Saturday matinee at the Palace Theatre, where the audience consisted of Aunt Tilly and the kids?"

By 1979, most were able to overlook Jessel's politics. They remembered him for his comedy, for his songs and for his charity work. They remembered him as a Jean Hersholt Humanitarian Award winner, and they remembered an anecdote about him from years back:

Jessel was escorting a young Lena Horne into the 21 Club. But the doorman gave them a hard time. These were the days when blacks could still be restricted from entering a well-known, respected niterie. The doorman continued to stall Jessel and Horne.

"Do you have a reservation?" the doorman asked.
"Yes," Jessel answered.
"Who made it?"
"Abraham Lincoln, you son of a bitch!"

The 81-year-old entertainer received one last honor before his death. On May 5, 1979, Mayor Tom Bradley proclaimed "George Jessel Day" in Los Angeles.

WILL JORDAN

"Will Jordan exaggerates my mannerisms until he is more like me than I am myself," Ed Sullivan recalled. "When he does me he changes his voice until it's right on the button. I can close my eyes, stand off in the wings, and tell myself I am hearing my own voice."

Will Jordan did more than that. "The mimic doesn't just exaggerate the character, or just find the highlights," Will Jordan explains, "he invents! This carbon copier is also creative. Did Ed Sullivan ever say 'R-r-really big sheew?' You're wrong. He never said it. I invented it for him. . . . I also invented the famous knuckle cracks, eyes upward roll and crazy body spins. . . ."

Back in the 1950's, when Ed Sullivan was the host of the most influential variety show on television, Will Jordan was the nation's top mimic. He startled audiences with his ability to transform himself facially into caricatures of Sullivan, Clark Gable, Charles Laughton and Edward G. Robinson. And he improved on simple mimicry by doing bits of vocal transmogrification, showing how Clark Gable sounded like Robert Preston who sounded like Dale Robertson who sounded like Dwight Eisen-

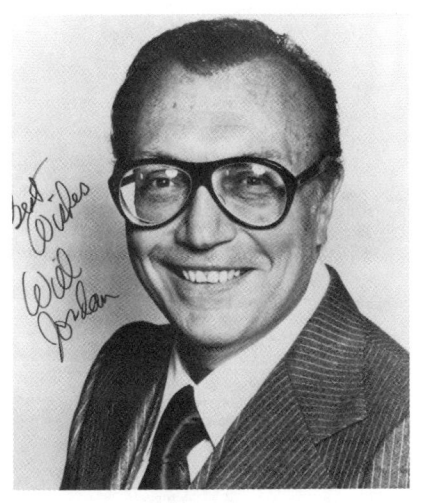

b. July 27, [1930], New York, New York

Records:
Ill Will (Jubilee 2032), Sick Magazine's Record (Amy Sick #2), All About Cleopatra (Topical T1001), The New First Family (Verve 15054), Tapped Wires (Roulette R 25204).

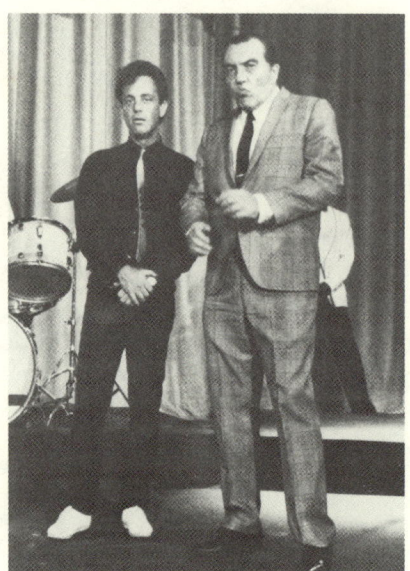

hower. He had astonishing skits where he combined Ed Sullivan and Jack E. Leonard (a car accident led Jack to donate some of his acid blood to Ed) and he amazed a *Playboy* writer by doing "Boris Karloff and Bela Lugosi as Martin and Lewis. Jordan doesn't simply impersonate Boris Karloff and Jerry Lewis, he impersonates Boris Karloff impersonating Jerry Lewis."

Jordan was also capable of original comedy concepts that had nothing to do with mimicry. He did sketches with sound effects, the kind of things Jonathan Winters would later become famous for, and a bit about Adolf Hitler going into show business, a concept later used by both Mel Brooks and Lenny Bruce. Bruce was only one of many comics influenced by Will Jordan's hip, often "sick" humor.

"Ill Will" convulsed ringsiders with his parody of hunchback Dwight Frye in "Frankenstein" (who, turning into a grotesque-nosed Dick Haymes, sang "Why Was I Born, Why Am I Living"), his report on an RAF flyer who heroically flies into German territory only to reveal later "I'm totally blind" and a routine about a Shakespearean actor attempting to do stand-up. Even his throwaway jokes were pretty solid: "My father's the head of the underground. You'll know him as soon as you see him— his clothes are filthy."

When Jordan cut his album for Jubilee around 1961, Hugh Hefner noted that "We've known Will as a close personal friend for several years, since before our friendships with either Mort Sahl or Lenny Bruce began." For the general public, though, the "Ill Will" side of Jordan was not seen as often as his more standard impressions.

Jordan first appeared on Sullivan's show in 1953, but nothing happened. He'd taken it easy, didn't want to satirize Sullivan fully. But the next year he went all-out with his manic version of the corpse-like emcee, and he was on his way. That year, 1954, Eddie Cantor called Jordan "the best mimic these eyes of mine have ever seen."

Ten years later, Woody Allen guest-hosted "The Tonight Show" and brought on Will, saying, "Having you on was my pleasure," calling him "a genius at mimicry."

But along the way, others were mimicking the mimic. Other comics began doing the Sullivan impression, and new impressionists coming up naturally added Sullivan to their repertoire. The impressionist who creates something new has "cracked the code." Like a caricaturist, he has given his audience those swift few magical lines that are the essence of the caricature. Now, not everyone can draw a picture of Alfred Hitchcock; but almost anyone can trace that famous caricature side-portrait of "Hitch." So it was that others imitated not Sullivan, but Jordan doing Sullivan. And only occasionally was he given credit.

Shecky Greene called attention to Jordan's dilemma by saying he was "the greatest of mimics," and also "the creator of comedy routines about Sullivan, Sabu and Hitler that were taken by Lenny Bruce and Jack Carter." But, as with many creative people, there was a fragility in Will Jordan, a sensitivity. The theft of his key impressions hurt him deeply and, naturally enough, he found it hard to think up new bits knowing these too would be stolen. So the man who did Ed Sullivan's offstage voice for Broadway's *Bye Bye Birdie* found himself unable to do Ed's show because the Sullivan impression had been worn out by other comics.

Through the late 60's and 70's Jordan staked out new territory. He began doing commercials, voice overs and special appearances at conventions, sales meetings and other functions where he imitated celebrities. He made more money in a month than he had during his hottest years. He could do straight mimicry for a convention of Ford Motor Company executives, and still bring an audience to its knees with laughter at a more free-form gig like a "Sons of the Desert" (the Laurel & Hardy organization) banquet.

The man who had made over 400 network appearances found a new, secure market. Remembering him as one of the pioneering "sick-nik" comics, journalists never ceased asking Will for his recollections of cohorts like Lenny Bruce. Albert Goldman interviewed Jordan extensively for his book on Bruce, and Phil Berger, author of *The Last Laugh*, also made extensive use of his interviews with Jordan.

The latter book included a virtually unedited transcript of Jordan describing his bitterness and his inability to write new material. As Richard Anobile did with Groucho Marx in *The Marx Brothers Scrapbook*, Berger produced a provocative work at the expense of the subject. Unexpectedly seeing himself made into a dramatic figure of tragedy only increased Jordan's legitimate feelings of being manipulated.

However, the "last laugh" was Jordan's. The book reminded some people that he was still around, and it perhaps won him some sympathy for the thievery he endured. Jordan is in greater demand than ever. He's done "hush-hush" work, like dubbing Robert Shaw's voice for *Force 10 from Navarone*, continues to entertain with stand-up at trade shows where he impersonates George C. Scott as Patton (lecturing salesmen on efficiency) and, with the revival of interest in rock, turned up in movies (*The Buddy Holly Story*, *I Wanna Hold Your Hand*) and rock video (Billy Joel's "Tell Her") as Ed Sullivan.

Although in the final editing some of his key material was removed, Jordan was also prominently featured as one of the veteran comics in Woody Allen's *Broadway Danny Rose*.

Impressionists usually rise with a specific, meteoric caricature that sets them apart. Frank Gorshin had his unusual Burt Lancaster–Kirk Douglas bit, David Frye had Richard Nixon, etc. Then either the star caricatured fades, or the novelty of the mimic's version does. And some impressionists, like Gorshin, John Byner, Larry Storch, etc., move on to something else. Will Jordan survived the eclipse of the Sullivan impression, endured, and is today as successful as ever.

JACKIE KANNON

Jackie Kannon had one aim, "taking comedy out of the nightclubs and putting it in sewers where it belongs!" In over a decade of working 40 weeks a year in his own club, "The Ratfink Room," he made New York funseekers come up to *his* sewer. Located atop "The Roundtable" and later "Upstairs at the Downstairs," patrons stepped up so they could be brought down.

A comic in the Joe E. Lewis tradition, cocky little Kannon favored snappy patter and risque songs. For the 1960's his snap included four-letter words and his songs were as high class as a limerick. Comedy writer Sol Weinstein said, "They come to hate him. The hard-bitten face evokes that sort of reaction ... yet when the last insults have been flipped, the last patron abused, the last ethnic group excoriated, the dazed clubgoers look at each other dumbly, still in shock. Hey, the little — is great. Great!"

Brash and aggressive, Kannon would end a show with lines like "You've been a great audience, but then again I've been brilliant." Never a household word, he nevertheless enjoyed his notoriety and the security of being the first comic successfully to set up and manage his own nightclub "home."

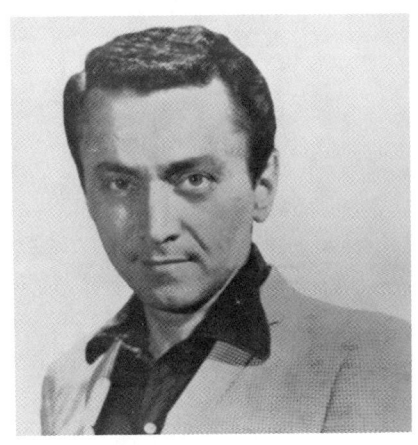

b. 1920 or 1926, Windsor, Ontario, Canada; d. February 1, 1974

Records:
Songs for the John (Roulette R 25187), Live from the Ratfink Room (Roulette R 25312), Prose from the Cons (Roulette R 502), Poems for John (Swan 503), You Don't Have to Be Jewish (Kapp KL 4503), Music for Rat Fink Lovers (Ratfink LP 1313).

Books:
Poems for the John, The JFK Coloring Book, Happiness Is a Rat Fink.

"I wouldn't want to be [a big star] if I had the chance," he said. "I'm content going along at this pace. Every big star I know suffers from an incurable, insufferable disease—humility. I learned a long time ago, it's easy to be humble when you're successful, the trick is to be arrogant when you're a flop."

A former shoe salesman, Kannon toiled in small clubs, steeling himself to failure and firing back one-liners.

"Why did I choose show business? In one word, greed. Also, I wanted to sleep late. I've always wanted to be in this as long as I can remember." In 1944 he was a shoe salesman, waiting for something better. Finally he decided to make it happen himself: "I went to a strip joint in Battle Creek, nearby, during lunch one day, and I told the owner I was a nightclub act from Chicago. I was put on for $75 a week . . . meanwhile I went to see other comedians in other joints and I copied down their material and used it." He went to the Coast for two years at Billy Gray's Band Box, but clicked back in Detroit at the Club Gay Haven in 1949. He stayed there for years, eventually getting his own local TV show over WXYZ.

By 1952 he was invading the Latin Quarter in New York. The 5'7" son of a rabbi made heads turn with his hip humor: "I crossed marijuana with menthol so you can be high and cool at the same time. . . . If her lips are on fire and she trembles in your arms, forget her. She's got malaria. . . . Wild horses couldn't drag a secret out of most women. Unfortunately they seldom have lunch with wild horses. . . . How about the Irish woman who prayed 'God have Murphy on me'!"

He did anything—parodies, whiz bang ("If all the beans are in Boston, how come Long Island has the sound?") and insults ("That's a suit? It looks like a Rayco seat cover. I know that girl, kid, and you're a cinch to get rid of the pimples"). He never crossed over into Lenny Bruce-type controversial material: "My theory is that there are too many serious things going on today to get serious about humor. Humor should be used to relax from the everyday worries, not to remind us about them."

In 1959 he and printer Alexander Roman formed Kanrom, a successful publishing company that handled Jackie's novelty books and the short-lived *Ratfink Magazine*. It was in 1963 that he first opened his "Ratfink Room," becoming an established part of the New York nightclub scene.

When he became ill in 1972 with polyps on his vocal chords, he quipped that his doctor had just the solution: "I know your material, my doctor told me. You'll be the only comedian in the business who'll have his throat treated by Preparation H."

Married with four sons, the comedian was happy with the security of the club, but was always brimming with other ideas. While the club gave him the chance to give other comics a break, he recorded a unique album, "Prose from the Cons," that gave prison inmates a chance to try stand-up comedy as a career. Utilizing material written by the inmates, Kannon and Eli Basse, it proved Ed Wynn's contention that anyone with a good script could be a comic—but that few were gifted with the ability to "say things funny" instead of "say funny things."

The busy nightclub owner/publisher/novelty book author/comic died suddenly of a heart attack. The age he generally quoted to interviewers was picked up by the *New York Times*: 48. Other sources, including *Variety*, gave it as 54. His comedy style is best exemplified in the album he recorded at his home base, "The Ratfink Room." As he said, "I couldn't get much TV work because of an outmoded concept called good taste. . . . At The Ratfink I can swing like I want to."

GABE KAPLAN

"I wasn't one of the loudmouth trouble-makers," Gabe Kaplan recalled. A graduate of Erasmus Hall High School in Brooklyn, he described himself as "a quiet underachiever." But in his quiet way, Kaplan became a major achiever in stand-up, and later a star of his own TV show about high school, "Welcome Back, Kotter."

Kaplan's initial ambition was to play professional baseball. He tried out for the minor leagues, but "there were no designated hitters then. I was all hit and no field." He took a job as a bellboy at a hotel in Lakewood, New Jersey, and it was there that he began to watch comedians at work.

"The hotel booked stand-up comics two or three times a week. It just hit me that to be a comic you didn't have to be an extrovert, you only had to have a funnybone basically and the presence to perform."

The shy, serious young man studied the comics and, with a handful of standard patter jokes in their style, decided to take a shot: "Without telling me, my mother wrote to Woody Allen. She told him that she didn't think it was the profession for me and asked him what to do. Naturally she and my father wanted me to go to college and be a C.P.A. or a dentist or something like that. Woody wrote back a very nice note. He said if I didn't have any success I'd probably give it up inside a year."

But by year's end, Kaplan had tasted some encouraging $100-a-week bookings. The 21-year-old comic was far from the big time, though. He spent five years on the road, working in small clubs, emceeing strip shows, trying to develop his own style. The new comedy showcases and emerging hip comedy clubs around town helped. "I started going to comedy clubs like The Comedy Workshop, and began to learn what's funny and what isn't funny." At the Bitter End in 1968, *Variety* reviewed his act. But they weren't sure he knew what was funny yet.

Kaplan persevered, developing a promising bit, an Ed Sullivan impression with a neat twist. He portrayed a drunk Sullivan, insulting his guests, up to and including Kate Smith. He also began to develop a more informal stance on stage, less the deadpan comic with the glazed eyes.

While he still tended to erect a wary wall between stage and seats, Kaplan broke the ice with recognition comedy, amusing local audiences with "When I was a kid" stuff, drawing on the Brooklyn characters he knew in school. He began to share his comedy with the audience rather than simply deliver gags.

The momentum was building. Kaplan wrote material for David Frye's comedy albums, and in 1972 a "Tonight Show" talent coordinator saw him at The Comedy Workshop and signed him for an appearance. More television work followed, and in 1974 he recorded the album "Holes and Mellow Rolls," which included an extended routine about high school and "gross out" humor.

The bit was a slice-of-school-life sketch about a nerd named Arnold Horshack, the type who would actually *ask* for homework if the teacher hadn't thought of assigning any. His witless put-down to his tormentors was, "Up your hole with a Mello Roll—and twice as far with a Hershey Bar."

Others easily topped him: "Why don't you shove a stick up your ass and go to a masquerade party as a Fudgicle!"

Eventually a "ranking" contest ensues, in which the sharpest kids begin knocking each other. One says, "I heard your mother is like the Pennsylvania Railroad—she's been laid all over the country." The other answers, "Your mother on a recent trip to Washington gave the Lincoln

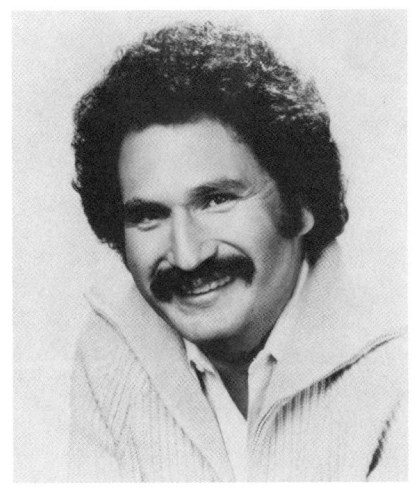

b. March 31, 1946, Brooklyn, New York

Record:
Holes and Mellow Rolls (ABC 8125).

TV:
Welcome Back, Kotter (ABC 1975–79).

Films:
Fast Break, Nobody's Perfekt, Tulips.

Video:
Catch a Rising Star 10th Anniversary (RCA Video).

Memorial a hand job." The insults get worse. They even use celebrity impressions to drive them home. Finally, in desperation, one of them ends up using "Up your hole with a Mello Roll"—to the amusement of nobody. Nobody except Arnold Horshack.

Kaplan had many more routines about school life. He did a bit about a gym teacher who used the euphemism "family jewels." He insisted the boys wear jock straps to protect "the jewels." One day, after Kaplan's put his watch and mezuzah away, the teacher stops him and says, "Did ya take care of the family jewels?" The guy faints as Kaplan says, "Yes—I put them in my locker!"

Also in 1974, producer Alan Sacks happened to catch a Kaplan performance at a West Coast comedy club. There to see Freddie Prinz, he ended up responding to Gabe's nostalgic bits that captured the rowdy humor of a Brooklyn classroom. Sacks, Kaplan and comic-turned-producer James Komack developed the nightclub routine into a situation comedy.

"Welcome Back, Kotter" was not an easy sell. Many still felt Kaplan lacked warmth, including Komack: "I thought Gabe was the strangest man I had ever come across. It was his inarticulateness socially that got to me." Kaplan was so quiet he seemed embalmed. But later Komack came to know Kaplan better: "He's direct, says what he means, and is a man of his word. He doesn't try to hurt people. He's a nice man and I like him very much. Gabe has very few friends. I consider myself one."

The loner agreed. At the time of the show he said, "I'm inhibited and shy. I'm only me when I'm performing. I don't have time to make friends or meet people or do anything. But I enjoy working." To an extent he has remained the loner, and remains unmarried.

"Welcome Back, Kotter," with Kaplan and a classful of comic characters including one played by John Travolta, was a major hit that ran for four years. In 1979 Kaplan was groomed for movie stardom, but although *Fast Break* grossed $30 million he has made only a few films since.

An avid poker player, Kaplan found a new diversion. Aside from simply playing Las Vegas, he played cards there, turning pro and winning the World Series of Poker in 1980. He hosted celebrity poker tournaments as well, many for the aid of cystic fibrosis sufferers. He served as honorary chairman for the Cystic Fibrosis Foundation for three years. Kaplan enjoys less sedentary sports too, especially tennis and basketball.

Kaplan has continued to entertain in clubs. In 1983 he and Groucho Marx's son Arthur put together *Groucho*, a one-man show, similar to previous shows about Mark Twain (Hal Holbrook) and Will Rogers (James Whitmore) but with a difference. In addition to witty Marx monologues *Groucho* included biographical material, and a metamorphosis as Kaplan changed from the brash young Groucho of the movies to the mellow host of "You Bet Your Life" to the wavery-voiced but puckish old man who turned up so often on "The Dick Cavett Show." Kaplan, like others, was adept at mimicking Groucho, but he went beyond that. His transformation into the 80-year-old man was not only accurate but eloquent. In 1983 the show was taped as an HBO special. Kaplan continues to tour with it, perfecting it into a classic.

ALAN KING

He strolls on stage in a vested suit, smoking a cigar, a disdainful curl to his lip, looking like a typical middle-class businessman with an ulcer. And his act is indeed one long kvetch: doctors! the telephone company! the gardener! the airlines!

At times, Alan King sounds like an executive on his psychiatrist's couch. Here he rants about his interior decorator:

"Interior decorators are the greatest fraud ever perpetrated on the American public. We've had seven decorators in four years. No furniture, just decorators! My wife found two boys on Madison Avenue. They're the last of the original Jesse James gang. If you don't watch them they'll take your eyeballs outta your head, put 'em on a piece of driftwood, hang 'em over the fireplace and charge you for it!"

When the comic lashes out, his audience laps it up, laughing, oohing and aahhing each time King, the average man, takes on one of these giant targets of frustration.

To his middle-class audience, King is Lenny Bruce. Never mind dirty words, Religions Inc. or Jackie Kennedy—did you ever try to get your luggage back from an airline?

King rose to fame by touching on what was occupying the minds of suburbanites, and it was for them that he played the resorts and casinos, and for them that he wrote such books as *Anyone Who Owns His Own Home Deserves It*, collections of comic essays that sold nearly a million copies to his affluent fans.

But oddly enough, Alan King was far from affluent when he began in comedy. He grew up in tough ghetto neighborhoods on New York's Lower East Side and in the Williamsburg section of Brooklyn: "I don't honestly think that an absence of money is funny. We went on relief when I was three years old and for nine years my father couldn't get a job in his trade."

He had seven brothers and a sister. As the youngest child, he recalled, "too much was expected of me. I had to go to the same schools my brothers graduated from . . . I wasn't a drop out from Boys High School of Brooklyn, I was a throw out. I majored in truancy and class-cutting."

Expelled from school, he found other diversions. He sang on street corners, and as a drummer he joined "Earl Knight and His Musical Knights" to play weddings and bar mitzvahs. He toured with amateur shows, ending up in Canada, and literally fought his way back home with a brief foray into boxing.

King began his comedy career in the Catskills and in New York's demanding burlesque houses. He developed a cocky style that sometimes got him into trouble: "I was fifteen when I got my first job. It was a tryout on the Decoration Day weekend. I slept in a room that was a deflated closet and I was promised that if I made good it meant the whole summer. Anyway, I stood there on the stage of the Hotel Gradus and cleverly opened with, 'When you work for Gradus, you work for gratis!' So, overnight I was out of work."

Like Lenny Bruce, who appeared on the "Arthur Godfrey Talent Scouts" with an innocuous routine, King turned up on the "Major Bowes Amateur Hour": "I came in second. The guy who won was a bald-headed guy who took his knuckle, banged on the top of his head and accompanied himself doing 'The Bells of St. Mary's.' You can imagine how good I had to be to come in second."

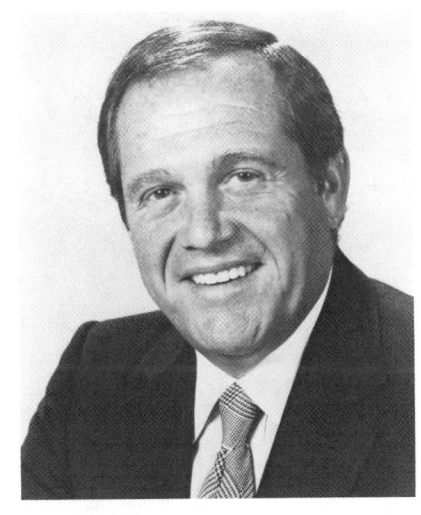

b. Irwin Alan Kniberg, December 26, 1926, New York, New York

Records:
The Best of Alan King (Bronjo BR 109), Alan King in Suburbia (Seeco SAW-2101).

Film:
Just Tell Me What You Want.

Video:
Alan King Stops the Press (Video Yesteryear).

Books:
Anyone Who Owns His Own Home Deserves It, Help I'm a Prisoner in a Chinese Bakery.

Still in his teens, King became a regular at Leon & Eddie's cabaret in Manhattan, at 22 he made it to The Paramount, and in 1956 he was "discovered" when he opened for Judy Garland at the Palace Theater. "I've been on Broadway for 15 years, but they discovered me last night," he said at the time.

King was an iconoclast even then, and he would sometimes run into guys like Lenny Bruce socially. Perhaps it was environment that caused these two men to diverge so dramatically, with Bruce hanging out with a more daring, hungry crowd and King encouraged by the more middle-class audiences he began attracting.

Lenny was encouraged to go beyond all bounds of taste. King trained his acerbic wit on the icons his particular audiences liked to see smashed. By nature prone to the humor of hostility, he just had to find the right targets. His audiences responded to the doctor jokes, telephone company bits and airline routines. Through the 1960's he became a favorite on "The Ed Sullivan Show" as well as in nightclubs.

Over the years, he has remained a cranky comic with a glumly truthful edge to his humor: "I'm 57 now. Everybody tells me I'm 'middle aged.' But I don't know many people who live to be 114. So what's 'middle age'?" And his nostalgia routines are a lot more peppery than Sam Levinson's: "My mother was the worst cook in the world. Everything had to cook for four days. She never believed the butcher killed it! My mother made chicken soup with fat on the top—it used to congeal and you could skate on it."

Irony and cynicism mixed with the humor: King recalled his mother, who fled Russia during the terror-reign of the pogroms: "I never knew I had such a good time as a girl, she said, till I saw 'Fiddler on the Roof.' Who had time for dancing? We were always hiding."

While King is still a favorite among the elders and affluents who people the Vegas and Atlantic City casinos, he has branched out considerably over the past two decades. As a performer, he has appeared on the stage, earning praise for his role as Nathan Detroit in a New York City Center revival of *Guys and Dolls*. In 1980 he got the chance to star in a movie, *Just Tell Me What You Want* with Ali MacGraw. It was hardly his first movie role.

In 1955 he was in *Hit the Deck* and the following year in *The Girl He Left Behind*: "I played soldiers in two movies. I was the guy who is always telling his buddies about all the dames he knows. Then I got a part in *The Helen Morgan Story* and I thought I was on my way. In my fourth picture I was cast as a soldier again and after that I said the hell with it." He has appeared in films sporadically since, in *Bye Bye Braverman* and *The Anderson Tapes*, and has appeared in a few films following his 1980 starring role. "I'm in New York. Anyone makes a picture in New York, they can buy me cheap."

The comedian works more often behind the scenes in the movie world. His production company has been involved with several TV shows and films including *Happy Birthday Gemini* and *Wolfen*. He's produced Broadway shows including *The Lion in Winter*, *The Investigation* and *Dinner at Eight*. In his spare time, King has a lively interest in fine cuisine and in tennis.

Although he has spent years knocking what is wrong with the world, King has also done a lot about it. He's been the recipient of over one hundred philanthropic awards and has donated his time and energy to a long, long list of charities. He founded the Alan King Diagnostic Medical Center in Jerusalem, endowed a scholarship fund for American students at the Hebrew University of Israel, and helped raise money for the Nassau Center for Emotionally Disturbed Children.

"The bottom line is security," says King. "I'm still crazy, that's for damn sure. But when you can look back 50 years and say 'You know something—I made a lot of mistakes but I'm not a bad guy'—that's security. I don't know if I've enjoyed myself, but I've had a lot of fun."

GEORGE KIRBY

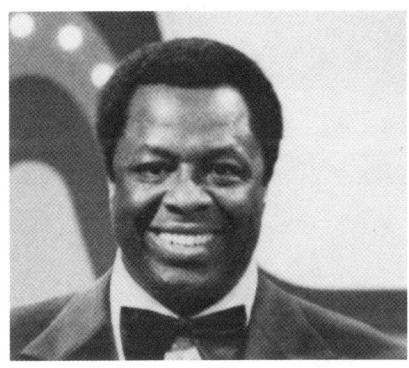

George Kirby began his career as an impressionist early: he would go to a movie and then describe it for his friends, playing every character and even imitating the sound effects. Part of a show business family, he studied some of his subjects firsthand. Louis Armstrong was a frequent guest at the Kirby house, and young George learned to do a perfect copy of Armstrong's singing style.

Working as a bartender at a Chicago club, Kirby persuaded the owner to give him a chance on stage. It led to a year-long engagement. "A mimic is born, not made," says Kirby, "it's a god-given gift, and all the teaching in the world won't do a bit of good if you aren't born with it."

Following service in the Army during World War II, Kirby toured with Sophie Tucker, one of the first stars to give Kirby a break. He added more and more famous names to his catalogue, from Wallace Beery and Sidney Greenstreet to Humphrey Bogart and Walter Brennan. He often did straight impressions, without jokes. Other times, he acted as "straight man" to a star:

"I checked into a very nice Hollywood hotel, and I happened to see an old friend of mine, Peter Lorre. I said hello, Peter, how do you feel? 'I don't feel so good.' Why, what's the matter? 'Well, I've been in this hotel for two weeks and I can't get any sleep. There's a dead bedbug in my bed.' Peter, you mean you can't sleep on account of one dead bedbug? 'It's not the one dead bedbug that bothers me. It's the fifteen hundred that came to his funeral.'"

In 1948 Kirby began a series of guest shots on Ed Sullivan's "Toast of the Town," becoming well known for his songs sung as Nat King Cole, Pearl Bailey and others. He also demonstrated versatility, with the audience never knowing whether his performance would be straight mimicry, joke mimicry, song mimicry or just plain jokes like this one:

"Next door I heard a loving couple in their room. They were carrying on! I heard him say, 'Oh my dear, what gorgeous shoulders you have. When we get back to Manchester, I'm going to have those chiselled in stone.' A few minutes later he said, 'Oh, my darling, what lovely lovely hips you have. When we get back to Manchester I'm gonna have those chiselled in stone.' I couldn't stand it no longer, I got up and knocked on the door. He said, 'Who is it?' I said, 'I'm the chiseller from Manchester!'"

Kirby was one of the first black stand-ups to speak without a dialect or Southern accent, and his elegant style made him at home in fine clubs in America and Europe. But he could also rock audiences at The Apollo and similar venues. And his act was also a balanced mixture of jokes, songs and mimicry. But then the delicate balance was wrecked.

"I tried the hard stuff," Kirby recalls. "I got hold of some powder, thought it was cocaine, and sniffed it. But it was heroin. Oh, it was

b. June 8, 1924, Chicago, Illinois

Records:
Night at the Apollo (Vanguard VRS 9093), Night in Hollywood (Dooto DTL 250), The Real George Kirby (straight songs; Argo 4045).

Compilation:
Best of Party Fun (Dooto DTL 274).

TV:
Half the George Kirby Hour (syndicated 1972), Rosenthal and Jones (CBS 1975).

Film:
Oh Dad, Poor Dad. . . .

terrible. I vomited, throwin' up my guts. But then I got this kind of floating feeling, and I said: 'Well, that's all right. . . .'"

Kirby was eventually arrested in a drug raid, and voluntarily committed himself to a drug rehabilitation clinic. Three years later, he made a comeback, and rose to star status in Vegas casinos and clubs. In 1966 he began getting movie roles, and television audiences saw him regularly in a series of specials, "The Kopycats," part of the "ABC Comedy Hour," starring a half-dozen mimics including Rich Little, a star Kirby had counseled years earlier.

Kirby had his own TV show in 1972, a syndicated series from Toronto featuring a new young comic named Steve Martin. A few years later he and Ned Glass co-starred in a short-lived situation comedy for CBS, "Rosenthal and Jones."

In the late 70's, Kirby's star began to wane. He could do a perfect imitation of Bill Cosby, but couldn't get the same kind of bookings. He wasn't working the Vegas casinos, and believed the reason was a "Catch-22" situation: he wasn't strong enough to attract crowds as the headliner, but he was too strong and threatening to be an opening act.

"I found myself about to lose my home," Kirby recalls. "I got involved in a deal which I had no business doing. A friend got me into it. It was an opportunity to get some money to catch up on my bills." In 1978 Kirby was sentenced to 10 years in prison for trafficking in cocaine and heroin. "I'm embarrassed and ashamed," he told the judge. The judge regretted having to pass sentence, saying, "I have appreciated and enjoyed very much the great talent Mr. Kirby has. It could be he has more intelligence and talent than anyone else in this courtroom."

Prison life was harsh. A chance to produce a radio show from prison was turned down. The 50-year-old comic was sent to a vicious federal prison where there were riots that could easily have ended his life. But as Kirby told interviewer Tony Brown, the experience brought him closer to God:

"It's a good lesson. As a matter of fact, there are a lot of people I know out here in the street should go in for a year so they'll appreciate the little things out here . . . you don't miss the big cars, the lavish house, the material things I was trying to hold onto . . . what I missed was opening a door because I wanted to open it, close it if I wanted to, eat what I want to eat when I want to eat, sit up and see the sunrise. . . ."

Once a prison guard heard him laughing and worried that Kirby had gone stir-crazy. "It's just a joke between me and the Lord," Kirby explained. "When I first started in show business, I was a porter. I had a mop and a bucket. And here I am—with a mop and a bucket again." He felt that he had strayed from his commitments to perform for churches and benefits, strayed from spiritual goals, and that it was only natural the Lord "knocked him to his knees."

Paroled after five years, Kirby found not only his wife waiting, but also his fans and many media supporters. He told his story to sympathetic reporters, and found work in clubs like Dangerfield's in New York. He brought with him a poem he had written decades earlier while in the rehab center: "King Heroin." He uses it as a closer for club dates and charity and school appearances.

"Behold, I'm King Heroin," Kirby intones. "I capture men's will and destroy their minds, and cause them to commit all sorts of crimes. . . . I can make a mere schoolboy forget his books, make a world famous beauty neglect her looks. I can make a husband forsake his family and wife and send a greedy man to prison for the rest of his life. . . ."

He describes every phase of heroin's blight, including withdrawal ("Now they must suffer. You see that's part of my game. They lay with discomfort and they squirm with the pain") and the temptation for more ("Oh they curse my name and defy me in speech . . . but they'd pick me up again if I were in reach"). It ends with a chilling challenge: "Are you my next victim . . . sucker?"

Kirby's face is contorted at the end of his long poem. It relaxes again only when Kirby recalls the sweetness of being out of jail and off the drug: "I tell the audience, you've seen many a performer come out on stage and say 'Ladies and Gentlemen, it is indeed a pleasure to be out here on stage.' You don't know if they're lyin' or not. But with me . . . you know I'm not lyin'."

ROBERT KLEIN

Robert Klein was caught in the middle. He grew up watching standard comics on "The Ed Sullivan Show," but when it was time for him to come out on stage, guys like Woody Allen and Mort Sahl had changed some of the rules. The result is an unusual hybrid, a hip comic square enough to appeal to middle of the roaders. Klein even had a routine illustrating the problems, a satire on people who can't even say hello because they don't know what kind of handshake to use, straight or freaky.

Klein shows the influence of old-timer Alan King, the way he takes to the stage with a pained expression, and with a middle-class stance attacks the things that irk him. "I'm not a teacher, preacher or prophet," Klein admits. "I look for laughs in things we accept without question." So, like King, he singles out irritating things like TV commercials ("Why is it that Robert Young has so many cranky friends? . . . Do you buy Carvel because you think Mr. Carvel is pathetic?") and brand names ("Hawaiian Punch is 10% fruit juice. What's the other 90%? You're better off with paint thinner"), annoying oddities ("I saw on the menu in Logan Airport, Boston, 'Potato Salad—in season'") and news quirks ("Why is it that flying saucers, without exception, land and expose themselves to total morons? Why don't they ever land in Carl Sagan's back yard?"). There are endless things about modern living that annoy Klein.

But, like more modern comics, Klein can flexibly shift to more personal humor, comedy with a hostile edge, describing what it was like to grow up as a "Child of the 50's" and deal with things like air-raid drills and strict teachers: "No talking," a teacher says through tight lips. "Take these tags home. They're to be used in the event you're burned beyond recognition in a nuclear holocaust! And *no talking* during a nuclear holocaust. I shall be taking names!"

He recalled odd things he learned in school: "Garfield was assassinated. Shot by a disappointed office seeker, right? Don't they always say that same sentence? It's crazy. Every time you read his name: James Abram Garfield: 'Shot by a disappointed office seeker.' That's all they can think of what he did in his short office. You look in the Encyclopedia Britannica under Garfield, James Abram. It says, 'See Office seeker, disappointed.'"

His best routines take the hard-gag approach of the old, and blend it with the improvisation and vocal dexterity of the new, as in his classic about panhandlers who seem to be part of a franchise, all dressed the same, crying out "Pleeeeeze," in the same heart-rending way.

Klein's first career goals were in theater, although after graduating from DeWitt Clinton High School, he enrolled as a pre-med student at Alfred University. From there he went to Yale Drama School and worked

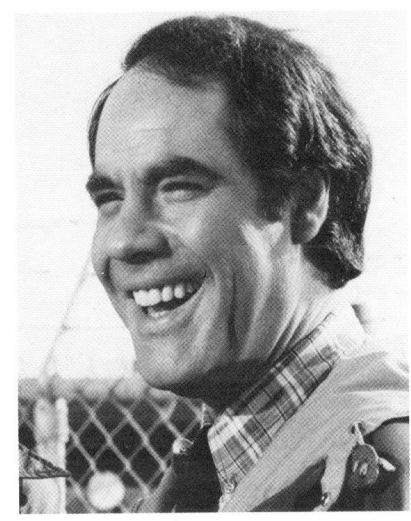

b. February 8, 1942, Bronx, New York

Records:
Child of the 50's (Brut 6001), Mind Over Matter (Brut 6600), New Teeth (Epic PE-33535), Howard Who? (Caedmon TC 9100), I Were a High School Graduate (Epic FLM 3312).

TV:
Comedy Tonight (CBS 1970), TV's Bloopers and Practical Jokes (NBC 1984).

Video:
Nobody's Perfekt (Columbia), Saturday Night Live 1979 (Warner), Child of the 50's, Man of the 80's (Thorn-Emi).

in summer stock, playing such diverse roles as Freddy in *Pygmalion*, Poobah in *The Mikado* and Benvolio in *Romeo and Juliet.* He appeared in industrial films like "How to Sell Shock Absorbers" and in 1963 was seen off-Broadway in *Six Characters in Search of an Author.* He supplemented his $5 a week salary by teaching.

On a questionnaire he completed for a prospective press representative, he mentioned (under "additional useful information"), "Before entering show biz full time I was a school teacher. Several times, former students have recognized me, in a theatrical capacity, as their former teacher. While taking my bows at a matinee of 'The Apple Tree' a girl in the first row screamed and pointed for all the world, I had him in history!"

It was while appearing in Broadway's *The Apple Tree,* following a stint at Chicago's Second City, that Klein began to build comedy routines and work on them at local improv clubs. "I was cocky," he recalls, "but of course you have to be. To get up in front of people? It's excruciating."

By 1967 Klein was working top clubs like Mr. Kelly's, but also encountering frustration. He was booked for "The Dean Martin Show," his big TV break, but the show's producer decided he wasn't funny: "That crushed me. They had to pay me, yes, but that wasn't the important thing. . . . I had told my family and friends about it and it was very embarrassing. Six months later, on January 19, 1968, I got my first TV spot on the Carson show."

He did the same routine he'd auditioned live for Dean Martin's producer—and it went off without a hitch. Klein would add another 50 "Tonight Show" appearances to his credits, reaching "headliner" status in clubs by 1970, the year he starred in "Comedy Tonight" for CBS. He'd come a long way from the days when he was with "The Teen Tones," auditioning for the "Ted Mack Amateur Hour."

Earning $200,000 a year, Klein won Grammy nominations in 1973 and 1974 for his first two albums, and his struggle to make it in show business was covered in *The Last Laugh,* an in-depth profile of a typical new young comic. By decade's end he earned a Tony nomination for his return to Broadway in *They're Playing Our Song.*

Despite his versatility as an actor, radio show performer and "personality" (his "Streets of New York" segments for "TV's Bloopers and Practical Jokes"), Klein continues to find the time for stand-up and cable TV comedy specials, which now concern new wrinkles like fatherhood, mellowing and aging. "What makes people laugh? It's not universal. The Marx Brothers? Laurel and Hardy? Slip on a banana peel? I have a good deal in common with the biggest clowns like Milton Berle. We started as one. We're comedians. Me, I have reached a plateau in my work where I fall into rhythms I developed long ago. I can make strangers laugh on my own terms. Which means I am universal enough, I am communicating enough. It's a very high calling, you know, making people laugh."

EDDIE LAWRENCE

In comedy he will be forever loved as "The Old Philosopher," but Eddie Lawrence is a Renaissance man who has had great success also as an actor, author and painter. In fact, over the past decade his main interest has been painting:

"As far back as I can remember, I was always a painter and a comedian. I always painted. When you're an actor, you have time to do other things. Some actors are in business—dry cleaning chains, photography developing—I'd rather spend my time in other ways. I always had a studio."

Lawrence was a stand-up comedy veteran by the time he put on shows for the troops in World War II, earning a bronze star in addition to the applause of his fellow soldiers. He wrote sketches for such touring performers as Leo Durocher and Humphrey Bogart, and supported them on stage.

He met actor John Marley during the war, and they teamed for many shows. After the war, they starred in their own radio show. "We did a lot of stuff similar to Monty Python," Eddie recalls. "We were always bucking the establishment with our comedy and with our attitudes." The boat-rocking team even fought with their director over matters of artistic freedom, and eventually found themselves out of work. But their unusual skits were so impressive that 25 years later, reviewing Bob and Ray, Jack Kroll of *Newsweek* mused about that "mysterious pair of now-forgotten geniuses."

Marley went on to become a popular character actor. Lawrence continued to pile up versatile credits, using his comic voice to narrate the Blondie movies, starring in 25 shorts for Paramount which he also wrote, and finally starring in radio's "The Eddie Lawrence Show." But always there was his other love, painting. Despite his agent's pleas, Eddie left show business at the turn of the 50's and went to Paris.

Many stars are known as painters—largely thanks to their publicists. In Lawrence's case, he is a genuine artist of enormous talent. In France he studied under Fernand Léger, and using his real name, Lawrence Eisler, has won critical praise for his one-man shows in America and Europe. While in Paris he also wrote and starred in a few films.

"When I came back I worked on the Kay Kyser Show, then I both wrote and acted on the Victor Borge Show. After that I was booked to do another show at a tremendous salary, but I had the beginnings of an ulcer, so I went back to Paris and painted. A few years later some jobs in America came up and I decided to go back."

Lawrence was called to Broadway, where he appeared to rave reviews in *Bells Are Ringing*. As a stand-up, Max Gordon booked him into the Village Vanguard where he amazed audiences with his bizarre comedy ideas and with his classic character, the Old Philosopher.

The character was a descendant of "Sentimental Max, a character I did when I was in the Army. People laughed at the voice," which was sorrowful, blubbering and comically woeful, wavering through a sorry report of sad-sack troubles. "When you go to parties, and get a little drunk, you start ad-libbing. And out came the Old Philosopher. These things are not planned. How can you plan a character like that?

"Times weren't very good," Lawrence adds. "I met this guy on Broadway once, an actor, and he told me so many terrible things—his voice was cut out of a cartoon short, and the next day he bit his tongue—all these things on top of each other—we both started to laugh."

The Old Philosopher is pure characterization, a sappy and sympathetic voice that intones outrageous, irritating problems and then dismisses them with a sudden hysterical burst of positive-thinking blather.

"Hey there, bunkie," he might begin, "You say you had your nose fixed, and it's bigger now? A friend calls to tell you he's got you a swinging blind date, and it turns out to be your wife? And your shoelace just busted? And your mother got arrested on a raid on a dry goods store with a bookie in the back? And your automobile horn just got stuck in a

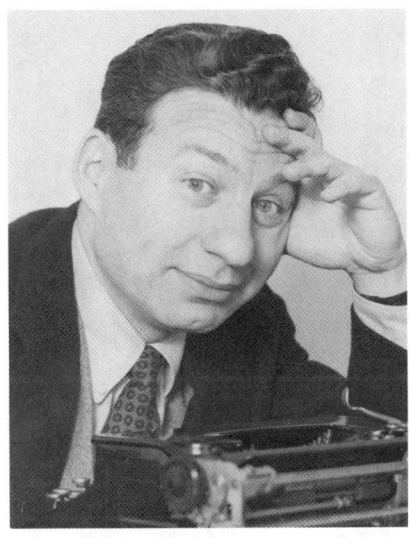

b. Lawrence Eisler, March 2, 1921, Brooklyn, New York

Records:
The Old Philosopher (Coral CRL 57103), Eddie Lawrence (Coral 57155), Side Splitting Personality of Eddie Lawrence (Coral CRL 757371), 7 Characters in Search of Eddie Lawrence (Coral CRL 57411), The Garden of Eddie Lawrence (Signature SM 1003), Is That What's Bothering You, Bunkie? (Epic LN 24159).

Plays (as actor):
Bells Are Ringing, Threepenny Opera.

Plays (as author):
Kelly, Animals, The Beautiful Mariposa, Adventure of Eddie Greshaw, Louie and the Elephant.

Films (as actor):
The Night They Raided Minsky's, Act of Love, Somebody Killed Her Husband.

Film (as author):
The Ladies and the Men.

hospital zone? And your sweatsocks are disappearing into your shoes? Is that what's troublin' you, cousin?"

Eddie shifts into hysterical high gear: "Well, lift your head up high! Take a walk in the sun with that platitude and fortitude and show the world, show the world where to get off! Never give up! Never give up! Never give up—that ship!"

The odd little philosopher with his hapless luck and mindless pluck had some kind of existential appeal for all those who heard it. Lawrence, a Brooklyn College graduate, even amazed educators and psychiatrists: "One night on a talk show I heard a group of psychiatrists talking. They said the old philosopher is right—a little thing can send you right over the line."

As a stand-up comic, Lawrence had many bits as bizarre as his many Old Philosopher routines. He was an impressionist with a twist: "On stage I did Ronald Colman held up in a dark alley . . . I did songs with comedy lyrics, a bit about a Hollywood writer trying to sell a script to a producer who couldn't read . . . and 'People to Stay Away From'—anybody with a raincover on his hat is dangerous. Psychiatrists who come to the door naked—that's trouble."

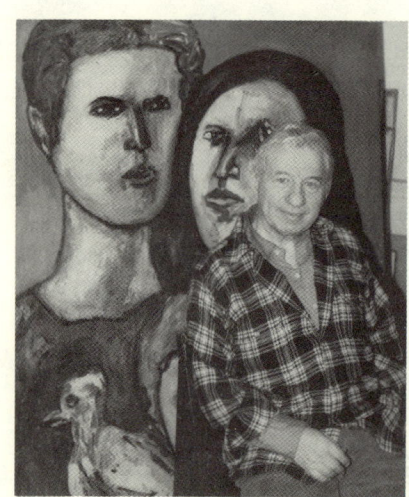

"I used to love the audience at the 2am show," he recalls. "They were a little dazed, high, and I used to do my good stuff then. But I'm not a nightclub person. It's a difficult life. I got tired of that. I had a lot of fun in those days, but when you get a little older you don't want to kill yourself out there on stage."

Lawrence's "The Old Philosopher," released in 1956, was one of the first of a pioneering group of comedy singles. "Getting comedy to stick on wax is one of the toughest jobs in the disk biz," wrote *Variety* that year. "Eddie Lawrence, however, seems to have found the formula." The record cost $200 to make, and sold 150,000 copies.

The seven lp's Lawrence made are among the most valuable collector's items in the comedy catalogue. Some 20 years before Firesign Theater, Lawrence was bringing people close to their stereo speakers to hear the sound effects, throwaway lines and unusual flights of fantasy in bits about celebrity chicken-plucking contests and Viennese travel.

Lawrence's technique, learned from the days when he wrote for Victor Borge, is to write the script, then polish it and watch it grow through rehearsal. Of a routine like "Old Old Vienna" he says, "I wrote, rewrote, wrote and rewrote. I believe what George S. Kaufman said about working a damn long time on a line. Sometimes one word makes the difference and gets a bigger laugh."

Lawrence wrote a Broadway musical with Moose Charlap (the man who also did *Peter Pan*). *Kelly* had the unfortunate fate of being a great success on the road but a flop when it opened. On its way to Broadway it was tampered with, and the comedy was largely removed by humorless prevailing powers. A song from the score, "Never Go There Anymore," has become a pop vocalist standard. He's written many more works for the stage, notably *The Beautiful Mariposa*, which Tyrone Guthrie called "a fascinating and powerful play."

These days Eddie can usually be found at his studio in New York's Union Square, painting. He also continues to write, and has recently released a book of audition monologues for actors (with an introduction by Jason Robards). But with over 30 "Mike Douglas Shows" and 40 "Tonight Shows" to his credit, Eddie is still willing to take time off now and then to meet the demand for the Old Philosopher.

"I've done a lot of benefits recently. The other day I rewrote ten pages of a play, and today I'm framing paintings for a one-man show.

People say, 'You gotta make up your mind, do one thing.'" Why? Married to an actual descendant of Captain Bligh, a father, and a painter, writer, actor, comedian, Eddie Lawrence is living proof of his own philosophy: "Do what you feel like doing!"

TOM LEHRER

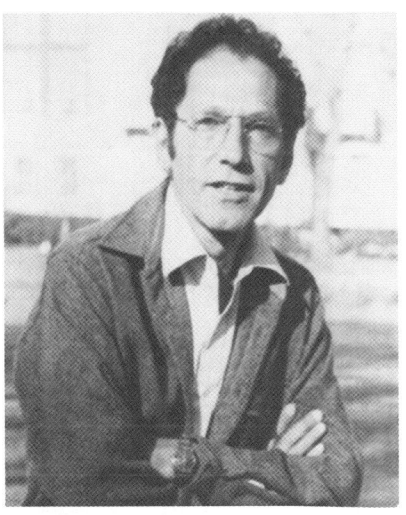

b. April 9, 1928, New York, New York

Records:
Songs by Tom Lehrer (Lehrer TL 101, Reprise RS 6216), More of Tom Lehrer (Lehrer TL 102), An Evening Wasted with Tom Lehrer (Lehrer TL 202, Reprise RS 6199), Tom Lehrer Revisited (Lehrer TL 201), That Was the Year That Was (Reprise RS 6179), Tomfoolery (released in England, MMT LP 001).

Single:
Poisoning Pigeons in the Park/ Masochism Tango (with orchestra) (Capricorn C-451).

Book:
Too Many Songs (the *Tomfoolery* material).

The first authentic, admittedly "sick" comic, Tom Lehrer, and his unabashed sophomoric and gleefully shocking songs about pigeon poisoning, perverted boy scouts and sado-masochistic lovers, rocked the collegians at Harvard and his fame soon spread across the nation. These amateur exercises made a reluctant comedy star out of a proper but prankish professor.

Lehrer graduated from Harvard at age 18 and early in the 1950's turned up as a mathematics teacher there. He enjoyed the diversion of writing comic parodies like "Don't Major in Physics," "The Slide Rule Song" and "Fight Fiercely, Harvard." The latter was a wry satire of the university's prissy image, with such inspiring battle chants as: "Impress them with our prowess, do! Oh, fellows, do not let the crimson down, be of stout heart and true." The professor was the life of the party when he sat down at the piano and sang "The Elements" (from antimony and arsenic to holium and helium, thorium, thulium and thallium) to the tune of Arthur Sullivan's "Modern Major General."

In 1953 he pressed 400 copies of a 10-inch album called "The Songs of Tom Lehrer," expecting to break even at best, and have some college souvenirs at worst. "Fight Fiercely, Harvard" was included, along with more biting undergraduate humor loaded with shock-for-shock's-sake grossness.

"My Home Town" splashed acid at the sentimental portrait of colorful villagers, with sketches of perverts, crooks and the druggist Dan: "He was swell. He killed his mother-in-law and ground her up real well. And sprinkled just a bit over each banana split."

"Be Prepared" gleefully misdirected boy scouts: "Don't solicit for your sister, that's not nice. Unless you get a good percentage of her price."

"I Hold Your Hand in Mine" took the concept literally. Lehrer the lover tenderly sings, "I hold your hand in mine, dear, I press it to my lips. I take a healthy bite from your dainty finger tips."

The disc became a campus phenomenon, reflecting the hip tastes of the college crowd that would shortly be raising comics like Mort Sahl and Lenny Bruce to national prominence. A second album was quickly pressed and received even greater acceptance. Lehrer's spirited nasal tenor relished each line's new atrocity, his enthusiastic piano playing underscored favorite lines.

Lehrer was rarely subtle, which probably accounted for his early negative reviews from critics accustomed to Cole Porter. But college audiences loved his ax-blade cynicism and his grinning-skull satire. In a song about pollution: "Wear a gas mask and a veil, then you can breathe long as you don't inhale." In a cheery, pre-Strangelove song about the bomb, "We Will All Go Together," "We will all fry together when we fry, we'll be french fried potatoes bye and bye. There will be no more misery when the world is our rotisserie, yes we'll all fry together when we fry." And in an anthem to graduates, "Bright College Days," he stopped the show by telling the students to look forward: "soon we'll be sliding down the razor blade of life."

He seized on the most highly prized taboos of his time (most are still with us) and smashed them with contagious zeal. Was it satire, or just bad boy iconoclasm? Whatever the motivation, Lehrer made the most of anti-Christmas carols, songs about incest and parodies of true love.

As the demand for his albums reached the 10,000 mark, the surprised scholar was called upon for concert appearances. He took a short leave of absence from his research to appear at the Blue Angel in New York. "I'm completely happy at my research job [at Boston's Baird Associates]," he told the *New York Times*. "I'd almost hate to be a success in comedy." But the very fact that the *Times* was covering his debut suggested that his success was assured.

Lehrer was evidently so amazed by the audience's response that his next two albums were merely his first two, rerecorded in front of an enthusiastic crowd. The only difference was the addition of Lehrer's shyly enunciated and carefully rehearsed throwaway jokes and introductions.

The *New Statesman* said Lehrer was "on his way to becoming a Noel Coward of the 50's . . . in his inimitable and ghastly way . . . he has a kind of genius." But the majority of critics held an opposite view. Lehrer delighted in putting these bad notices on his next album jacket: "Vulgarity," *Pittsburgh Sun-Telegraph*, "More desperate than amusing," *New York Herald-Tribune*, "Obvious, jejune, and remarkably unsophisticated," *London Evening Standard*.

Lehrer's first real brush with controversy came during his 1960 Australian tour. He had trouble with censors in Adelaide who banned such numbers as the boy scout parody, "Be Prepared."

"I thought that democracy here was ruled by the majority," he said. "Nothing like this has ever happened to me before. I have sung these songs before many well known Americans and also before members of the British family."

In 1967 the part-time performer once again ran into trouble. He sang "The Vatican Rag" on an educational TV channel's fundraiser special in New York. Critics were aghast and the song was banned in a New York Public School until the Board of Education overturned the ruling.

The song took the timely subject of the church's revision of hymns from Latin into English a step further. "To really sell the product," Lehrer suggested these hymns be updated to such popular forms of music as ragtime jigs. To a fast, uproarious ragtime tune, Lehrer imagined his flock following his instructions: "Get down upon your knees, fiddle with your rosaries, bow your head with great respect and . . . genuflect! Genuflect! Genuflect!"

Using his favorite technique of the wacky near-rhyme, he continued, "Do whatever steps you want if you have cleared them with the Pontiff. Everybody say his own Kyrie Eleison, doin' the Vatican Rag."

This bold, nose-thumbing parody may not have had the same intent as the sort of morally outraged religious satire of Lenny Bruce, but its friskiness raised the subject of . . . "bad taste." Lehrer answered nonchalantly, "Certainly [the lyrics] are. They're in very bad taste. Now someone should come along and write a pro-Catholic song." But he insisted, "the song only makes fun of the rituals, not the beliefs."

Lehrer, more than a decade earlier, had seemed to ask Lenny Bruce's question, "what's wrong with appealing to prurient interest?" When his audience cracked up over one of his shocking lines, he'd smile and say, "You people are sick, you know." In fact, he'd even written an anthem about his favorite cause, "Smut." But he wasn't about to take too many risks to preserve the first amendment. One reason was that he was obviously being offensive for the fun of it, throwing mud pies, not bombs. For another, he was a professor first, a performer second.

A star who never even put a photograph of himself on an album cover, Lehrer said, "I've always been indifferent to the actual work [on stage]. I'm not a performer by instinct, I'm a writer, and I just like to play the songs once to see if people will laugh. The main reason I always played was to put some money aside so I could do what I like—teach and continue writing and lie down a lot and just enjoy myself."

The life-long bachelor taught at M.I.T. through the 1960's and then moved out to the University of California in 1971. Aside from contributing songs to "That Was the Week That Was" and later making the 1965 album "That Was the Year That Was," Lehrer performed sporadically, and then abandoned performing altogether. The shows were "just a chore. The fact that I could earn a year's teaching salary in a week as a performer wasn't very important to me. I happen to enjoy a low standard of life. . . . I hate show business. I don't have much in common with the people. There's no real satisfaction in it."

In later years, Lehrer found little satisfaction in writing comedy. He found little that was funny in the world: "I used to pick up the newspaper and laugh. I'd say, isn't that ridiculous or silly. Now I pick up the paper and I have to wait till breakfast is over because it's just going to ruin it. . . . I don't know why I've become more serious. I wish I could tell you."

In 1980, 27 of his songs were put together for the *Tomfoolery* revue. The comedian, who over the past decade had written only a pair of tunes, and those for the PBS children's series "The Electric Company," was not part of the cast. The show received good notices, but in interviews, Lehrer insisted that he was not going to write more comedy, that today's complex issues and morality had blurred his satiric edge: "There were a whole group of people who agreed on everything, like 'lynching is bad.' Issues that have come along since are a lot more complicated. So I just am not sure about where I stand about some things anymore. Life was simpler then."

But Lehrer's songs remain and, in complex times, retain their bite. Whether for a grisly chuckle or a cynical smirk, they are still powerful. As Lehrer has often said, "If after hearing my songs just one human being is inspired to say something nasty to a friend, or perhaps a loved one, it will all have been worthwhile."

JACK E. LEONARD

Would nightclub patrons pay good money to be insulted? Instead of jokes directed at mothers-in-law, politicians or plumbers, would they allow a comic to whip his quips at *them*? It was an outrage! But Jack E. Leonard was outrageous. And he was the first comic to make a career playing with his audience instead of indulging in self-abuse.

At first Leonard was a standard comic who made the world and himself the targets. "I was on the bill ahead of Tony Martin," he recalled, "and all the ladies were too busy looking at each other's clothes to pay attention to me. Until I told them, 'When you cross the George Washington to go home, I hope the bridge falls.'"

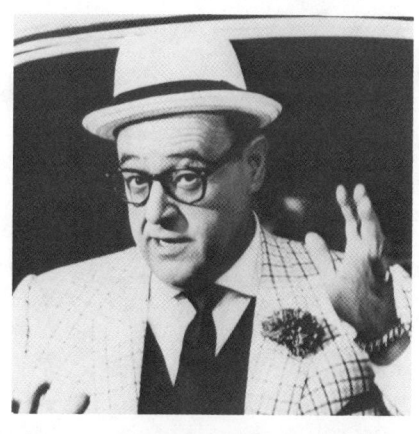

b. Leonard Lebitsky, April 24, 1911, Chicago, Illinois; d. May 11, 1973

Records:
Jack E. Leonard's How to Lose Weight (RCA Victor LPM 2892), Rock and Roll for Kids over 16 (RCA Victor LX 1080), Scream on Someone You Love Today (Verve V6-15056).

Films:
Three Sailors and a Girl, The World of Abbott & Costello, The Fat Spy.

Video:
The Arthur Godfrey Show (Video Yesteryear).

From there, Leonard crossed over from brief heckler squelches to a full-time barrage. Leonard not only found that his muttering, mumbling, sneering style of delivery was well suited to these venomous asides to ringsiders; lacking really good comedy material, he sometimes had to come up with these insults in self-defense.

By 1943, Leonard was making $1,000 a week for his daring, outrageous nightclub act. In the 1960's, he was earning $250,000 a year. For that kind of money, his targets had to be big. He told the Duke of Windsor, "You've been in this country so long, you should have your second papers by now." To Perry Como: "You have a very fine voice. Too bad it's in Bing Crosby's throat." A regular on "The Ed Sullivan Show," he stung the stone-faced host with: "Don't worry, Ed, someday you'll find yourself—and you'll be terribly disappointed. . . . There's nothing wrong with you that reincarnation won't cure."

Leonard could tell a one-liner ("Remember the words of Norman Vincent Peale who said, 'A family that plays together will certainly be talked about' "), but after a while would revert back to the insults. In fact, often he couldn't wait. He'd set them up. To Jackie Gleason, he offered a pleasant, "Where are ya livin', Jackie." Gleason, sensing something, cautiously answered, "Mt. Kisco." "You look like you swallowed it!"

Of course, obesity was one of his own problems. He joked about it: "You look like a nice bunch of people," he'd tell the audience, "and I'm a nice bunch of people, so maybe we'll have a good time." Once, squeezing himself into a taxicab, he told the driver, "Take me to a larger cab." In 1955 he managed to reduce from 350 pounds to 200.

Leonard had a philosophy about success with insult humor: "An insult is only funny if it's really ridiculous, and if it's aimed at some really big shot. You can't kid a woman like you can a man. With a woman you have to wait until everybody starts hating her. Then you can get her: 'the next time you go on a Halloween tour I hope your broom breaks.'"

Leonard's japes were often genuine insults with little humor or wit evident when set down in cold type on a page. But in the proper psychological setting, a nightclub, and given the comic's backhanded delivery, they worked. They deflated the pompous, shocked the shy and brought out the wicked little kid in anyone who wanted to point at someone and offer a surprisingly honest observation.

"You can't work all the best places with the insult act," Leonard admitted. "They're afraid to book me 'cause they don't know what I'm gonna come up with." But in one club, the joke was on him:

"I devastated myself in Miami one night with a one-liner I'd been using for ten years. I was working a nightclub and I said, 'There's my boss sitting out there with his wife—and his girl friend.' The gag got a remarkable reaction. I got fired." His boss *was* sitting out there—with his wife and his girl friend.

The tough insult comic who grew up in a tough Chicago area ("When my father got a $5 raise we moved to California Avenue, a better neighborhood about a mile away . . . there I met a boy who became famous later as Baby-Face Nelson. That was the better neighborhood we moved into"), Leonard rarely veered away from the nightclub scene.

His few movies were failures, although as a character the big, dome-headed, egg-shaped Leonard had promise. His gruff mumble was a favorite of impressionists, and to show how lovable the grousing bald bird could be, a Leonard-inspired bald eagle turned up in a Beany & Cecil cartoon. There were several other impressionist tributes like that.

Obviously lovable to someone, Leonard was married for 22 years to Katherine (Kay) Dillon. She died in 1967. In 1970 he remarried. Leonard was still active, though eclipsed by the younger, brinier Don Rickles, when in April of 1973 he underwent open-heart surgery. He died a few weeks later.

SAM LEVENSON

Sam Levenson was a naturally funny man, a raconteur and a storyteller, the kind who is always told, "Gee, you're funny enough to go on stage." He fulfilled the dream of every such amateur storyteller: he went on stage, and then on television, and on to become a beloved star.

One of eight children, Levenson grew up in a tenement nourished by love more than money. He worked in his father's tailor shop but found time to earn a B.A. in Spanish from Brooklyn College. In 1934 he became a Spanish teacher, spending eight years at Brooklyn's Samuel J. Tilden High School. Along the way, he tried to make learning an exciting experience, giving digressive "lessons in life" with the schoolwork.

He began performing at informal school functions. He was often a master of ceremonies, livening things up in the auditorium with anecdotal humor. He spent a few summers in the Catskills, earning money as a musician in an all-teacher orchestra. He also performed comedy, and discovered that light, warmly human stories about personal experience worked better than gags.

He gradually found himself in demand for school affairs, fundraisers and other events. He began to arrange local bookings, and in 1946 took a sabbatical to pursue comedy full time. In 1949 he got a major break: an appearance on Ed Sullivan's TV show "The Toast of the Town."

The humorist's style of gentle jests and recollections of family wit and wisdom made its mark almost instantly. In an era where slow-paced Jack Benny and unassuming George Gobel were among the top comics, Levenson fit right in. In 1950 he was the lead-in for Jack Benny, doing a 15-minute show. In 1951 he had his own series, and in 1955 hosted another series, "Two for the Money."

From a $20 a night lecturer, Levenson advanced to earning $2,000 a night. From a $3,000 annual teacher's salary he skyrocketed to $150,000. Typical of his one-to-one style of informal, conversational monology is this opening from a "Two for the Money" broadcast:

"Good evening. It's nice to see you here. Somebody wrote me a letter the other day and asked me how my mother managed to feed eight kids on my father's income.... It was very easy. It is still being done around America in some places. My mother used to buy one pound of meat and make three pounds of hamburgers. You know how? We had a slogan in our house. It said 'old rolls never die.' Everything went into a hamburger. After a while, my mother learned to make chopped meat completely without meat and I liked it that way. Of course, there is a matter of living costs that comes in today. Isn't that right? In the old days, if you bought an order at the butcher's he threw in the liver for the cat. You remember? I will tell you the truth. We didn't always have a cat but we always had liver ... you are looking at the family cat...."

Levenson could put over quickies, too: "You know what my mother's attitude was toward raising children? She used to say to my father, 'Go outside and see what Sammy's doing and tell him to stop.'"

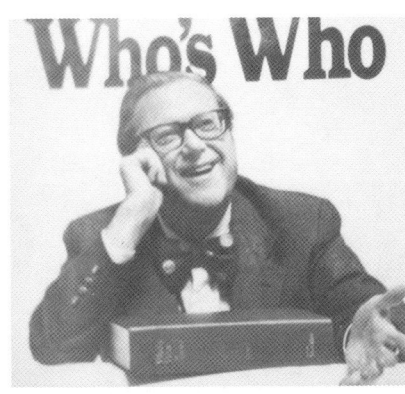

b. December 28, 1911, New York, New York; d. August 27, 1980

Record:
But Seriously Folks (Signature 1026).

TV:
The Sam Levenson Show (CBS 1951–52), This Is Show Business (CBS 1951–54), Two for the Money (CBS 1955–57).

Books:
Meet the Folks, In One Era and Out the Other, Sex and the Only Child, You Can Say That Again, Sam, You Don't Have to Be in Who's Who to Know What's What.

The humorist appeared on game shows and talk shows like "Arthur Godfrey Time," where he became known as a raconteur who mixed humor with social observation. He was especially prone to giving advice on raising children and teaching them. "In Russia," he said, "they teach a child what he'll die for. I would really love to teach a kid what he's got to live for."

Back in 1946 Levenson wrote his first book, *Meet the Folks,* a small volume of Jewish lore, humor and standard jokes, like the one about the husband who mutters about his wife, "There's no end to it—all the time she keeps nagging me for money, money, money and more money." "And what does she do with all the money?" "Who knows. I never give it to her."

In the 60's Levenson began to turn out more books, but these were based on the index cards and notes he'd used for his lectures, not well-known jokes from others. The world according to Levenson, the books were all solid sellers, right up to 1979's *You Don't Have to Be in Who's Who to Know What's What.* In that one, Levenson covered both familiar topics, such as kids ("Between the ages of 12 and 17 a parent can age thirty years") and new subjects such as women's liberation ("You've got to look like a lady, act like a man and work like a dog").

JOE E. LEWIS

Joe E. Lewis was making $650 a week in a Chicago nightclub called The Green Mill. When a rival club offered $1,000, Lewis accepted the offer. What happened next was one of the goriest incidents in the history of show business.

The owner of The Green Mill put out a contract on Lewis. Machine Gun Jack McGurn vowed to extinguish the young comic's rising star. The fearsome killer, who had already ended the lives of many with his Thompson submachine gun, approached Lewis with a warning.

"I start at the Rendezvous November 2nd," Lewis told him.

"You'll never live to open," McGurn replied.

The gutsy comedian ignored the threat and began his stint at the rival club. But a week later, McGurn's henchmen attacked. It happened suddenly, in mid-morning. Lewis had been warned by a bodyguard not to open his door to anyone, but out of habit, he did.

"Just one favor, Joe," said one of the three men who burst in on him, "don't yell." In his book *The Joker Is Wild,* Art Cohn describes what Lewis recalled of the incident:

"An horrendous blow struck him from behind. He turned as he fell and saw the man with the .38 raising his arm to clout him again. The third assailant was unsheathing a hunting knife. Pain coiled around his brain, tighter, tighter, and sank its fangs deeper and deeper. A searing, blinding flash, and he felt his head being torn apart. The two gunmen used the butts of their revolvers. They hammered his skull until he was unconscious, and they continued pounding. The knifeman went to work. He punched the blade into Joe's left jaw as far as he could, ripped his face open from ear to throat, and went on cleaving impassively, like a butcher. Joe did not yell."

Half-paralyzed, his face lathered in blood, Lewis made a long, agonizing crawl to the nightstand. But the nightmare wasn't over. His torn tongue and broken jaw could not form words. He slumped the telephone back. His vocal cords were severed. He crawled to the door, the

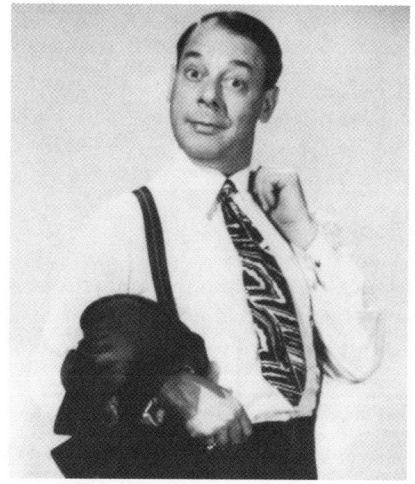

b. Joe Klewan, January 12, 1902, New York, New York; d. June 8, 1971

Record:
It Is Now Post Time (Reprise R/RS 5001).

Video:
TV Variety (Shokus Video).

Bio:
The Joker Is Wild.

carpet sopped with blood, the doorknob so slippery with red that it wouldn't turn. He crawled down the hallway to the elevator, and to help.

It had taken more than a half-hour of torture to get help. And after, it took months of recuperation. Dozens and dozens of stitches sewed his mouth into a permanent grin. Bits of skull were removed from his brain. And it took seemingly forever before he found himself able to speak and to relearn the alphabet that was literally smashed from his memory.

But Lewis was tough. He was a tough kid from the Lower East Side of New York, determined to make something of himself. Early on, he knew he wanted to be in show business.

"I was going to DeWitt Clinton High School and rehearsing for a burlesque show at the Strand Theater," he recalled. "I was a real third wheel. I was the comic, singer and straight man in this cheap burlesque. I loved to be with the old hags. Then my mother found out and took me out of burlesque. I was so damn mad I went down to 14th Street and joined the marines."

After his hitch in the service, Lewis returned to show business, at first with partner Johnny Black, hitting Chicago in 1925 as "The Dardanella Boys." In those days Lewis was a fair singer, with standards like "Macushla" to his credit. But it was as a solo comedian that he discovered his ticket to fame.

The scars from the savage beating he took were still red and visible when Lewis heroically took the stage once more at the Rendezvous. But his voice was only a croak. Curiosity seekers came at first, but before long the house was empty. It looked as if his career was finished. Early in his life he had worked as a haberdashery salesman. Funds were raised so he could return to the quiet life of a shopkeeper. Meanwhile, the three men who had attacked Lewis were found dead, their bodies strewn in different Chicago locations.

Lewis regained his voice and returned to show business.

In 1933, after grim years of struggle, Lewis found the key to his return to fame. It cost $25. A novelty tune called "Sam, You Made the Pants Too Long," based on the song "Lord, You Made the Night Too Long," it was a risque number with lines like, "I get the damnedest breeze through my BVD's. My fly is where my tie belongs . . . Sam, you made the pants too long."

Time has lessened the appeal of the song, but it was certainly an improvement on the novelty pieces Lewis had used earlier. Lewis became known for sophisticated, sexy song parody and one-liners about his drinking and gambling. In 1940 he was headlining at the Copa, spending half the year there to the delight of the city's racy clientele. He had dozens of winning wisecracks to offer:

"I don't like to drink. It's just something I do while I'm getting drunk. . . . I broke my toe at a Christmas party. I saw a spider on the ceiling and tried to step on it. . . . If I had my life to live over, I wouldn't have the strength. . . . In high school I was voted most likely to dissolve."

Raising a glass, he would say, "It is now post time," and launch into his routine. He never accepted offers for a TV series, and did few movies or even guest TV appearances. He enjoyed the nightlife, and the environment of the clubs. And he enjoyed the easy access to women, booze and bookies.

When urged to quit drinking, he'd say, "I know more old drunks than I know old doctors." Or, acknowledging his poor health, "I passed on years ago but nobody had the heart to tell me." Once he admitted, "I'm beginning to see the handwriting on the floor."

For hecklers he had dozens of quick comebacks. He could be tender: "I don't mind you snoring, but you hurt me when you didn't say goodnight." He could be tough: "When you use your brain it's a violation of the child labor law."

Lewis influenced many young stand-up comics. Eddie Lawrence recalls, "It was his timing—he took his time. He didn't feel you had to fill up every second jabbering. He had a great delivery."

In 1953 the star was saluted in *Variety* on the 30th anniversary of his show business career. 23 solid pages were packed with congratulatory advertisements from well wishers. His life story was brought to the screen with Frank Sinatra in the lead. Lewis quipped, "I sometimes think Sinatra had more fun playing my life than I had living it."

Lewis was forced to relive the nightmare of his speech loss when, in 1966, he suffered a stroke that left him in almost the same condition as the Chicago attack. He couldn't remember words and couldn't speak them. But he came back, once again. At first his speech was slurred. "They think I'm drunk," he told a reporter. "What a bum rap. I work sober for the first time in 40 years and everybody thinks I'm plastered."

The beloved legend of comedy did not stay down for long. Soon the quips were coming, fast and glib, old and new: "A race track is where the windows clean the people. . . . There are a lot more important things than money. Trouble is, they all cost money." Audiences relished the definitions, the parodies, the drinking and gambling lines, all delivered with great timing and flair. "You're my kind of people," he told his audience, "drunks!"

Even today some Lewis lines are frequently quoted. In 1984 Senator Alan Cranston campaigned against his image of being too liberal, with "both feet firmly planted in mid-air." He quoted Lewis: "Show me a man with both feet on the ground and I'll show you a man who can't put his pants on."

In 1970, at a Friar's Club roast, Lewis delivered an off-the-cuff toast: "As I approach the final curtain—I leave my broads to Richard Burton." Then he collapsed. This time there were no comebacks. Lewis rallied briefly, but died the following year.

As Earl Wilson recalled, his "was one of the most remarkable funerals I ever attended. It was about an hour late getting started. Presently the funeral hush was broken by soft laughter. As they waited, people began quoting their favorite Joe E. Lewis line. All over the chapel people were chuckling about Joe E.'s jokes. It didn't seem sacrilegious to say he left us laughing."

RICH LITTLE

"I think you can be funny without being cruel," says Rich Little. And he's proved this philosophy by remaining the nation's top impressionist for over a decade. While many mimics antagonize their subjects, few stars have objected to Little's view of them, a view that generally comes from total adulation: "I think the voices I do best are the people I admire most. Nobody has ever told me they don't like me doing them. Most people consider it an honor, I guess."

John Wayne once ambled over to him and said, "Little, let me see you do that walk." Rich regained his composure and did his version of the John Wayne strut. The Duke paused a moment and said, "I'm glad you've still got it. I'm losing it." Cary Grant used to get a kick out of

Little's impressions, and, the essence of humility, would sometimes ask, "Did you do me tonight? Do you think they really remember?" One of the few less than enthusiastic stars was Tony Randall, who simply told the young comic, "You're terribly hopeless."

If Little's Tony Randall has not been his strongest impression, few would deny the accuracy of some of the Little standards: George Burns, Johnny Carson, Ronald Reagan and Jimmy Stewart. The most flexible mimic of all time, he can rattle off over 150 successful impressions. Perhaps his greatest artistic triumph was duplicating with absolute fidelity the narrative style W.C. Fields used on his "Temperance Lecture" 78 rpm single, in order to show how Fields might have read sections from his book, *W.C. Fields for President*. This version of Fields is quite different from the "standard" one Little uses for live shows, with which audiences are more familiar.

Little has been doing impressions all his life, but insists his motivation has never been to escape personal unhappiness. "When I was going to school that was the only way I could get dates. Rich Little couldn't get anywhere," he says. He'd find out a girl's favorite actor, then call her up imitating him. He flustered his teachers by mimicking them, but it was less an act of rebellion than a desire to show off his skill.

The young mimic began making money as a performer when he was 17, appearing on local talent shows. He was helped by George Kirby, who told him to do offbeat, unusual impressions, and Will Jordan: "Will Jordan helped me when I was younger. I stole his Henry Fonda. He put it on tape for me." As with most young impressionists, only some of his comic portraits were original. He could imitate someone else's caricature, but hadn't yet perfected the ability to find the key himself: "I imitated Vaughn Meader imitating [John] Kennedy," he recalled.

It was Mel Torme who got Little his first American exposure, on "The Judy Garland Show" in 1964, at a time when Little's specialty was doing 103 impressions in under four minutes: celebrities calling out their names.

Unlike most mimics, there was never much malice in Rich Little. He was also nice-looking, with an affable personality. Early on, in 1967, he learned what can happen to comics who dig too deeply with their wit. Nancy and Frank Sinatra had a hit with "Something Stupid," and Little parodied it, with Lyndon and Lady Bird Johnson singing, ". . . and then you go and spoil it all by saying something stupid like Vietnam." A newspaper columnist launched a long, snide attack insinuating Little was a communist sympathizer. The Copacabana terminated the mimic's contract.

By 1969 Little was a regular on "The John Davidson Show." Of the other top impressionists at the time, Frank Gorshin and David Frye, he insisted, "They go for impressions while I like to capture the person without exaggerating him. I can't just do a reaction and let that suffice."

Little became the most successful mimic because of his talent, but also for what he did with it. An impressionist offers a vicarious thrill twice removed. People fantasize about being stars, and they enjoy watching someone like them actually turn into a star before their eyes. Most mimics do this with exaggeration and cutting humor, but Little keeps the fantasy alive by revelling in being these stars, communicating with mild humor his own joy in mimicry. Whereas Gorshin and Frye had intensity on stage, Little prided himself on his cool.

As Little's star grew, he mirrored changing times. After Frye's grotesque Johnson and Nixon caricatures, here was Little doing mild Gerald Ford. Referring to a Little appearance on TV, President Ford "found [the impression of him] very enjoyable and relaxing." Little had even greater

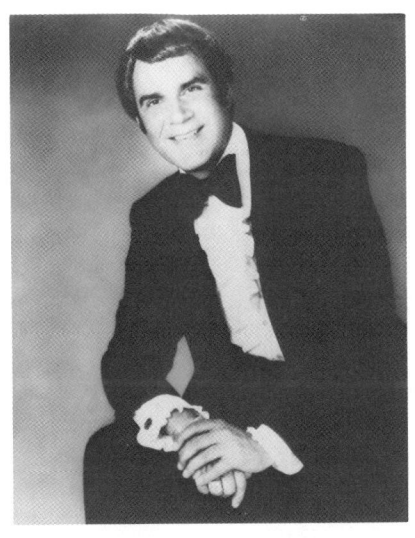

b. November 26, 1939, Ottawa, Canada

Records:
My Fellow Canadians (Canada/Capitol T 6028), Scrooge and the Stars (Canada/Capitol T 6049), Politics and Popcorn (Mercury SRM 1-617), Rich Little's Broadway (Kerr SPL 800), Rich Little in Concert (Much CHLP 5004), The New First Family (Verve 15054), The First Family Rides Again (Boardwalk NB1-33248), W.C. Fields for President (Caedmon TC 9101), Earle Doud's Celebrity Workout (Capitol XT 12312).

TV:
The Rich Little Show (NBC 1976), You Asked For It (syndicated 1982).

Video:
Rich Little's Hollywood Trivia Game (Vestron).

success with other "pleasant" politicians, Jimmy Carter and Ronald Reagan. Little also did Nixon, but in puffy-cheeked cartoon, not shadowy jowled caricature.

In 1976 the impressionist had his own show on NBC. Aside from comedy impressions, he began to do morbidly accurate "tributes," straight acting as a famous star. He'd dress up in a trenchcoat and pretend to be Bogart doing a mini-"one man show" of his greatest scenes. He even injected some straight singing into his act, and took straight acting roles on such shows as "Police Woman."

A superstar and Vegas headliner, Little would eventually announce, "My big goal now is to let the fun come through." He hinted that he was tiring of mechanical "technical accuracy," and it showed. Many mimics "lose it" through boredom, or by finally allowing their own strengthened personalities to shine through the charade. One thing that always showed through with Little was his Canadian accent. Nearly every star in "Hawlywood" used the Ottawan pronunciation of "O" that came out "Aw." Now once-perfect impressions began to get ragged, although the public didn't seem to care.

Of his Atlantic City audiences Little says, "Humor there has to be pretty broad. You're not playing to high society or anything. In fact, most of the audience seems to be wives. I guess their husbands are out gambling."

Little has produced a series of very successful TV specials, both live concerts and such productions as "Rich Little's Christmas Carol" in which through telemagic he is the entire cast from Scrooge (W.C. Fields) to the ghosts to Bob Cratchett (Paul Lynde). He has virtually no competition as an impressionist, and evidently no sympathy for other mimics. When old mentor George Kirby was imprisoned for dealing drugs to keep up payments on his house, Little remarked, "What a waste. I guess he's getting a great chance to do James Cagney convict routines."

Married since 1971, with a daughter, Bria, Little lives in an oceanfront home in Malibu. In addition to his sojourns to Vegas and other venues around the nation, he plans more specials and more fantasy shows like his "Christmas Carol," where to the amazement of many and the vicarious thrill of all, he is not just one star, but everyman playing every star.

PAUL LYNDE

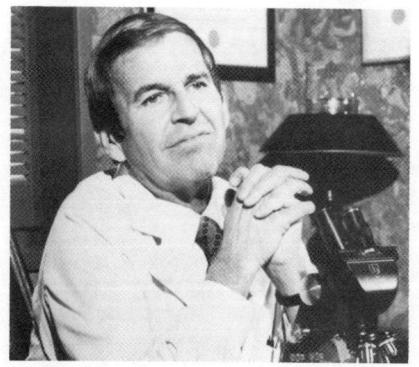

b. June 13, 1926, Mount Vernon, Ohio; d. January 9, 1982

A beloved "sick" comic who made kink a comical topic for mid-America, Paul Lynde grew up physically unhealthy and emotionally traumatized. With one brother a better athlete, the other a superior scholar, Lynde recalled being "lost in the middle," unable to compete for his parents' affection. He had a childhood bout of peritonitis and was then overfed into embarrassing obesity.

In high school Lynde spent his time writing out fantasies. After school, reality involved working at his father's store killing and plucking chickens. A childhood romance with a young girl failed, and the sensitive Lynde claimed never to have gotten over it. Family traumas further scarred the inhibited young man: while he was a student at Northwestern University, his favorite brother was killed in World War II, and his parents died three months later.

Lynde's desire to become an actor seemed just a dream. He wanted to act in serious dramas at school, but was always cast in comedy. "I made up for my weight by being a silly goose. That's what my teachers called me," Lynde recalled, and it was as silly comedy characters that he received some attention.

After graduating from Northwestern in 1948, Lynde worked at various sales jobs in New York while hoping for a break. "Those years left me a shambles," he said. "I lived next to the telephone, fed on rumors and died several deaths." He couldn't even secure fat-man character roles. Eventually he began the task of dieting down from 260 pounds to 180.

He wrote monologues for himself, and one, "The African Hunter," clicked when he performed it in an amateur contest in 1950. He began to make club appearances, and won a slot in the Broadway revue *New Faces of 1952* with "The African Hunter." He also performed the monologue on "The Ed Sullivan Show." He played a delirious tourist lecturing on his recent trip:

"Our destination for that first day was the source of the Nile, the longest, and I might add the dirtiest river in the land. Oh, but it was stinkin'! Our pack mules fell down and played dead when it came time to water 'em!" With a manic smile and an even more demented laugh, the trauma-shocked tourist recalls, "We'd only been tramping on the trail four or five hours when my wife began to complain of her feet. The only shoes she had with her were those high-heeled sling pumps! Ha ha, she just couldn't take it . . . so we had to leave her there out on the trail. On the way back I found this piece of her dress and to this day I don't know what happened to her! Heh heh."

He showed snapshots of the trip, including one of a native girl: "The day after the picture was taken she got caught in one of those sucking bogs . . . she was completely submerged in 57 seconds! Luckily I had a picture to give her mother, and she was very happy about that and made me a necklace out of lovebird's feet. The mother was later taken by black rot. . . ."

Early on, Lynde demonstrated the ability to win laughs with grim material, and to find humor in Charles Addams–type characters and poetry like this:

"There are roses in bloom in my hospital room. Hear the bird in my window singing its song: 'Chirrrup! Cheer up! You haven't got long.' Don't sob my pretty roses, I feel no pain. While fishing in Maine I was struck by a train. The doctor says I'm as fit as a fiddle. But everyone knows they lie just a little. I don't even know if I'm in bed. Because I don't have a head. Cheer up, cheer up, you haven't got long."

Lynde enclosed himself in tightly written sketches or comic lectures, most of which featured the smiling-skull grimace and sardonic edge of one determined to be cheerful under the most hideous of conditions. He began to win more praise, and was prominently featured in *New Faces of 1956*. But offstage Lynde was miserable. At a dinner party he suddenly said, "I haven't heard one word you've said all evening. And I love you all too much to inflict this on you." He began seeing an analyst.

Even so, Lynde continued to find performance a trial. In 1960 he made a major stride forward playing the harried father in Broadway's *Bye Bye Birdie*, but in 1962 he could still say, "I have never gotten over being terrified in front of an audience. Oh, I know most performers get the jitters before they go on. My reaction is more like nervous collapse. I'm in awe of people who can't wait to get out there. I've never been like that. I have to be shoved."

Once Lynde experienced the actor's nightmare: while doing a stock

Record:
Recently Released (Columbia CL 1534).

TV:
The Paul Lynde Show (ABC 1972–73), Bewitched (ABC 1965–72), The Hollywood Squares (NBC 1968–72; syndicated 1972–82).

Broadway:
Bye Bye Birdie, New Faces of 1952, New Faces of 1956.

Films:
Bye Bye Birdie, Send Me No Flowers, Rabbit Test.

Video:
Alan King Stops the Presses (Video Yesteryear).

show in Pennsylvania he forgot his lines and left the stage. He came back a few minutes later and finished the show, receiving a tremendous ovation at the finale. He became a popular character comedian in the movies, and was grateful to leave stand-up behind. Referring to his friend Jonathan Winters, he said, "I'd end up on a flag pole too if I kept playing them [nightclubs]. All you can talk about is the bathroom, sex or golf. Those are the only subjects the audience can understand."

Lynde restricted his monologues to television, where he was a frequent guest through the 60's, appearing in sketches that he often found difficult: "Guesting with other people you have to say what they write for you and you wish you could avoid it. It isn't just a line here or there, it's whole sketches such as one of those things on the 'Dean Martin Show' where you say to yourself, if you're going to take the money, you better do it."

In 1965 a 24-year-old actor, clowning and drunk, fell from Lynde's hotel window in San Francisco. The fatality was just one of a series of miseries that seemed to dog Paul Lynde. Also that year, however, he began what would become a semi-regular role as the warlock Uncle Arthur on "Bewitched."

Two years later Lynde became a panelist on "The Hollywood Squares" and, encouraged by a growing cult of fans, began confidently to expand on his sassy sick-nik character. From 50's black humor he turned to kink, giving comic answers to straight questions like these:

"What's the best way to keep two-year-old children from biting their fingernails?" "Make them change their own diapers." "What happens usually when a man takes female hormones?" "Is it hot in here, or is it just me?" "According to Poor Richard's Almanac, you should dress to please others but do something else to please yourself. What?" "Undress others." "According to the classic old song, when should you button up your overcoat?" "When the movie is over."

Audiences were shocked and delighted by Lynde's kinky, misanthropic, misogynistic, sick and just plain weird answers, delivered with feverishly staring eyes, an icy grin and an occasional breathy giggle of bemused malevolence. He was lovable, America's odd uncle, an eccentric who fascinated middle America, hinted of an exotic gender-bending lifestyle somehow more exciting than and superior to everyday life. Unfortunately Lynde didn't find himself as lovable as his fans did: "I look like an iguana," he said. "I'd rather not watch myself and I'm better off."

Through the 70's Lynde was making up to $325,000 a year. He remained the central star of "Hollywood Squares," but did not succeed with his own sit-com in 1972. As early as 1964 he'd begun making pilots for the major networks, but never did find the right character and supporting cast and environment that could sustain a weekly series.

Lynde's body was weakened by his determined dieting, and in 1979 he suffered a bout of hepatitis. The man who would go back to Ohio in the summer to do the stage plays he loved at least died a romantic, movie star's death. He was found in a posture similar to the dramatic demise of Marilyn Monroe: nude, in bed, with drugs nearby. In his case, the drug was butyl nitrate, ingested in an amount the coroner declared insufficient to be lethal. He suffered from acute hardening of the arteries and death was from a massive heart attack.

MOMS MABLEY

"I think of the audience as my children," Moms Mabley used to say. The feeling was mutual. "She has the face and all the charm of a real mother," Redd Foxx insisted, "all that warmth that a mother has, plus she always tries to help all of her children."

Coming out center stage in outlandish, loose-fitting outfits, lecturing in a gravel-voice, she had a presence that transcended her material, much of which was lightly sexy anecdotal stories that (by now) are familiar to readers of *Playboy*–type joke anthologies.

Like a feisty lecturing grandmother, too excited and involved even to put in her false teeth before setting on her young charges, Moms would offer earthy reflections that garnered huge laughs. The following lines were punctuated by laughter so long you could count the seconds. If they don't seem hilarious, then the magic of Moms' raucous delivery and the charm of her comic character will be even more apparent:

"Love is just like a game of checkers, children. You sure got to know which man to move! (laughter) 'Cause if you move the wrong man (laughter) and he jump ya (laughter) tear your Mason and Dixon line up! (laughter, applause)."

Another typical joke: "A drunk comes up to this man on the street and says, 'I want your daughter for my wife.' And he said, 'You go home and tell your wife she can't have my daughter!'"

Black poet Langston Hughes tried to explain huge laughs and small jokes, and the atmosphere of the legendary Apollo in Harlem: "the nuances of some of the Apollo's funniest comedy is, on occasion, likely to be entirely 'en famille,' and rather hard to explain to strangers without going to great lengths. But, mostly, it has the gusto and openness of the humor of unabashed burlesque without seeming off-color even when it is. For example, Jackie Mabley once said, 'I've been reading in the papers about Mother England. There's a mother for you.' It was five minutes before the show could continue."

She had the audience on her side. Very few comedians have her kind of presence; most must win an audience over, but Mabley exuded warmth and good humor, more like a neighborhood character than a professional performer, and the audience was with her immediately.

Of her start in show business she said, "I didn't pick it. I was pregnant and I didn't believe in destroying children. And I prayed and it come to me more a vision than a dream—go on the stage." She used the name Jackie Mabley. "Jack was my first boyfriend. I was real uptight with him and he certainly was real uptight with me, you'd better believe. He took a lot off me and the least I could do was take his name."

She was discovered by the dance team of Butter Beans and Susie and came to New York in 1923. Appearing first at the Cotton Club and the Apollo, where she played dates with Jimmie Lunceford's big band and others, she went to Broadway with *Swinging the Dream* and *Blackbirds*. She appeared in two films during the 1930's, *The Emperor Jones* with Paul Robeson and variety shows on film like *Boarding House Blues*.

She evolved the unique character of "Moms" fairly early: "I had in my mind a woman about 60 or 55, even when I first came up. She's a good woman, with an eye for shady dealings . . . she was like my granny, the most beautiful woman I ever knew."

She had the costume down pat in the 1940's: a loose-fitting dress,

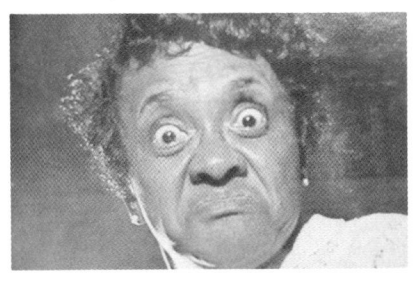

b. Loretta Mary Aiken, March 19, 1894, Bravard, North Carolina; d. May 23, 1975

Records:
Funniest Woman in the World (Chess 1447), At the UN (Chess 1452), At the Playboy Club (Chess 1460), Funny Sides (Chess 1482), Best of (Chess 1487), Young Men Si (Chess 1477), Breaks It Up (Chess 1472), Man in My Life (Chess 1497), I've Got Something to Tell You (Chess 1479), Moms Wows (Chess 1486), Moms the Word (Mercury 60907), Now Hear This (Mercury 61012), Out on a Limb (Mercury 60889), Live at Sing Sing (Mercury 61263), Her Young Thing (Mercury 61205), At the White House (Mercury 61090), Abraham, Martin and John (Mercury 61235). With Pigmeat Markham: One More Time (Chess 1504), Mabley and Markham (Chess 60009).

Films:
Killer Diller, Boarding House Blues, Amazing Grace.

floppy hat and a set of slightly suggestive anecdotes and novelty songs. Typical of her humor from the Apollo era is the following, where she tells a woman in the audience,

"Honey, you'll have to laugh a little louder. Mom can't hear you up there. That's it . . . thank you. I can't hear very good. Moms tell you how that happened. They sent for me to come down to Washington in an airplane. I ain't scared of an airplane. I'm no square. . . . Sure enough, no sooner I got in the plane they strapped me down. The stewardess come by I say honey, my ears is all stopped up. Both ears stopped up. Ohh, I was so sick! She say, 'here's some chewing gum.' I chawed that. That ain't unstopped 'em. I got right limp. I said do something for me honey, I'm dyin'. She said 'Drop your *jaws!*' And I misunderstood her . . . they grounded me in Baltimore. . . ."

At first her delivery was a bit stilted, leaning toward recitation, and she tended to act out the lines as if she were performing before children. But as she aged, she simply got funnier and funnier, more seasoned, very loose and confident. She did many one-liners on her penchant for young men, delivered with a raucous, now-toothless rasp: "The only thing an old man can do for me is to get on a bicycle and bring me a message from a young man!" She'd say, "A woman is a woman until the day she dies. But a man's a man only as long as he can!"

She lectured on world affairs as only a mother can, promising that if she were in office, she'd straighten out the mess made by the young kids playing with their dangerous toys. About the only person who was beyond help was Richard Nixon: "Even Old Moms couldn't do nothin' for that man 'cept give him a few licks upside the head."

The 1960's proved to be a peak for Moms, after many years of struggle. White comics had stolen jokes from her, and black comics were no great help either: "They promised when they got up there, they'd help me. But they sure didn't. They put their feet on me." It was Harry Belafonte in 1967 who helped secure nationwide TV exposure for her. There followed a new explosion of Moms Mabley records, which were curiously successful despite the difficulty of understanding her toothless delivery. A few years later she starred in a movie, *Amazing Grace.*

This was the story of a tough, religious old woman battling corrupt politicians in Baltimore. Like George Burns, Moms was now revered in old age, about to be given a rebirth in movies. But unlike Burns, Moms' movie was not a beginning but a signal of the end.

During filming she suffered a heart attack. "I weighed 161 when I went into the hospital, and 116 when I came out. You can't tell in the movie, because I don't wear tight clothes. I was in misery. I couldn't get my breath good, but my doctor fixed me up." She returned to the set with a pacemaker.

She had to take it easy after that. "I'd be all right except for them Ritis Brothers," she said. "Arthritis, Neuritis, Peritis and all those other Ritis." When asked if she was bitter that it had taken her so long to attain national prominence, she answered that she always tried to look on the positive side. "Ain't a person in the world I don't love," she'd say. "Nobody ever gave me nothing, and I ain't ever asked, either."

Success didn't spoil her simple tastes. Although she could afford a maid and a Rolls Royce, and had these luxuries, she remained in touch with her friends from decades earlier. For 25 years she was a parishioner at the Abyssinian Baptist Church in Harlem, where she would sometimes rise to recite her favorite passage from the Bible, the 27th Psalm. When she died, it was there that thousands came to pay their respects to a memorable performer, a friend and a woman who wanted to be Moms to them all.

CHARLIE MANNA

"There are two varieties of comedy. Funny and not funny." Charlie Manna's comedy, like his view of humor, is deceptively simple. Manna was underrated during his ten years of TV and nightclub popularity. Although he never failed to make the audience laugh, he also never made a strong impression, largely due to his pleasant, slightly bland appearance.

He had little to identify him. He was a nice-looking, well-mannered gentleman with no particular facial or vocal mannerisms for audiences to remember. He didn't do ethnic, beatnik or sicknik material, nor did he take the other extreme of broad slapstick or one-liner and wife jokes.

Manna performed cleverly crafted, polished sketches. He did situation comedy bits on universal subjects, including one about a troop of Brooklynites flying to the moon on their home-made rocket ("Keep contact with earth at all times—who brought the extension cord?") and one on an astronaut who refuses to begin his mission unless he can take his crayons with him.

One of his best monologue sketches was a trip inside the human body, to view the head of the central nervous system, who, like the captain of a ship, gives orders: "Pretty girl coming! Now hear this: all glands, secrete! Connect me with the stomach—any butterflies down there? Connect me with the unconscious please. Well . . . keep ringing!"

Each organ has a different voice, from the obviously stuffy nasal cavity to a puckering lower lip that sounds like Maurice Chevalier. The routine builds with throwaway jokes ("Captain?" "Yes, what is it, corpuscle?") to intrusions from the mighty brain ("This is the brain! B-r-a-n-e . . ."). There's an all-out alert when the pretty girl slaps the face after the central nervous system has urged a pass. The body isn't sure what to do next until the subconscious suddenly wakes up and shouts, "Hit her!"

Manna enjoyed performing musical comedy, and used to do musical monologues like "Alcatraz," where he not only played all the characters in his prison movie parody, but interrupted for comic songs, too. Another favorite was his version of "The Barber of Seville," singing a stanza of straight opera and then translating the barber's dialogue into a series of quick gags:

"Hey, Figaro, I can't stand this part in the middle of my head. Move the part from ear to ear." "You crazy—do that and people will whisper in your nose!"

"Hey, Figaro. I just met Cardinal Siccola, he's a smart man, he's gonna be Pope someday." "No, how would that look? Pope Siccola?"

After graduating from James Monroe High School, Manna majored in voice at The Music School and studied opera. He spoke fluent Italian and could play the piano by ear. After World War II he was a member of a musical trio.

He was a natural comedian, though, and when Carl Reiner saw him at a private party, he urged Charlie to try comedy as a career. Reiner

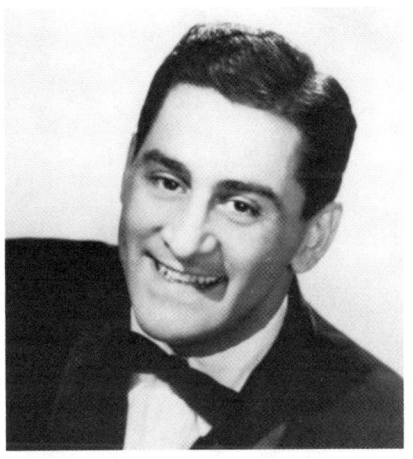

b. October 6, 1925, Bronx, New York; d. November 9, 1971

Records:
Manna Overboard (Decca DL 4159), Manna Live (Decca DL 4213), The Rise and Fall of the Great Society (Verve 15051).

Book:
A Loser Is. . . .

helped him to get some bookings, and in the Catskills in 1954 Manna began to try out material and perfect his technique. His straight singing talent helped him get work along the Strawhat Circuit as well. In addition to appearing in musical revivals, he attracted attention for his work in the *Shoestring Revue* of 1957.

At first Manna utilized one-liners, things like, "It's not who you know that matters, but it's how your wife found out" and little gags from real life: "I was a precocious child. I could sing before I could walk. When I was 16 my mother told me, 'Charlie, stop singing and learn how to walk.'"

It was in 1961 that he recorded his first album and his astronaut routine caught on. The bit was so successful, and timely, that when Commander Alan Shepherd entered his capsule for that first mission barely a month later, someone handed him a box of crayons. "That was a real tension breaker," the astronaut recalled.

Manna's appealing albums and pleasant personality made it look easy, very easy. But he took his craft seriously. "Audiences are different and the comedian today who takes any gags for granted as sure-fire is deluding himself," he once wrote. "Very often ... a comedian has to have at the tip of his tongue 'the topper' ready to spring, the minute he finds he has drawn a blank. The little remark over the 'bomb' just laid often gets the laugh intended for the original."

Called by *Variety* "a clever comic with an essentially softsell delivery," Manna continued to make frequent appearances on TV and in clubs, always inoffensive and, unfortunately, indistinctive. "There was a funny comic on the Sullivan Show last night—can't remember his name. But he was good"—that was too often the reaction to Manna.

Following his initial success with monologue sketches, and not having made much of an impression with political satire on an album for Verve, Manna began to incorporate "loser" gags into his act. In 1971, the year of his death, he published a book of these, titled *A Loser Is....* It contained lines like "A loser is ... a guy who plays hide and seek and nobody looks for him." That kind of material eventually worked when spoken in the first person, by someone who looked the part: Rodney Dangerfield.

Still fresh, still funny, and certainly classics, Charlie Manna's two Decca albums remain as entertaining now as they were over 20 years ago.

PIGMEAT MARKHAM

When audiences saw Sammy Davis, Jr. cutting up on NBC's "Laugh-In," trucking and quipping "Here come de Judge, here come de Judge," a new catch-phrase was discovered. And a few months later, so was Pigmeat Markham—who had invented the routine nearly 40 years earlier.

"I wrote 'Here Come the Judge' in 1928 when I was doin' stock at the Alhambra," Markham recalled. "We kicked it around through burlesque."

Markham's "Here Come the Judge," in which various wacky defendants appear before a comically bewildered and outraged jurist, was as familiar to black audiences as "Crazy House" or "Slowly I Turned" was to whites. When Davis used it as a throwaway on "Laugh-In," he was using it the way a white comic might throw in a snatch from "Who's on First"—with fondness and respect.

Originally a tap dancer, Markham is credited with creating several dances, including "The Boogy Woogy" and "The Chuck." Like Lou

Costello, the hefty but graceful comic was a natural for fast-paced knockabout and soon shifted into comedy full time. For one burlesque routine, typically on the bawdy side, he dubbed himself "Sweet Papa Pigmeat" and the name stuck.

His real name was Dewey, but the comic said, "I hear it so seldom, I almost don't recognize it. Even my kids don't use it. They yell: 'Hey, Papa Pigmeat.'"

For Pigmeat and other black performers, the "TOBA" or Theater Owners Booking Agency had another meaning: "Tough on Black Actors," and he worked the "Chitlin' Circuit" of black burlesque as well as carnivals and minstrel shows.

According to Langston Hughes, "For a long time most black comedians felt that in order to be funny, they had to work under cork. The strangest paradox of them all was Pigmeat Markham, one of the funniest and most popular of black comedians. For years on stage his makeup was burnt cork. When changing times after the second world war caused him to stop blacking himself up, his audiences were amazed to discover that in reality Pigmeat was himself darker than the burnt cork he had been using."

By this time Pigmeat's eccentric dances, clowning and blackout sketches were familiar to audiences at the Apollo Theater and other Northern spots. In 1944 *Variety* covered an Apollo show and noted, "The guy has much talent and could get by with cleaner stuff. However his bluest gags garnered the biggest bellies so that's probably what's keeping him in that groove."

Pigmeat agreed. He was going for laughs—big belly laughs: "Listen to Mort Sahl, say, and then listen to Red Skelton. Then you'll get what I mean. Man, I could never work for giggles."

Markham's antic routines and double entendres began receiving attention from white audiences. At least, there were *some* whites who ventured to the Apollo. Pigmeat vividly recalled seeing one fellow who stood out for two reasons. He was white, and he was writing Pigmeat's jokes down on a pad. His name? Milton Berle.

The Markham brand of free-for-all burlesque was brought to "The Ed Sullivan Show": "I had a sketch, I'd see a ghost, and yell 'WOW' and go right through the roof on a piano wire. The piano wire broke and I broke both my legs."

In 1967, when "Here Come the Judge" brought him into the spotlight, Markham and Bill Levinson produced a paperback version of the routine. Although Shorty Long beat him to the airwaves with a "Here Come the Judge" single that reached the Top 10, Pigmeat's version cracked the Top 20 a few months later and he loaded the comedy racks with his albums. George Kirby wrote the liner notes for one:

"I know only too well the hard knocks, the trials and tribulations the older comics had to go through to become stars, especially the negro comics. So many had that taste of stardom just once but one of the greatest, who has brought laughter to millions, has a new birth of stardom. Yes, this comic was one of the few greats who walked in the back door so that we young comics of today could walk in the front, and thank god he has a chance to walk in the front with us. It is not what he has, nor even what he does, which directly expresses the worth of a man, but what he is. And Pigmeat Markham is the greatest. . . ."

As in many burlesque and vaudeville routines, the humor rests more with the comedian than the material. Pigmeat's "Here Come the Judge" was great fun because of Markham himself as he'd roll the lines out with lusty, blustery delight: "The judge is *high* as a Georgia *pine*! Everybody's goin' to jail today! And to show you I don't mean nobody no good this

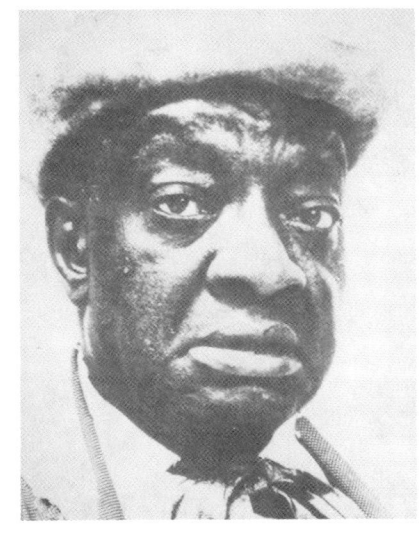

b. Dewey Markham, April 16, 1904, Durham, North Carolina; d. December 13, 1981

Records:
The Trial (Chess 1451), Anything Goes (Chess 1467), Crap Shootin' (Jewel 5007), Would the Real Pigmeat Markham Please Sit Down (Jewel 5012), World's Greatest Clown (Chess 1475), Tune Me In (Chess S 1526), This'll Kill Ya (Chess 1500), Save Your Soul, Baby (Chess S 1517), Open the Door, Richard (Chess 1484), Mr. Vaudeville (Chess S 1515), Mr. Funny Man (Chess 1493), If You Can't Be Good Be Careful (Chess 1505), Here Come the Judge (Chess S 1523), Bag (Chess S 1534), Hustlers (Chess S 1529). [Most of these discs were recorded between 1964 ("Open the Door, Richard") and 1969 ("Hustlers").] With Moms Mabley: One More Time (Chess 1504), Mabley and Markham (Chess 60009).

morning I'm givin' *myself* six months! And if I'm gonna do six months, district attorney, you can imagine what *you're* gonna do!"

His courtroom (where "your honor" became "you ornery") saw all kinds of defendants including a man accused of being a nudist. "I've got 12 children," the defendant begins. The stunned judge immediately decides the case is closed: "This man is not a nudist! *This* man hasn't had *time* to put his clothes on!"

The thundering voice of Judge Pigmeat, brimming with exaggerated righteousness, can be heard on many albums containing a variety of routines. Usually the themes are blue, but sometimes a joke is in vivid black and white. "Knock knock." "Who's there?" "Ize!" "Ize who?" "Ize yo' next door neighbor!" Markham's albums are loaded with slang and strong Southern accenting, a vivid Negro speech pattern that was out of favor during the sensitive civil rights period but pridefully came back some time later.

Like most of the old burlesque stars, Markham knew only one way to be funny: pulling out all the stops and going full tilt. And he continued on through the late 60's, commanding $1,000 or more a night, a famous star at last. He retired to Co-op City in the Bronx. He was invited to nearby Lehman College to lecture on the history of black entertainment in America, and fulfilled many such speaking engagements. His funeral in Harlem was a major event, attended by many of the greats he had worked with over his long career.

MARTIN AND LEWIS

They were a phenomenon. In July of 1951, Martin and Lewis were in such demand they were performing six shows a day for a two-week run at the Paramount Theater. In addition to doing 84 hour-long shows in those two weeks, the duo gave dozens of ad-libbed performances for the crowds who gathered in the streets, under their dressing room window, and wherever they went. It was hysteria.

Hysteria was what the team of Martin and Lewis was all about. Their humor was fast-paced slapstick, with the incorrigible, unstoppable Jerry Lewis frantically breaking it up with every zany old trick he knew and many he invented on the spot. The act was simple enough: looney comic keeps interrupting his singing straight man's act, then demolishes the orchestra and finally even the audience.

Lewis would mug behind Martin's back, make faces, do eccentric dances, use prop buck teeth for a gag, spill food and dunk audience members' cigars in their drinks: anything for a laugh.

Audiences responded to the spontaneity of Jerry Lewis, a new character for a new age. He was the 1950's personified: awkward, young, energetic, uncool and totally jerky. He was more imbecilic than any "dumb" comic yet seen, more rubber-faced, more infantile than previous "little boy" manics like Lou Costello.

Lewis's young years in Newark were marked by loneliness. His parents were entertainers, and they often left their son with relatives. To gain attention he would contort his face, do slapstick shtick and try to perform all sorts of crazy stunts. Skinny, sickly and, as far as his schoolmates were concerned, ugly as well, Lewis joked his way out of trouble most of the time. When he was attacked not by brainless youths but by hostile adults, he fought back fiercely.

In high school, the increasingly defensive, rowdy Lewis was called

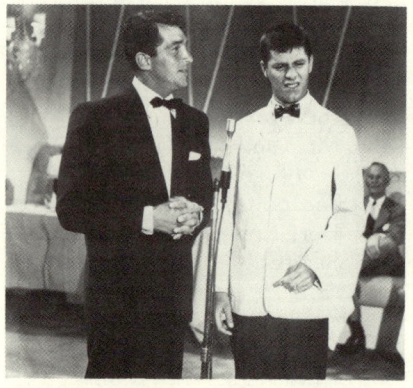

DEAN MARTIN b. Dino Crocetti, June 7, 1917, Steubenville, Ohio
JERRY LEWIS b. Joseph Levitch, March 16, 1925, Newark, New Jersey

Records:
Martin and Lewis on Radio (Radiola MR 1102), Martin and Lewis (Memorabilia MLP 714).

Films:
At War with the Army, Sailor Beware, Scared Stiff, Living It Up, Pardners.

Video:
Colgate Comedy Hour (Video Yesteryear), Muscular Dystrophy Telethon 1951 (Budget Video).

before the principal. The man looked disdainfully at the freshman student and said, "All Jews are stupid." The boy lunged forward, toppling a huge wooden desk onto the man. It ended the taunts and, shortly thereafter, his school years.

Lewis put together a pantomime act in which he would make outrageous faces to popular songs and opera recordings. He began to develop a dazzling talent for physical comedy. It was only a matter of time, some thought, until he became a top comedy star.

Dean Martin's early years were spent in the tough steelmill town of Steubenville. At 14 he was prize fighting, scraping through more than 30 fights for dubious prizes like watches and pens, which he would pawn for a few dollars. A few years of this, and the broken-nosed boxer was ready to try something else. From making about $2 a fight he switched to making $2 an hour in a local steelmill.

Other professions were still more lucrative. Martin joined a gang, stripping cars and shoplifting from stores. His pals affectionately nicknamed him "Punchy," but "Punchy" was smart enough to get into other rackets. He made money delivering bootlegged liquor and later dealt cards expertly in the backroom of a local cigar store.

Martin admired Bing Crosby, and imitated him for his own amusement. Friends were impressed by Martin's voice and encouraged him to perform, and one night he was discovered by a bandleader who needed a new singer. Martin wasn't really interested—the salary was much less than he was used to—but his friends encouraged him and vowed to lend him any extra money he might need. He also got a nose job.

In 1946 Martin and Lewis teamed up in Atlantic City at the 500 Club. "I'd like you to meet Dean Martin," Lewis would say, "one of the greatest singers in the country. I don't know how he'll do in the city, but anyway, here he is." Mayhem would follow, as the stooge got the better of the straight man during an hour of prepared gags and spontaneous buffoonery. The duo were an almost instant success, becoming the most talked-about nightclub act around, getting their own radio show in December of 1948, and making their first film the following year.

With the aging Abbott & Costello hardly a threat, the new comedy team was netting millions from TV, films and club dates. Most felt that it was in the nightclubs that Martin and Lewis were at their best, their act thriving on audience reaction, fueled to new highs by laughter. Of course, there were those who felt that Lewis's antics were silly, and Martin bland, and that at their best they were not so hot. Huffed Jack E. Leonard, "This is a nothing act. What Martin and Lewis do isn't basically funny, but nobody else has the gall to do it in a sophisticated cafe."

Some critics, though, found themselves helplessly overpowered by the energy of Jerry Lewis. Martin evidently was similarly affected. It was tough being a straight man to all that nerve-shattering slapstick, and to be prodded by a workaholic partner toward an exhausting schedule of appearances.

Martin began to feel the burden of being an offstage "big brother" figure to Lewis. The comics' wives didn't get along. Artistic friction developed and the pace was murderous.

A 1953 film, *The Stooge*, underlined another problem: Dean Martin's sublimated ego. In a story about an ordinary singer (Martin) who refuses to acknowledge the greatness of his comedy partner (Lewis), Martin had an opportunity to sing some songs and do some straight acting, but he was also forced to deliver this speech after his character bombs in an attempt to be both singer and comic on his own: "I want to apologize," he tells his audience, "I'm only half an act. The fellow that made the act work isn't here tonight. I can play an accordion and sing a song, but I need that spark . . . that something . . . I bored you and imposed upon you . . . I humbly apologize."

It would soon be demonstrated that in reality Martin didn't need Lewis, and vice versa. On July 24, 1956, the team appeared in a nightclub for the last time, delivering a brilliant performance of rowdy gags and spontaneous destruction. Fans urged the two to reconcile. Lou Costello published an open letter to the team in a newspaper, but before an answer could be given, Costello was performing as a single without Abbott.

The "divorce" was bruising for both men. Professionally, Martin had a tough time at first, but with his friend Frank Sinatra he scored impressively in the 1958 film *Some Came Running*. Lewis brooded over his future, but found his fears unfounded when he substituted for Judy Garland on short notice and received his quota of laughter and cheers.

Eventually both men found their identities emerging to the fullest. Martin developed his flair for comedy, and enjoyed veering off course, changing lyrics to songs like: "You made me love you . . . you woke me up to do it." He starred in a popular TV variety show in the 1960's and has continued to be a favorite when he chooses to perform.

Lewis's first movie on his own was a hit, and his fans have remained with him through his long, undisciplined and critically controversial film career. As a solo on stage, there's no question of his charisma and ability to bring instant laughter from his bag of slapstick tricks and shtick.

While it's doubtful that the 1950's Martin and Lewis films will emerge as "classics," many are still amusing, suggesting the excitement and spirit the team brought to stand-up in the postwar era. Given the subsequent success of the two as solos, many look upon the crazy comic bits from Lewis and snippets of song from Martin as only a portent of the things to come.

STEVE MARTIN

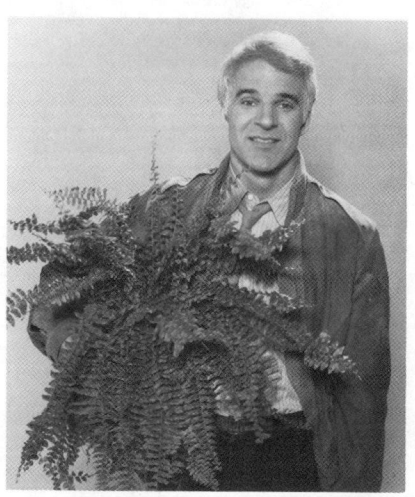

b. August, 1945, Waco, Texas

Growing up conservative in Orange County, California, Steve Martin recalled, "We were very middle-class. My whole orientation to comedy was very secret. I think that's the premise of my whole act. You're laughing with a close friend at some nuance or subtlety. But you can't *explain* it to someone."

Proving that it's hard to explain Martin's comedy, he added, "It's about the way people are in the ten feet that surround them. It's about what people think, not about what businesses do, or what governments do. It's about individuals and how distorted their thoughts can get just being alive in the world, and how you have to completely become crazy in order to survive . . . of course, it varies from that just to get laughs."

Influenced by the standard comics of the era, like Red Skelton and Jerry Lewis, Martin worked at Disneyland and at Knotts Berry Farm, playing the banjo, performing magic and telling jokes. It was probably in this atmosphere that Martin's smile turned steely, the jokes delivered with a huckster's sense of put-on and his personality sealed with a protective hipness.

A philosophy major in college, by 1967 Martin had shifted to theater arts. The combination of these two interests could be seen in some of his later throwaway lines, like the giddy, "We're having a great time, considering we're all going to die someday."

In the late 1960's, the Smothers Brothers were looking for a specific type of writer: young. 21-year-old Steve Martin got a break and later won an Emmy for his work on their series. He moved on to write for shows hosted by Sonny and Cher, Pat Paulsen and Dick Van Dyke, earning $1500 a week. He quit the "Glen Campbell Goodtime Hour," according to his publicists, "not because of censorship, but because he thought it was so dumb."

Dumbness. Jerks. From gawking geeks watching him play the banjo at Disneyland to pseudo-hip geeks lounging in hot tubs and eating granola bars, Martin had seen it all. He began to parody some of the egotists, the emotionally barren status-seekers, the thick-skinned hedonists and the show-biz hucksters. And, seemingly from out of nowhere, audiences were suddenly overpowered by a new type of comic: a jerky, artificial, egocentric cornball comedian in a blazing white suit, with blazing white hair and shining pearly teeth. He looked like a pitchman in a bleach commercial. But instead, he blitzed the crowd with his eccentric brand of comedy.

Performing as an opening act for rock groups only toughened up this exaggerated character. Privately Martin resented the "blithering idiots and acid casualties" in the audience, but it was in front of them that he developed a penchant for inane, self-involved, demented one-liners ("I do terrible things to my dog with a fork!") and bizarre drug humor.

One of his classic bits was "Let's Get Small," wherein he insinuates, with all the intense glee of an addled addict, how great it is to take a "forbidden" drug that makes your body shrink instead of your mind expand. It's a double-edged parody: recognition comedy for everyone who has ever deliberately set out to get smashed in order to look at the world through warped vision, and yet a devastating put-down of such thrill-seeking and ultimate emptiness.

Martin cartooned his physical movements, coming up with a silly walk, a cheesey smile and a set of arm and finger movements Joe Cocker would've thought strange. He added geek-pleasing balloon animals and arrows-through-the-head gimmicks, and ushered in a character of awesome insincerity and obnoxiousness, so incredible as to be laughable.

By 1976 this strange new comic was well known through his appearances on "Saturday Night Live." He even had some catch-phrases. As the most incompetent of doltish dates, he would describe himself with a wide grin as "a wild and crazy guy." And when his conceit and "me-generation" inanities were not appreciated, he'd huff a snide and outraged "Well, excuuuuuuuuse me!"

His "non-comedy" style included parodying the awkwardness of traditional stand-up comedy and the artificiality of stepping up and making people laugh. He experimented with making an audience laugh at the very paucity of jokes. Many other comics would attempt comedy based on an obnoxious character or parodies of 1980's-generation vapidity and self-involvement, but none managed to pull it off with the elan of Steve Martin. Probably that's because none had Martin's background as a legitimate comedy writer who knew the mechanics of making *anyone* laugh.

In private, Martin was anything but hip, egocentric or loud. Serious, down to earth, even conservative, his coworkers noted that Martin's wild and crazy ways started only when the spotlights splashed over him and his $600 white suit.

Martin's first album, "Let's Get Small," won a 1977 Grammy and sold over 1.5 million copies. His second album had similar million-selling success. Martin-mania reached a peak the week of April 3, 1978, when his staring eyes, gritted teeth, wildly gesticulating arms and bent forward legs were splayed over the cover of *Newsweek*.

Records:
Let's Get Small (Warner BSK 3090), A Wild and Crazy Guy (Warner HS 3238), Comedy Is Not Pretty (Warner HS 3392), Steve Martin Brothers (Warner BSK 3477).

Films:
The Jerk, Pennies from Heaven, Dead Men Don't Wear Plaid, The Man with Two Brains, All of Me.

Video:
Funnier Side of Canada 1974 (IUD), Saturday Night Live (Warner Brothers).

Book:
Cruel Shoes.

Bios:
Steve Martin (Lenberg), Steve Martin (Daly).

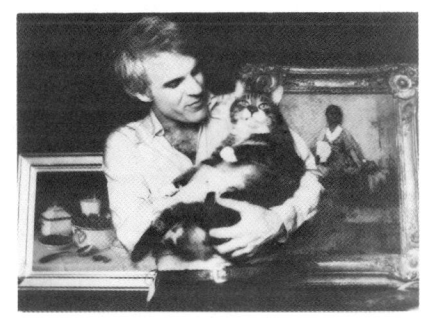

"All Steve Martin asks is that everyone have a good time," *Newsweek* reported. "Martin is part of a counterrevolution in American comedy: white and middle-class in appearance, mock arrogant in posture and unthreatening in its message." Martin did fit in with the mock-arrogant "Saturday Night Live" crew of Chevy Chase, John Belushi and, later, Joe Piscopo, but his underlying message was not quite so light-headed and light-hearted.

One of Martin's most popular stand-up bits was a mock-furious discussion of cats. With huffy breaths, pauses for overemphasis and great indignation, Martin asked,

"How many people have cats? Now let me ask you this—do ya trust 'em? Because I've gotta get a pair of cat handcuffs and I gotta get 'em fast! I found out my cat was embezzling from me! You think you know a cat for ten years? He pulls something like this. I found out that while I was away . . . he would go out to the mailbox . . . pick up the checks . . . take 'em down to the bank and cash 'em . . . disguised as me! I wouldn't have caught him, but I went out to his house, outside where he sleeps—and there was about three THOUSAND dollars worth of cat toys out there! And you can't return 'em, 'cause they have spit all over 'em!"

The love/exasperation/confusion critics felt toward Martin was summed up in a review of *Cruel Shoes*, a 128-page book that had an advance sale of 200,000 copies. The *New York Daily News* reported, "Steve Martin has written a series of cocktail napkins and called it a book. . . . At this point in his career, Martin could sell his two-day-old dental floss and it would go platinum inside a week. Which is one way of saying that Martin's legion of fanatics is not the most demanding on this planet. At the mere sight of their hero, they are rendered helpless with giddiness. It doesn't really matter if Martin says or does anything funny; just out of habit the audiences will scream, shriek and generally act like total imbeciles. I know because I am one of the afflicted."

Cruel Shoes was a bewildering series of surreal, tongue-in-cheek anecdotes and nonsense. But for the average, uninitiated listener, 1977–78 Steve Martin albums are equally strange, loaded with seemingly inappropriate laughter over non-jokes. A viewing of old videotapes also doesn't quite capture the flavor of the Steve Martin phenomenon. Martin's third album, "Comedy Is Not Pretty," is probably the most coherent, with bits of verbal whimsy that don't need an interpreter or a fan saying, "you hadda be there."

He talked about basic subjects, like sex: "I actually learned about sex watching neighborhood dogs. And it was good. Go ahead and laugh. No, go ahead! I think the most important thing I learned was—never let go of the girl's leg no matter how hard she tries to shake you off." He offered sage advice: "I'm not into that one-night thing. I think a person should get to know someone, even be in love with them before you use and degrade them. . . ."

Just as Martin moved away from TV writing, he decided to step out of the spotlight. He learned, "you can't tour forever, and even if you could, you won't be successful at it forever." He quit while he was ahead, "retiring" from stand-up in 1980 to pursue a film career.

With two Grammys and an Emmy, all he needs is an Oscar. He's already been nominated (for a short subject, *The Absent-Minded Waiter*). He's made quite a few important films, after a shaky start with films that were either overtly commercial (*The Jerk*) or the opposite (*Pennies from Heaven*). Teamed with Carl Reiner as director, he starred in *Dead Men Don't Wear Plaid*, an inventive comedy exercise in which he was cut in and out of classic old detective movies, and *All of Me*, his most perfect vehicle, allowing him to be believable *and* wild and crazy. Most important, in that film he was wild and crazy with a purpose (his body was half taken over by a recently deceased woman).

GROUCHO MARX

There were six Marx brothers in the family that lived on East 93rd Street: Leonard, Adolph, Manfred, Julius, Milton and Herbert. Manfred died at age three; the others were directed toward careers in show business.

"Our mother's brother was Al Shean, of Gallagher and Shean, and he was pulling down $150 a week," Groucho recalled. "Mother knew a good thing when she saw one." With Leonard (Chico) and Adolph (Harpo, who later changed his name to Arthur) working at odd jobs, it was Julius who was first prodded toward the footlights.

He answered an ad for a boy singer, auditioned and won the job. Over the years Groucho remembered his employer's name variously as Le May, Larong and Le Roy, but one thing never changed in his memory: "he was a fag." The act featured the man, Groucho and another boy in drag, flouncing about singing "I Wonder What's the Matter with the Mail" and other gems.

This first job took Groucho on a grueling cross-country railroad tour. In Denver the other two stole Groucho's money and left him stranded. He raised the fare home by riding a horse-drawn grocery wagon over mountainous terrain and through the aptly named Cripple Creek.

Shortly thereafter he teamed with Lily Seville, whose gorgeous body made up for her lack of talent. His tour with her ended when she disappeared—after stealing his money. These incidents made the serious and studious young man a bit cynical: "I was an innocent boy! Why, it wasn't until the following year that I got gonorrhea from a hooker in Montreal."

Eventually Groucho chose slightly less larcenous company: his mother and brothers. In 1909 they were called "The Four Nightingales," then "The Six Mascots," depending on how many relatives showed up. Groucho always had a few solo songs, either as a German or Jewish comic. One had lines like this: "It's better to run to Toronto, than to live in a place you don't want to."

Through arduous tours over nearly a decade, the Marx Brothers evolved into a raucous, breakneck comedy act that would do almost anything for a laugh. Their first major vaudeville sketch was "Fun in Hi Skule," with Groucho as teacher, the others as unruly students.

Groucho developed his ad-libbing and the humor that twisted his serious side into zaniness, his cynicism into feisty wisecracks and his hostility into insults. He even attacked the audience. One night, during a dreary performance in Nacogdoches, Texas, he shouted, "Nacogdoches is full of roaches!" But, as would be the case for 50 years, the eye-rolling, funny-voiced wiseguy made them laugh at the outrage. "We played in towns I would refuse to be buried in," Groucho said, "but when you're young, you're not afraid. You don't know any better."

Other sketches followed, including "Home Again" and "On the Mezzanine," and the troupe even toured England. They finally hit Broadway in 1924 with the polished *I'll Say She Is*. The show ran for two years

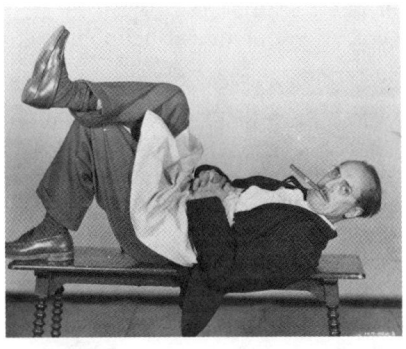

b. Julius Henry Marx, October 2, 1890, New York, New York;
d. August 19, 1977

Records:
An Evening with Groucho (A&M 3515), Hooray for Captain Spaulding (Decca DL 5405; more readily available as a British import, Ace of Hearts 103), The Mikado (Columbia OL 5480), My Favorite Story (20th Century-Fox TFM 3106), Face to Face (Decca DXD-166), Groucho on Radio (Radiola MR 1072), Groucho! (Mark 56 #758), You Bet Your Life (Golden Age 6A 5021), Groucho on Radio (Memorabilia MLP 73), Marx Movie Madness (Radiola MR 1097), Marx Brothers Voicetracks (Decca DL 79168), Three Hours, 59 Minutes of the Marx Brothers (4 lps, Murray Hill 931680), Cocoanuts (Sandy Hook 2059).

TV:
You Bet Your Life (NBC 1950–61).

Films:
Cocoanuts, Animal Crackers, Monkey Business, Horse Feathers, Duck Soup, A Night at the Opera, A Day at the Races, Room Service, A Night in Casablanca, Copacabana, Double Dynamite, Mr. Music, A Girl in Every Port, Skidoo.

Video:
You Bet Your Life (Video Yesteryear), NBC Comedy Hour 1956 (Video Yesteryear).

Books:
Beds, Many Happy Returns, Groucho and Me, Memoirs of a Mangy Lover, The Groucho Letters, The Marx Brothers Scrapbook, The Secret Word Is Groucho, Groucho Phile.

Bios:
Hello I Must Be Going (Charlotte Chandler), Life with Groucho (Arthur Marx), Son of Groucho (Arthur Marx), Groucho (Hector Arce).

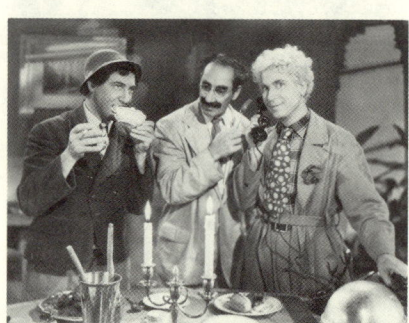

and was followed by more hits. Groucho was always the leader, and often delivered monologues. His most famous was in *Animal Crackers*, when he portrayed eccentric explorer Captain Spaulding:

"Africa is God's country, and He can have it. Well sir, we left New York drunk and early on the morning of February 2. After fifteen days on the water and six on the boat, we finally arrived on the shores of Africa. The first morning saw us up at six, breakfasted and back in bed at seven. This was our routine for the first three months. We finally got so we were in bed at six-thirty. . . . One morning I shot an elephant in my pajamas. How he got in my pajamas, I don't know. Then we tried to remove the tusks, but they were embedded in so firmly that we couldn't budge them. Of course, in Alabama, the Tuskaloosa. But that's entirely irrelephant to what I was talking about. We took some pictures of the native girls—but they weren't developed. But we're going back again in a couple of weeks."

Always independent, Groucho was evidently the star of the lost Marx Brothers film *Humorisk*. He told the first Marx biographer, Kyle Chrichton, that the film represented "humor with pathos. Like Chaplin. I was going to be great, get rid of those dopey brothers and be famous." Late in life, when Chaplin expressed admiration of Groucho for his ability to speak in the movies, Groucho began to get the idea that he might indeed be greater than The Little Tramp.

One thing is certain. He's had as much influence as Chaplin on upcoming comedians. They admire his wit, his cadence, his voice, his cocky attitude that acknowledges cynicism and corruption and treats it with deflating darts, zany outrage or even sassy spitballs. His humor was a crazy quilt of iconoclasm, pure punnery, silliness and satire. Even his famous insults (which defied any attempt at a comeback) were delivered in a variety of styles.

One of Groucho's techniques was to underplay a line with a cynical slur, a runaway aside: "You've got the brain of a 4-year-old boy," he begins, then slides, "and I bet he was glad to get rid of it." Another was the straight challenge: "Why don't you bore a hole in yourself and let the sap run out?" And in the surprise shot, he begins in neutral, then suddenly delivers a blow: "I've got a good mind to join a club and beat you over the head with it."

Groucho, for good or bad, was always "on" in private life. Some of the results are legendary. He quit the Friars Club, writing, "Please accept my resignation. I don't want to belong to any club that will accept me as a member." When he got married, the jokes were still flying. "We are gathered here to join this couple in holy matrimony," the judge began. Groucho interrupted, "It may be holy to you, but we have other ideas!"

In 1930 Groucho wrote his first book, *Beds*, containing the famous line: "Anything that can't be done in bed isn't worth doing at all."

Groucho didn't even take himself seriously: throughout his career he wore a greasepaint moustache. "In good times or bad, Father was never without his insecurity syndrome," his son once wrote. He was "never an optimistic man by nature," and the 1929 stock market crash confirmed his cynicism. Then, after he and his brothers turned out five of the greatest comedy films ever made, they were dropped by Paramount.

Groucho and Chico appeared on radio in "Flywheel, Shyster and Flywheel" in 1934. Fortunately the next year the brothers signed with M-G-M and rebounded with some of their finest films. They were toasted as zany anarchists, as outrageous comics, and while the general public thought of them as three hilarious characters, intellectuals could dissect them as the ultimate satire of humanity's body (Chico), intellect (Groucho) and id (Harpo).

Their fortunes waned again by the time of *The Big Store* in 1941. Groucho wrote, "I'm happy to escape from this kind of picture . . . acting in the movies no longer interests me." He recalled, "Writers thought because they wrote long speeches for me and had me talking fast and using a lot of non-sequiturs and silly puns, that was all there was to it. That's my style all right, the trouble is a lot of writers forgot to be funny along with it."

Groucho found he could be freer on radio. He also made some records, singing his classic novelty songs, some from movies ("Lydia the Tatooed Lady"), some that never made it in ("I'm Doctor Hackenbush"). He also wrote a second book, *Many Happy Returns*, attacking the tax system. He was still the iconoclast on paper, if he couldn't be in movies. "So far as I'm concerned," he wrote in the introduction, "you can slip this book into your pocket when the dealer isn't looking."

In 1947 he appeared on a show with Bob Hope, and the two tossed their scripts away for a 20-minute ad-lib spree. The performance astounded John Guedel, who produced "People Are Funny." He knew the combination of Groucho and people would be funnier.

"I wasn't particularly proud of doing a quiz show," Groucho recalled, but "You Bet Your Life" was a smash hit on radio and TV through 1960. His son Arthur said it springboarded him "to more fame and money than he had ever had before." As a solo he topped even the fame of the Marx Brothers. He signed a $760,000-a-year contract, and on December 31, 1951, was on the cover of *Time* magazine.

Each week on "You Bet Your Life" Groucho unleashed a flurry of fresh gags, along with old gags given a new twist. A contestant gushed about her many, many children and said "I love children and I love my husband." Groucho cracked, "I love my cigar, but I take it out of my mouth once in a while."

Of the show, Groucho said later, "It was some of the best stuff I ever did. I really had to think. I never worked so hard." He added, "People have no respect for comedy. They think it's easy, but very few people have made a living doing comedy."

People had great respect for Groucho. In later years he appeared often on "The Dick Cavett Show," offering reminiscences that were almost monologues, including this one about fans:

"A woman came up to me the other day and said 'Aren't you Groucho Marx? May I kiss you?' I said feel free. I was feeling free at the same time. She invited me up to her room but I didn't want to go. She was an old babe. She was about 24. In the Plaza Hotel once, when I was doing the quiz show, there was a priest in the elevator. I hope you're not offended by this—I'd tell a story about a rabbi but it doesn't fit—and neither did the rabbi and they finally threw him out of the synagogue. Anyhow this priest says to me 'Aren't you Groucho Marx?' I said yes. He says 'Gee, my mother's crazy about you.' And I said 'Really? I didn't know you fellas had mothers.' I had a priest stop me in Montreal some years ago. He came up and said 'Aren't you Groucho Marx? May I shake your hand?' I said fine. I shook hands with him and he said 'I want to thank you for all the joy you've put in this world.' And I said 'I want to thank you for the joy you've taken out of it.'"

Fans and interviewers flocked to hear Groucho's views on people and current events. "Even when I'm kidding I tell the truth and that's no joke," he once said. In 1972 he performed a one-man show on tour. In

1974 he was given a special Academy Award, and his 85th birthday was proclaimed "Groucho Marx Day" in Los Angeles as over 200 guests, including Peter Sellers and Jack Lemmon, came to Groucho's home to toast their aged but unbowed hero.

Asked what he'd do if he could live his life over, Groucho said, "Try more positions."

"Groucho Marx was the best comedian this country ever produced," Woody Allen once wrote. "I can't think of a comedian who combined a totally original physical conception that was hilarious with a matchless verbal delivery. I believe there is a natural inborn greatness in Groucho that defies close analysis as it does with any genuine artist . . . his outrageous unsentimental disregard for order will be equally as funny a thousand years from now."

JACKIE MASON

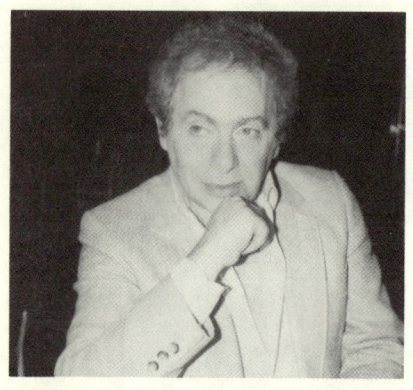

b. Yacov Moshe Maza, June 9, 1930, Sheboygan, Wisconsin

Records:
I'm the Greatest Comedian in the World . . . (Verve 15033), I Want to Leave You with the Words of a Great Comedian (Verve 15034).

Films:
The Stoolie, The Jerk, The History of the World, Part II.

Broadway:
A Teaspoon Every Four Hours.

Book:
Jackie Mason's America.

It was like "The Jazz Singer," only in comedy. Jackie Mason wanted to make people laugh, but like his father and brothers, he became a rabbi. He grew up on New York's tough Lower East Side, studying Jewish laws and principles, imbued with a sense of morality that was unshaken by poverty and temptation, a sense of justice and a vow of nonviolence sorely tested in such a fierce environment.

He graduated from City College and held forth at a synagogue in Weldon, North Carolina. The young New Yorker's humorous sermons won them over. "You should be a comedian," they told him.

After Mason's father died in 1957, Jackie decided to give show business a try. He became a social director in the Catskills, putting on amateur shows, performing comedy and discovering how quickly his funny lectures were used up. Facing the same crowds each night, he couldn't do the same gags over and over.

Mason bounced from hotel to hotel. Along with his misery he was plagued with a deeper sense of doubt and guilt: the rabbi had left his congregation. Was this failure part of the punishment? He sought psychiatric help in dealing with his insecurities. In the meantime he tested his material in nightclubs and even in strip joints where his clean comedy and Jewish accent got him nothing but jeers.

In 1960, Mason made a name for himself at the Slate Brothers Club in California. "At the beginning all I heard is why I wouldn't make it," Jackie recalls. "I sounded too Jewish. But here I was in front of the elite of show business. Bing Crosby, James Stewart and Stanley Kramer were there. I said if these people find me so funny, you mean to tell me some unfortunate soul in Utah sitting on top of a pound of potatoes next to a dump truck—that guy won't like me? And if he won't could I be that bad anyway?"

Steve Allen signed him immediately: "Right after that first six-minute spot on his show my price went up from $300 a week to five thousand. Gentiles hired me—Garry Moore, Perry Como, Ed Sullivan, Jack Paar. And Jews kept telling me how Jewish I was."

Some Jews were sensitive about the Jewish image Mason was portraying. Part of his comic presence was a brash impudence. Before Muhammad Ali, Mason was saying, "I'm the greatest comedian in the world—only nobody knows it yet." He joked about governmental bureaucracy, sex, money and power, but with his thick accent, Jewish agents and fans felt Jackie's sniping sounded like a Jew being a troublemaker. Most of the criticism was unjust, but an occasional line did cut close:

"Money is not the most important thing in the world, love is. Fortunately, I love money." It was a cute throwaway line, but coming from a Jew?

"I wasn't saying it as a Jew," Mason says. "I'm saying it as a person. Everybody could identify with that joke. Generally my jokes are of the opposite nature, that show up the stupidity of thinking money is everything and humanity is nothing."

But even his gentlest jests made some of his Jewish friends uneasy. And even today, there are those who see in Woody Allen and Mel Brooks an ugliness that encourages anti-Semitism. Says Mason, "Jews have been persecuted for so many years—it's not an illusion. But to give up your identity plays into the hands of anti-Semitism." Better to look Jewish, to act Jewish, to keep the accent. "I think it's a kind of rebelliousness, a way of showing that you're proud of what you are, that it is a source of pride. It's a defiant symbolism. You better respect me for what I am and I'm not ashamed of it, I'm proud of it, I'll dance with it, I'll fly with it, I'll make an issue of it whether you like it or not. The worst thing you could do as a Jew is to assimilate and lose your identity."

Discussing the large number of Jewish comics, he adds, "If you feel persecuted and left out you're looking for ways to achieve attention, to be somebody. Jews accentuated education and developed verbal and intellectual talents for comedy, but it's an emotional need. Nobody feels more vulnerable than a comedian and takes more of a chance to be destroyed emotionally. And still the Jew is more likely to become the comedian because he's willing to suffer the price to achieve that much attention."

He's aware that "every actor is on an ego trip. I'm not that sick that I think I'm an exception, but if you understand the sickness that drives you and put it in the proper perspective you can then do good, and not harm." Part of the acceptance even extends to cases like Don Adams's well-known use of Mason's jokes word for word. When asked about it, he says, "It's offensive—I don't know why somebody as comparatively successful would steal so blatantly—but it hasn't hurt my career. Comedians fear somebody stealing their material. It's nonsense. A comedian starts off being insecure and fearful, he doesn't know where his career is going and imagines if somebody takes a joke he'll be wiped out. But the audience is buying our personalities. They get a kick out of you personally. They're not one tenth as familiar with your jokes as you think they are."

Much of Mason's material exists beyond gags. In 1960, along with Bruce, Sahl and others, he loaded his monologue with biting satire. "I have certain moralities and social issues I introduce in my act. I get very emotionally disturbed about fraud and fakery and people taken advantage of. If I can talk about it and it doesn't detract from the humor, I'll do it. As long as I'm hilarious." As with Bruce and Sahl, the hilarity is helped by a fascinating delivery and a rhythmic cadence.

He loves to perform intricately woven pieces that boil and bubble with irony and incongruity. Here are portions from his classic bit on psychiatry:

"I finally went to see a psychiatrist. I asked him 'What will this cost me?' He told me $75 a visit. I said, 'For $75 I don't visit, I move in.' For $75 I figured I'll drive *him* crazy. He said, 'What's bothering you?' I said, 'Your $75 fee for the visit.' He said, 'We have to search for the real you!' I said to myself, if I don't know who I am, how would I know what I look like? And even if I find me, how would I know it's me? Besides, if I want to look for me, why do I need him? I could look myself, or I could call my friends. They know where I've been! Besides, what if I find the real me, and I find that he's even worse than I am? Why do I need him? I don't make enough for myself, I need a partner?

"The psychiatrist said, 'The search for the real you will continue at our next session. That will be $75.' I said to myself, this is not the real me. Why should I give him $75? What if I find the real me and he doesn't think it's worth $75? Then I wasted my money for the real him. For all I know the real me might be going to a different psychiatrist altogether. In fact, he might even be this psychiatrist himself! I said to him, 'What if you're the real me? Then you owe me $75.' He said 'If you promise never to come back we'll call it even.'"

George Burns said of Mason, "He's a funny man." Asked if Jackie was as funny as Lenny Bruce, Burns paused. "Funnier." Mason did neurotic jokes before Woody Allen, and social satire at the time of Bruce, yet hasn't been elevated to their level. To an extent this is because he's not a figure the critics or youth can rally behind. He looks square and still has the "Catskill" image, a bit to the left of Alan King. But imagine Lenny Bruce doing these 1960 Jackie Mason lines:

"There's a double standard about sex. Our father or mother becomes our father or mother. Beautiful. The arrival of a child is celebrated. But how that child was created and arrived is something that is cloaked in secrecy. They're ashamed of it. They thought it was pretty clever when they did it. . . ."

In 1964 Mason achieved Lenny Brucean notoriety when he was accused of having been deliberately obscene in front of a national TV audience. Guesting on "The Ed Sullivan Show" Jackie was machine-gunning through his bits when Sullivan signalled with a finger: one minute to go. Mason ad-libbed and began pointing too. To Sullivan it seemed that Mason had flipped the forbidden third finger, although he hadn't.

Sullivan made a tremendous scene backstage and the young comic received enormous publicity which, amazingly, helped his career instead of hurting it. But a short time later he was hurt and almost killed because of his antics on stage.

Like many comics, he did Sinatra jokes. He spoke of the "sickness" of a man going from woman to woman in a need for conquest. "Do you think Sinatra is really happy?" Mason would ask. "I happen to know—he's *very* happy." These and other mild jokes were met with bullets that tore into his hotel room, narrowly missing him. Later there was an assault, punches thrown at Mason as he sat in his parked car.

Despite the passing years, Mason is as brash and opinionated as ever. When Jimmy Carter said he'd whip Senator Edward Kennedy's ass in the primaries, Mason joked, "Do you expect the President to use a word like that? A man with hemorrhoids yet should have the right to say this? Carter couldn't take care of his own ass and he's after Kennedy's already?" On Ronald Reagan: "At the age of 73 the only job you can get in this country is President. He couldn't be a plumber. For that you need qualifications. At least President Reagan is happy. He can't remember how he got the job or what he's supposed to do, so he laughs."

Periodically Mason has shifted from stand-up to other areas. His Broadway play, *A Teaspoon Every Four Hours*, set a record: 99 previews, one performance. It was a sweet, good-natured show with a lot of laughs, but as he says, with justification, "The critics were waiting for me: who is this gross Jew from the mountains, he doesn't belong on Broadway. They had to preserve their semi-homosexual atmosphere of arrogant social elegance, the Noel Coward set walking and talking in their own language, living in an Ivory Tower of 'Theater' with all the pretentious nonsense it's supposed to represent."

The reviews were better for *The Stoolie*, a film that despite good notices received limited distribution. Now he's "optimistic—the time is right to make more films. And I've made a few TV pilots." Whatever Mason does in the future, he has a great deal of support—certainly from himself:

"Above all, I want to wish myself the best of luck. I sincerely hope that I should have whatever I want. And whatever you want, I should also have. In case you want something I never heard of, why should I be left out!"

VAUGHN MEADER

Comedy is often built on irony and the laughter fed by tragedy. A young comic named Vaughn Meader found himself bathed in irony and tragedy. It was no joke, and there was absolutely nothing he could do to avoid becoming, like Sonny Tufts, Larry Parks or Richard Nixon, a living symbol of failure, a shivering reminder of what fate can do. In some perverse way, the harder he tried, the more the public blanched, and the deeper entrenched his image became in disaster.

Meader's first ambition was to become a lawyer, and he fantasized about it as he watched courtroom scenes in movies. His father died when Meader was one year old, killed while doing a high-dive act. His mother worked as a waitress, and Vaughn helped keep the family afloat with a succession of odd jobs.

Interested in music, he amused friends with his imitation of twangy-sounding hillbillies. He joined the Army as a Petroleum Lab technician and was shipped to Germany where, in his leisure time, he played piano in a GI band. It was there that he met his first wife, a waitress who had come up to him to say a customer wanted to hear "Sawdust." Meader broke up, and the two shared after-hours jokes after the band played what the man was really after: "Stardust."

Stateside, supported by his wife, Meader struggled for six years, taking gigs as a musician and comic. In January of 1962 he brought his humor and his John F. Kennedy impression to Greenwich Village in New York. Political impressions were not new. Another comic, Elliot Reid, also did Kennedy. But Meader really looked like the nation's young president. In reviewing his 20-minute set at the Blue Angel in September, *Variety* reported that "the cerebral school of comedy seems to be gaining more practitioners." The critic noted that Meader had "a few other bits that register, but it's the JFK that gives him the top plateau."

Meader made it to TV's "Talent Scouts" and "The Ed Sullivan Show," and was picked by Earle Doud and Bob Booker for a proposed ensemble studio comedy album, "The First Family." It was recorded on October 22, 1962, and as Earle Doud noted, "It was the worst night possible. President Kennedy had just made his speech saying the Russians had missiles in Cuba." Meader recalled, "During rehearsals I snuck out to the hotel bar

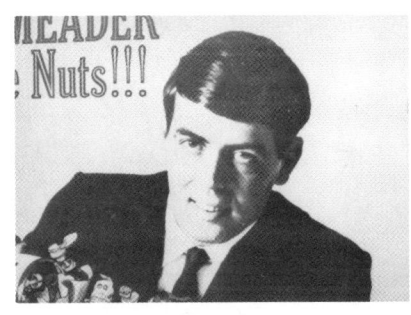

b. Abbott Vaughn Meader, March 20, 1936, Boston, Massachusetts

Records:
The First Family (Cadence CLP 3060), The First Family, Vol. II (Cadence CLP 3065), Have Some Nuts (Verve V 15042), If the Shoe Fits (Verve V 15050), Take That! (Laurie LLP 2035), The Second Coming (Kama Sutra KSBS 2038), The First Family Rides Again (Boardwalk NB1-33428).

to watch Kennedy. . . . Thank God he took a strong stand, or our record would have died right there."

The record died at MGM, Capitol and Mercury, but was released on the small Cadence label on November 7. It almost died shortly thereafter: in New York, radio station WOR immediately rejected the album on the grounds of "good taste," although the lp was mild, with gags about Kennedy enjoying a rubber duck in the bathtub and playing touch football on the White House lawn.

Fortunately, WINS and WNEW decided to play the "controversial" lp, and 50,000 copies of the first pressing were gone within days. By November 19, 1962, the *New York Times* was reporting on a phenomenon: 200,000 copies of a comedy album sold. During the Christmas season, that number ballooned to a staggering 2.5 million copies. In two months Meader's comedy disc sold more copies than "My Fair Lady" had in a year.

"For the first time since I was born I won't be owing anyone money," Meader remarked. "We didn't try to be vicious. Making fun of people in authority is very healthy. And I've never heard it said that the President doesn't have a sense of humor."

The 26-year-old comic hoped to get an audience with Kennedy, but the only comment the President gave on the album was a wry, "I enjoyed Mr. Meader's album very much. But I really think he sounds more like Teddy."

But for Vaughn Meader there was a slippery feeling at the top. Even as the lp became Guinness World Record material, a nightclub version of "The First Family" was bombing. Meader and the other principals would appear on stage, in spotlight, doing a "radio" version of the album. Meader failed in his home turf, Boston, lost money in Pittsburgh and had to cancel plans for a West Coast tour.

As a stand-up, Meader had better luck. He began pulling down $20,000 a week, varying the JFK impression with his other material. By his own estimate, he netted $500,000–$750,000 in 1962–63 from records and personal appearances. A second "First Family" record was released March 28, 1963, but Meader was already planning even bigger things.

In November of 1963, an enthusiastic Vaughn Meader made a new album, "Have Some Nuts," an excellent record of satiric sketches. He was phasing out the Kennedy bits, and there was nothing about the President on the album. In his liner notes on the precarious world situation and the satirist's role in it, he wrote, "I believe it was Shakespeare who said: 'All the world's a stage, and the only thing to worry about is falling off the edge.'"

The edge was much closer than Meader ever realized.

"JFK Record Is Haunting Vaughn Meader," the *New York Post* headlined. The article was about Meader's *new* record, and his problems shaking the Kennedy impression. Even though he was limiting the JFK portion of his act to just a 10-minute ad-lib press conference with the audience, people were identifying him only as an impressionist. Meader figured "Have Some Nuts" would change that. He said it "is the funniest album ever recorded. It's a satire of such groups as the John Birch Society and the Communist Party."

"JFK Record Is Haunting Vaughn Meader" appeared in the *New York Post*'s issue of November 22, 1963.

That same day, just a few hours later, the *Post*'s presses were running again for an extra edition announcing the assassination of President John F. Kennedy.

Vaughn Meader was not in New York that day. He was en route to a comedy concert in Milwaukee. He was so accustomed to the laughter, and to the fairy tale success he had achieved, that reality intruded with difficulty. A Milwaukee cab driver asked, "Did you hear Kennedy was shot?" Meader answered, "No, but how does it go?"

Meader cancelled his show that night and retreated briefly from public view. On January 7, 1964, he returned, hoping to find an audience for the non-Kennedy material he had been using all along. He did folk parodies on the guitar. He talked about his small town where the Howard Johnson stand had only one flavor. He did silly escapist bits like Dr. Bow-Wow, animal expert. In his ad-lib segment with the audience, someone asked the expert, "What can I do if my dog has ticks?" "Don't wind him," Meader answered.

But now everybody was escaping. In the 1980's, an assassination one day yields a dozen assassination jokes the next. But in the 1960's a shocked nation went into a period of mourning, and even the sight of Meader seemed too much. Newspapers were quick to call attention to the comedian's plight. Some tried to draw some conclusion through him that the important thing now was to persevere. America would survive, and so would young Meader.

Meader's "Have Some Nuts" lp was good, but it was ignored. A second album, a notch below the first, was also ignored. Meader did a revue, *The Populace*, and slid into summer stock with *A Thousand Clowns*. And slid into the late 60's when he and a generation of traumatized and disillusioned young people found what they thought was the answer.

"Turn on, tune in and drop out. That's just what I did," Meader recalled. He lived in the Bronx. He became an L.A. hippie living in a tepee. He lived in a log cabin in Maine. The money ran out quickly and Meader hit the gutter, literally, when he was mugged one night in Chicago.

Into the 70's, Kennedy's death became the subject of theories. Meader became a subject for the morbid. Periodically he was unearthed, checked for vital signs and buried again.

In 1971 Meader and old friend Earle Doud made an lp called "The Second Coming." Meader played Christ. "I didn't identify with JFK like a lot of people thought," he said at the time. "I never met him. It wasn't until Bobby was killed that the full impact hit me. I had a serious drinking problem. I lived in windowless shacks . . . it was through LSD that I found peace. It was a spiritual medicine but I no longer use it. . . . Jesus is the only sense I've been able to make out of this confused world. I'm a Jesus Freak."

Jesus was now a superstar. Meader was not. The pleasant, sometimes sharp lp described the problems Christ would have coming back to a cynical world. By 1972 Meader and his new bride were living in obscurity in Jefferson County where he briefly held a $7,500 a year government job. "In the final analysis," he said, success "happened too fast. It made me a big star and gave me a lot of things that weren't that good to begin with."

Through the 70's Meader made ineffective comebacks and remained a perennial "whatever became of" item. He turned up in the film *Linda Lovelace for President*. He tried selling country songs. In 1974 he planned "An Evening with Kennedy," a one-man show similar to those dealing with Will Rogers, Mark Twain and Clarence Darrow. He turned up as Walter Winchell in the movie *Lepke*. In 1976 he was again a small news column item when he announced plans to star in *When the Walls Come Tumbling Down*, a play about a reporter who goes insane and transforms himself into Kennedy while tracking down assassination clues. And in 1979 he wrote "I'm Getting Ready for Teddy," a campaign song for Edward Kennedy's proposed presidential race, with lines like "I've grown much smarter since I went with Carter." It wasn't used.

Ironies? In 1984 Earle Doud produced "The First Family Rides Again," a very mild studio album with President Ronald Reagan played by Rich Little. It actually duplicated the original "First Family" album cover. The tiny part of a reporter was played by the bearded Vaughn Meader, who can be seen in one of the small photographs on the back cover.

MORAN AND MACK

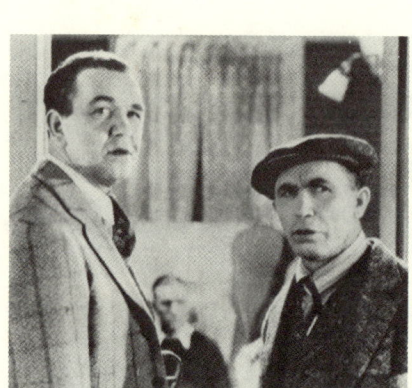

GEORGE MORAN   b. George Searcy, 1881, Elwood Kansas; d. August 1, 1949
CHARLIE MACK   b. Charles E. Sellers, 1887, White Cloud Kansas; d. January 11, 1934

Record:
Moran & Mack/Smith & Dale (Timestu TS 81600 aka: Bramel 59).

Films:
Why Bring That Up?, Hypnotized.

Walter Cronkite remembers the first record he ever bought: "It was the Two Black Crows. They were . . . pure ethnic humor, and you look back on it today with total embarrassment that it was considered funny. But it was the kind of humor that Blacks themselves did in the theaters back then, though these were two white men. But we thought at the time that it was very amusing."

Groucho Marx recalled, "They were great, one of the great ones that we ever had in vaudeville." And he could even recite one of their rather Groucho-esque gags: "One says, 'Good morning,' and the other one says, 'Good afternoon.' And the other one says, 'Good night.' And the other one says, 'Well, I'm glad *that* day is over.'"

Aside from Cronkite and Groucho, somebody else must've been buying Moran and Mack records. "The Two Black Crows" sold over seven million of them in the late 1920's.

Both were successful vaudevillians, singly and in teams, when they decided to form a duo. Within a few years they were starring on Broadway in *The Passing Show of 1921*.

Mack, the larger of the two, was the leader, the funnyman who mixed his dumb remarks with a slight dash of Southern commonsense wit. When Moran asked him if he knew what "alibi" meant, Mack would answer, "A alibi is proving that you was where you was when you wasn't and that you wasn't where you was when you was."

On center stage, their dialogue included these typical quick lines:

Moran: Do you believe in spirits, lazy boy?
Mack: I sure does. I went to de spiritualists last night. He's de feller made my boss Mr. Horowitz change his name.
Moran: How come?
Mack: Well, he conjured up a spirit for Mr. Horowitz, and right after that, Mr. Horowitz went by de name of plain Mr. Horror. You see, de ghost, he scared him out of his witz!

It was a naive age that found delight in this bit:

Mack: On our farm the white horses eat more than the black horses.
Moran: Oh, that's silly, why should the white horses eat more than black horses?
Mack: We tried every way to figure it out and we couldn't figure any reason unless it was because we had more of the white horses.

Much of the humor of the age was based on ethnic and immigrant stereotypes: Dutch comics, Jewish comics, Irish comics and so on. Audiences enjoyed laughing at the accents and appearances of the comedians almost as much as their jokes.

For such mild dialogue, the veteran Charlie Mack didn't feel a straight man had to do much except set up the lines. Besides, he could do some jokes without a straight man at all:

"One night I dreamed I was eating flannel cakes and when I woke up the blanket was gone. And I had another dream. I dreamed I was awake and when I woke up I was asleep."

As the team became more popular, the two men began to argue more. The year 1927 was a big one for the duo. An East Sider named Louis Sterling signed them to Columbia Records. In 1928 they had their own radio show. The following year they starred in the film *Why Bring That Up?*, the title based on their most popular catch-phrase. Their simplicity of wit sometimes earned them the approval of the sophisticates. Algonquin wit Franklin Pierce Adams adapted one of their lines: "About censorship we feel the way either Mr. Moran or Mr. Mack feels about piccolo playing. 'Even if it's good,' drawls the drawling one, 'I won't like it.'"

The uneasy partnership became strained. Moran resented getting $200 a week when he knew the salary for Moran and Mack was closer to $5,000. The straight man wanted a straighter deal, but it turned out he was in no legal position to get it. Mack owned the "Moran and Mack" name and was entitled to set the rates. When George Moran left the act, Mack continued with a less obstreperous Moran. In fact, he ended up with a series of new Morans.

As the Morans changed, so did the times. Amos 'n Andy became the top blackface act. Radio audiences developed a taste for fast-paced comedy. "Now the only comedians are nut comedians," remarked Lew Fields, of another old ethnic duo, Weber and Fields. "They roam around and are wild. We had to stick to ideas. The audience looked for the idea behind the pun, behind the action. They don't look for ideas anymore."

Nobody was looking for Moran and Mack. In 1932, George, the "original" Moran, was back for a reunion with Mack at the Palace Theater. They hoped to get a second chance, and at first there was some hope. They toured the following year with Fred Waring and managed to get some radio work. In October of 1933 the *New York Evening Post* summed up their latest radio appearance by reporting, "We were assailed with the suspicion that they had been brought on the program for the sole purpose of comparing the smoothness of the sponsor's product with goober feathers." The team "seemed to garner very few laughs" and their best jest was "so feeble we can't recall it."

The fortunes of Moran and Mack slid—then crashed. The team, trading in on their nostalgic former fame, was having some meager success in some low-budget Mack Sennett shorts when Moran, Mack and Sennett were involved in an automobile accident. It was the end of Charlie Mack, the only one fatally injured. It was not the end of Moran and Mack, though. Moran recruited another Mack and continued to work sporadically into the 40's when he died of a stroke.

MARTIN MULL

Some comedians have a sense of humor that works best when an audience is relaxed and receptive. Martin Mull knew how to make people feel at home. Billing his act as "Martin Mull and His Fabulous Furniture," he sat himself down in an overstuffed armchair on a set decorated with

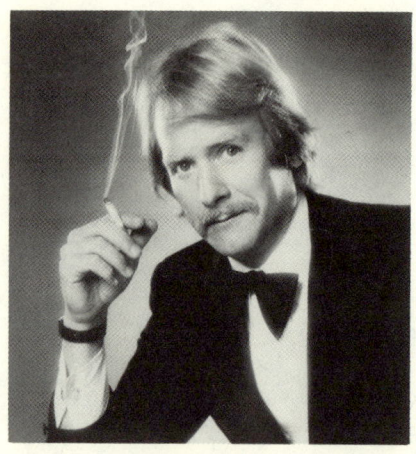

b. August 18, 1943, Chicago, Illinois

Records:
Martin Mull (Capricorn 0106), Martin Mull and His Fabulous Furniture (Capricorn 0117), Normal (Capricorn 0126), Days of Wine and Neuroses (Capricorn 0155), In the Soop (Vanguard 79338), I'm Everyone I've Ever Loved (ABC Records AB 997), Sex and Violins (ABC 1064), Near Perfect (Elektra 6E-200).

Compilation:
No Hits, Four Errors (Capricorn CPN 0195).

TV:
Mary Hartman, Mary Hartman (syndicated 1976–77), Fernwood 2-Night (syndicated 1977), America 2-Night (syndicated 1978), Domestic Life (CBS 1984).

Video:
Seals & Crofts with Martin Mull Live (Media Home Entertainment), Serial (Paramount), My Bodyguard (CBS/Fox).

homey antiques and sang his songs. It worked. The audience did feel at home. But they weren't laughing.

"I wrote my own music," he recalls, "songs about things I was interested in—midgets, people with missing fingers, families who live over their own gas stations. But when I'd sing these songs, the audiences would look at me like the porchlights were dim."

The material, which showed the influences of Randy Newman and Steve Martin, was subtle. There was the song about the poor guy who was in love with a ventriloquist: "Ventriloquist love, it ain't such a groove. Whenever I kiss you your lips never move." Or the fellow who's in love with Margie the Midget: "we go walking hand and ankle down to the dock . . . she's got her arm around my sock." And the one who sings: "I made love to you in a former life, why can't we do it right now?"

These songs, sung in a low-key country style with an occasional hint of 1940's pop, went over the heads of his listeners. His more obvious bits, like playing the theme from *2001: A Space Odyssey* in polka form, or turning "Dueling Banjos" into the liver-churning, gut-busting "Dueling Tubas," were merely deemed quirky.

Mull tried to guide the audience: "I realized I'd have to introduce the tunes, and my tongue sort of went into my cheek, because that's who I am. And out of that, certain things got great laughs and cumulatively built into an act."

While Steve Martin's frustration with his dim audience drove him toward a manic form of obnoxiousness, Martin Mull developed a sly and dry form of arrogance, a defense mechanism that allowed him to dismiss smugly the lack of appreciation from "the dumb-belt contingent." Some critics found the smug ego routine rather pointless, detracting from some of the more whimsical songs, but it certainly gave Mull what he needed to stand up to audience adversity. Slowly but surely, the crowd caught up with him and he developed a cult.

He began making records in 1972 and people were amused by things like "In the Eyes of My Dog I'm a Man" and "Dancing in the Nude" and low-key satires including the almost-serious-sounding "Livin' Above My Station," about a soulful gas station attendant.

His 1973 "Fabulous Furniture Album," with "2001 Polka" and "Ukulele Blues" (a piece for ukulele and baby bottle dedicated to the memory of bluesman Blind Lemon Pledge) helped solidify his reputation. The following year he released "Normal," with sharper satires on race ("The Blacks Are Giving Me the Blues"), religion ("Jesus Christ Football Star") and drinking ("Drunkard's Waltz"). But he didn't neglect a talent for subtle-but-nauseating puns ("I'd love to go to Holland, wooden shoe?").

By 1977 he was a smooth, established act catering to a hip young audience, the same audience that was making a hit out of a deadpan soap opera satire called "Mary Hartman, Mary Hartman." He joined that show in the role of a wife beater who was eventually impaled on an aluminum Christmas tree. He starred as host of the variety spin-offs "Fernwood 2-Night" and "America 2-Night," playing Barth Gimble, brother of the lately impaled Garth Gimble, a character Mull has described as "a guy with a lot of gaping holes in his knowledge. But he doesn't want people to know that, so he glosses them over, like an amateur carpenter using plastic wood."

Mull also turned up as a "Tonight Show" guest host and started making movies. He devoted less time to the satiric songs and albums, which were often more critically successful than financially rewarding. Most of Mull's associates saw the switch coming. Mull had always had a lot of different interests, and it was inevitable he could not be confined to three-minute songs about midgets. Mull had a lot of options right from the start.

Like Jonathan Winters, Mull grew up in Ohio, and the strange normalcy of life there gave him that super-normal twist. After living in North Ridgeville for 12 years, the Mull family made the big move: to North Olmsteed. Martin's father, who once broke an arm falling into a wheelbarrow full of cement blocks, and his mother, a director of community theater plays like *Happiness Is a Thing with Feathers*, were certainly major influences on his humor.

When the family moved to New Canaan, Connecticut, Martin was still living the dream of the All-American boy. A star place-kicker for the football team, he was also a champion pole vaulter. He could have gotten an athletic scholarship, but instead enrolled in the Rhode Island School of Design and spent several months studying art in Rome (the experience turned up in a song that went: "Go to Rome and study art, it seemed so good it seemed so smart. I hate the art I once adored. I'm in Rome and bored."). In 1967 he received his masters degree in painting.

Perhaps the first public sign of Mull's natural tendencies toward the peculiar was his appearance before his draft board. Determined to impress, he Vaselined his hair, brought a homely lunch with him (carrot sticks and celery stalks, each individually foil wrapped) and quaintly gnawed on his fingers while answering questions. When the subject of the draft was brought up, Mull abstractly muttered, "The draft . . . it *is* sort of chilly in here." The board didn't have to take a closer look at this dimwit in the too-tight shirt. They passed him by.

Mull was free to explore art and music. He was in several bands: the Double Standard String Band, the Magical Midget Band and Soup. He dabbled in the stuffy art world, raiding the Boston Museum of Fine Art's men's room and staging with five other artists a show called "Flush with the Walls, or I'll Be Art in a Minute." His paintings were never price-tagged at $200 or $500, but wore bargain tags like "$499.99." Today, Mull's paintings are respected by critics and command thousands of dollars each.

Encouraged by some success in the music field, Mull persevered. In 1970 he gave Jane Morgan a chance to answer "A Boy Named Sue" with "A Girl Named Johnny Cash." Fired from his job as a Warner Brothers songwriter, he had the last laugh, receiving critical praise for the music he wrote for the PBS series "The Great American Dream Machine."

Mull continues to explore the dual worlds of music and art. His comic Yuppie obnoxiousness has made him a natural for TV commercials where he's persuasively pitched soda and pizza. In 1984 he and executive producer Steve Martin cooked up "Domestic Life," a CBS show Mull described as "sort of like 'Leave It To Beaver' on acid. We don't have cars that talk, we don't wreck cars, we don't have wet T-shirt contests, anything you'd think you''d need for a hit." When it wasn't a hit, he moved on to HBO for cable TV specials like "White People in America," a sympathetic look at "the white Anglo-Saxon in his current state." He found that whites were "really just folks like anybody else." Meanwhile audiences have continued to shake their heads, realizing that Mull is like nobody else.

EDDIE MURPHY

The crowd is restless, chanting "Eddie! Eddie!" as he makes his way to the stage, flanked by an entourage of guards and friends. As he stands in the wings, he crosses himself. The crowd keeps chanting, clapping their hands over their heads. At last he runs out on stage, wearing a red

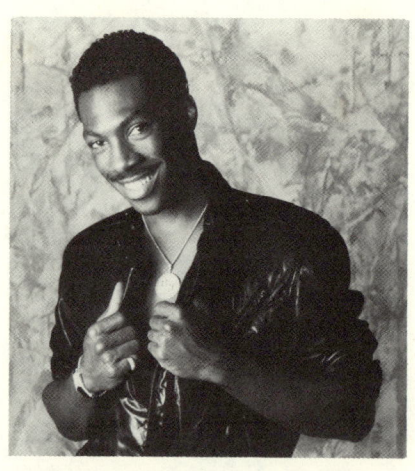

b. April 3, 1961, Brooklyn, New York

Records:
Eddie Murphy (Columbia FC 38180), Eddie Murphy: Comedian (Columbia FC 39005, also available as a picture disc).

Films:
48 Hrs, Trading Places, Beverly Hills Cop.

Video:
Delirious (Columbia), Best of the Big Laff Off (Karl).

leather body suit and gold chains that glimmer against his bare chest. The crowd is delirious. And Eddie Murphy flashes his brightest smile as he struts back and forth from one end of the stage to the other.

The newest heavyweight champ? The latest rock star? The reaction for Murphy, a *comedian*, reflects what can happen when a stand-up incorporates the slick moves of a sports champ, the cocky stance of a rock star and adds hip, good-natured comedy.

"I got rules when I do my stand-up," he tells the crowd. "Faggots aren't allowed to look at my ass while I'm on stage!" His bad-boy comic frankness and mildly funky delivery amuse an audience already on his side.

"That's why I keep movin' while I'm up here. You don't know where the faggot section is so you gotta keep movin'. . . . I'm afraid of the gay people, I'm petrified. . . . Imagine if Mr. T was a fag: 'Now come over here and fuck me up the ass! I'm gonna clench up my butt cheeks and rip your dick off!'"

Murphy starts riffing on sex: "Gonorrhea—your dick hurt, you took a shot. Herpes, you keep that shit forever like luggage. Then AIDS kills people. What's next? You put your dick in and it explodes!"

The comic touches lightly on the kind of minor topics that preoccupy modern comics: parodies of old TV shows like "The Honeymooners," quick impressions of celebrities, some mock-arrogant audience put-down. Then he weaves through more artistic material, from impressions of kiddie hysteria over ice cream to painless but funny jabs at white and black mannerisms. Writer Chet Flippo, commenting on these portrayals of timid whites and arrogant, angry blacks noted that Murphy "appeals to white audiences while doing routines that border on anti-white harangues. During the same act, he can play with hated black stereotypes and keep a black following."

Murphy's appeal is basically in his sense of fun, a stance free of bitterness and filled with honest observation. "Richard Pryor is my idol artistically," says Murphy, alluding to Pryor's fluid, loose style. He adds that he was influenced by Bill Cosby "morally. You never hear any garbage about Cosby. To have the best of both worlds would be ideal."

Murphy's father, a transit officer, and mother, a telephone operator, separated when he was three. His father was shot and killed in 1969 by a girlfriend. His mother remarried and the family moved to Roosevelt, Long Island, where Murphy had a comfortable childhood: "Being black has never been a hindrance to me," he says. "I've been called 'nigger' only once in my life. There's very little anger in my humor . . . my comedy's good-time comedy: conversations and fooling around with my friends, stuff that just happened to me. That's why I poke fun at everybody, 'cause I'm not a racist, I'm not a sexist, I'm just out there. I use racial slurs, but I don't hate anybody."

Some of his race routines are close to the kind of things one might expect to hear from friends goofing around, like his bit about Chinese men who "got little rice dicks." If there's any rap on Murphy, it's that much of his material has the insubstantial feel that is endemic to any "life of the party."

Murphy listened to Cosby albums and George Carlin lps, and at school he was the "life of the cafeteria" for his impressions of singers like Al Green, and for his ability to make up "rank jokes" on his schoolmates. His funny put-downs gained him an audience. By the time he was 15 he was hosting talent shows and trying out routines on stage at the Roosevelt High School Auditorium, youth centers and even local bars.

He began to do "A Tribute to Richard Pryor" as a good excuse for stealing entire routines from albums. Slowly he evolved into a Cosby-Pryor hybrid, and amused audiences with cool humor as well as some sting. Not that the hybrid was always appreciated—part of the Pryor side included a lot of cursing, and many have objected to that—even Bill Cosby, who warned him early in his career that it was unnecessary.

"I could do my stand-up without cursing," Murphy told Dick Cavett once. "I just like to curse. Not like to. That's the way I talk. It's not like I write a comedy routine and I need a word here and I say 'Mmmm, fuck would be nice.'"

Under his high school yearbook picture appear these words: "All men are sculptors, constantly chipping away the unwanted parts of their lives, trying to create their idea of a masterpiece." Murphy was a confident chipster. While still in his teens he went off to try his luck in such New York City comedy shops as "The Comic Strip." There he impressed club coowner Robert Wachs, who became his manager. "From his earliest appearances," Wachs recalls, "Eddie had an amazing confidence on stage, a tremendous smile, an infectious laugh, a vulnerability, a likability."

Wachs heard that "Saturday Night Live" was looking for one last addition to its cast. The only stipulation was that he be black. Murphy auditioned, and he was impressive by any criterion. He joined the show in the 1980–81 season at $750 a week. He caught on a few months later, growing into the show, getting a chance to perform some monologues.

One of the few bright spots on a deteriorating program, Murphy's lively humor was a stark contrast to the obnoxiousness of most other cast members. His parodies of Mister Rogers, Stevie Wonder and Gumby were cheered to the point where he became tired of doing them. The show's producer felt he was becoming conceited; or, putting it lower, he told Murphy, "Your butt's getting big."

Murphy answered, "That's 'cause I get fucked in it every night." He was tired of the show's 1pm–3am rehearsal schedule, more interested in doing stand-up concerts and films. In movies he scored immediately with *48 Hrs.* When Gene Wilder and Richard Pryor turned down *Trading Places*, Murphy and Dan Aykroyd turned it into one of the top-grossing hits of 1983.

"I can't wait to leave," he said of "Saturday Night Live." "I don't like the show. I don't think the show is funny. I hate it." He was receiving $20,000 per show when he left. With Paramount, he signed a five-picture deal for $15 million.

1983 was Murphy's big year. Aside from *Trading Places*, he earned two gold albums and sold out an 18-city, 37-show tour. His "anti-gay" cable TV special was controversial, but for most the sassy street-corner conman could do no wrong. Murphy sold the rights to a video cassette version for a quick $250,000. Most recognized that Murphy's gay remarks were simply part of his cheerful desire to outrage, the same way he was allowed to mock Stevie Wonder's blindness by describing a ride he took, supposedly telling the superstar, "Stevie, you don't impress me. You want to impress me, Stevie? Take the fuckin' wheel!" He made fun of people who called him tasteless. Imitating an angry brother's reaction to the Wonder routine, he caricatured the man's huffy "Yo! Quit fuckin' with Stevie man, I'm gonna fuck you up!"

Though Murphy's popularity turned into a delerious fad (there would be so much gratuitous laughter greeting him that he'd have to shout "Calm down, I ain't even said shit yet!") he's always had a less than delerious point of view about taking care of himself. He's serious about not smoking, not drinking and staying away from drugs. And he's aware that, like Steve Martin and Robin Williams, the fad appeal can end as easily as it began. He knows that no amount of audience euphoria can last without solid material to fall back on. With "unfunny stuff I have no tricks. I bomb. Everybody bombs. Your mood can be messed around that night. When you first come out the audience accepts you, but if you don't feel like performing, or you bomb, they start hating you."

Murphy's fans love him so much that they lined up all night for tickets to his series of concerts at Radio City Music Hall in February of 1985. The lowest priced ticket was $20, yet the mammoth Music Hall was sold out for five shows in less than one day. It was the fastest sale in the theater's history, outdistancing previous quick sell-outs for Diana Ross and Barry Manilow.

Beverly Hills Cop grossed over $150 million in 1985, though most critics agreed with Liz Smith that ". . . it's not even honestly very funny. The audience is laughing at Eddie Murphy saying 'Bleep!' and 'Man!' over and over and they're also laughing along with his famous hyena laugh." Meanwhile, Murphy was off trying to secure a more meaningful follow-up film. He negotiated with Charles Chaplin's widow for the right to re-make *The Kid*.

These days comedians wear out their welcome quicker than ever—almost as quick as flash-in-the-pan rock stars. But Murphy enjoys the pace of stand-up comedy, film work, even some rock singing thrown in. "Nothing's been happening so fast I can't deal with it," he says.

JAN MURRAY

"Tastes have changed," says Jan Murray. "Today many comics appeal to young audiences, and the material is, to me, unfortunately, often drug-oriented and sex-oriented. It's almost sadistic. The audiences are being put down. In my day put-down humor was mostly about ourselves—I'd do jokes about how thin I was, how dumb I was. Now it's directed at ethnic groups, other groups, politicians. My comedy has always been gentler."

Gentle, but with a bit of an Alan King-type sting, Jan Murray continues to find an audience in nightclubs and casinos, offering both standard wife, airplane and gambling jokes and topical humor: "Russia needs our wheat. After all, you can't expect them to invade a country on an empty stomach."

Murray's mother was often ill, and early on he discovered that comedy was a way to keep a smile on her face. He joked in school, too, but quit high school for a more lucrative occupation: Borscht Belt funnyman. He worked his way through the Catskill circuit where he did monologues and experimented with audience participation gags. One of the standards that Murray worked with an audience member was a waiter-customer bit. As the waiter, he would tell the good sport playing the customer, "We have two kinds of soup: chicken and pea."

The customer was told to first order chicken, and then change his mind. "I'll take the chicken soup," the customer would say. "Okay, one chicken soup coming up." "Wait—I've changed my mind. I'll have the pea soup." "Okay," Murray would yell offstage to the kitchen, "hold the chicken—and make it pea!"

Murray found himself ad-libbing and joking with strangers often: as a quiz show host. Although he had his own brief variety series, co-starring

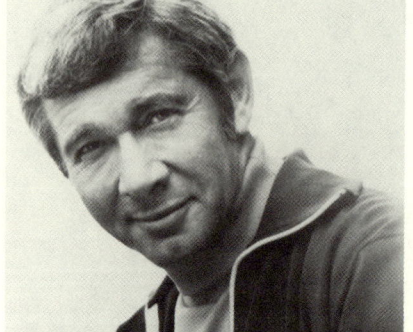

b. Murray Janofsky, October 4, 1917, Bronx, New York

TV:
Blind Date (Dumont 1953), Songs for Sale (CBS 1950), Sing It Again (CBS 1950–51), Go Lucky (CBS 1951), Dollar a Second (Dumont 1953; NBC 1954; ABC 1955–56; NBC 1957), Jan Murray Time (NBC 1955), The Jan Murray Show (NBC 1960–62), Treasure Hunt (ABC 1956–57; NBC 1957–59), Chain Letter (NBC 1966).

Films:
Who Killed Teddy Bear?, Thunder Alley, The Busy Body.

Tina Louise, it was in quiz shows that he was seen throughout the 1950's and 60's. Like other emcees from Johnny Carson to Garry Moore, Murray found that his background as a comic helped him succeed with game shows. He kept up light-hearted repartee and a feeling of good humor.

Over the decades practically every type of game show was hosted by Murray. In 1953 a woman could meet her future husband on "Blind Date," picking one of the offered contestants. In 1954 folks had to perform odd stunts if they missed a question on "Dollar a Second." In 1957 it was a "Treasure Hunt" for one of 30 boxes on stage containing a prize. And there were word quizzes and name-the-tune quizzes mixed in as well.

Meanwhile Murray maintained a steady stand-up career, was a safe and sturdy guest on TV variety shows and continued to be a consistent nightclub draw with jokes anyone could appreciate: "Sorry I'm late . . . that stupid wife of mine—she didn't shovel the snow from the driveway this morning. Forgot to put on the snow tires—and halfway to New York I realized she hadn't dressed me."

In 1965 he turned up as a detective in the lurid thriller *Who Killed Teddy Bear?* which offered the semi-dressed Juliet Prowse and peeping psycho-killer Sal Mineo. The film offered Murray a rare opportunity to play a leading role, and the ruggedly attractive Murray made the most of it, turning in a very credible performance. Unfortunately the film was apparently too offbeat and low-budget to gain a wide audience or lead to other major film roles.

Murray continues to fit firmly into the "rotation" of middle-of-the-road comics like Alan King and David Brenner, who appear regularly in clubs and casinos. His polished routines have made him perennially welcome.

BOB NEWHART

The late 1950's was the time for hip comics and sickos. Mort Sahl and Nichols and May were redefining the style for satire. Shelley Berman was studying Freud. Jonathan Winters was flying over the cuckoo's nest.

In Chicago, an accountant named Bob Newhart was supplementing his income by writing and performing comedy sketches on radio. One year he actually made a thousand dollars at this "hobby." He might have remained comfortably pigeon-holed on the anonymous airwaves of mid-America except for another 1950's phenomenon. Not only were comics big—so were comedy albums.

Newhart's radio style was a natural for records. His material was fresh and different. His "button-down mind" was creating cool, calculated and controlled sketches, satiric but in a new way. Newhart wasn't Lenny Bruce or Shelley Berman, shaking up or lecturing the audience. Newhart was part of the audience himself, gently mirroring the faults and foibles of the unassuming average man.

Few were more unassuming than bland Bob, who came from a stable Chicago household, attended St. Ignatius High School and graduated from Loyola University in 1952. When some of his comedy radio tapes found their way to Warner Brothers Records, Warners assumed Newhart was ready to become its star comic, opposite the Verve roster of wits.

But there was a problem. Newhart had never done stand-up before a live audience. It took persuasion and a push to get him before a hand-

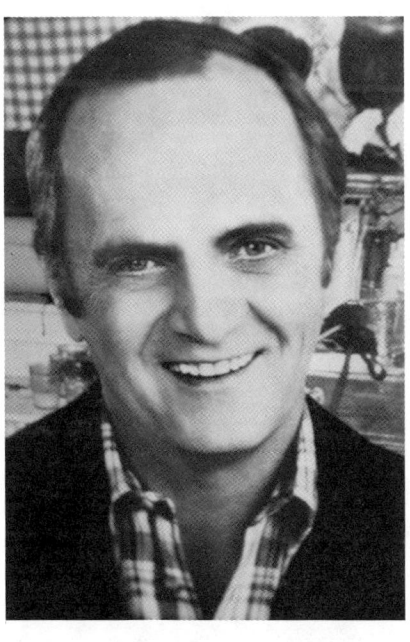

b. George Robert Newhart, September 5, 1929, Oak Park, Illinois

Records:
The Button-Down Mind (Warner Brothers W 1379), The Button-Down Mind Strikes Back (Warner Brothers W 1393), Behind the Button-Down Mind (Warner Brothers W 1417), The Button-Down Mind on TV (Warner Brothers W 1467), Bob Newhart Faces Bob Newhart (Warner Brothers W 1517), Windmills Are Weakening (Warner Brothers W 1588), This Is It (Warner Brothers W 1717), Bob Newhart Deluxe Edition (his first two lps with souvenir booklet) (Warner Brothers 2N 1399), Best of Bob Newhart (Warner Brothers W 1672), Very Funny Bob Newhart (Harmony 11344).

TV:
The Bob Newhart Show (NBC 1961–62), The Bob Newhart Show (CBS 1972–78), Newhart (CBS 1982–   ).

Films:
Catch-22, Cold Turkey, The First Family.

Video:
The First Family (Warner Video).

picked audience in the small Tidelands Club in Houston. Even then, it took a few tries to get a usable complete performance.

Newhart may have been a basket-case at the time, but it's hard to tell from the results. His characters were mildly nervous anyway. Hiding behind set pieces, going from routine to routine, his shyness was an endearing example of vulnerability. The audience responded, even under such awkward conditions, with loud, appreciative laughter. Newhart proved that with good material (and a bit of prior experience in radio) he could indeed make the transition to stand-up.

Released in 1960, Newhart's first album offered historical "what ifs," a favorite device of his. These included Abraham Lincoln coached for the Gettysburg Address, Abner Doubleday laughed at for inventing a complex game called baseball, and the merchandising of the Wright Brothers. Newhart's other favorite device, the nervous monologue sketch, was exemplified by the classic "Driving Instructor" routine, with Newhart as a harried man whose life is in the hands of an outrageously inept student driver.

Many of Newhart's sketches involved average men of the old generation trying to deal with the machinery of the brave new 60's: airplanes, advertising agencies, even unexploded bombs. He didn't attack modern times, like Shelley Berman. Newhart merely questioned modern times. A cop confronts a suicidal man on a building ledge with, "First time?" A hapless soul pinned to his chair by a huge dog asks his host, "You got him from the Army, did you? Whose Army?" And when that unexploded bomb appears on the beach, an official remarks to the frantic telephone caller, "You think that's unusual, finding a shell on the beach?"

The humor of these deadpanned questions was matched by the solutions. Trying to defuse the bomb, the official looks into a coffee-stained manual and mutters, "One wire is kind of a bluish gray, and the other . . . kind of a grayish blue." And as time ticks away, the bureaucrat tells his assistant, "If that thing goes off it's me they'll want to talk to, not you."

Only 15 gold records were issued in 1960, and Newhart had one of them. He was also voted "Best New Artist" at the Grammy Awards and his was "Album of the Year." Over a million and a half copies of "The Button-Down Mind" were sold, and his follow-up won a Grammy as well.

Newhart conquered most of his performing worries but remained uneasy with fame. The father of three lived a calm, quiet life, going on stage to portray the understated everyman caught in embarrassing situations, injecting strong satire into his routines about the ad men, PR men, and fools who would've interfered with the destinies of Lincoln and Sir Walter Raleigh.

Despite its weaknesses, his third album hit #12 on the charts. 1962 saw "The Bob Newhart Show" on NBC—briefly. He wasn't happy with the limits imposed by the network: "Those who control the medium are obsessed with the notion that if they offend even one viewer, they have one less customer. What the TV biggies don't know is that people like entertainment with bite. They want satire. The growth of the talking-record sales proves that. When the public couldn't get satire on TV it turned to records . . . satire on TV could be the next TV trend."

He was right, just eight years too soon. Still, his short-lived show won an Emmy, and the subsequent album of his TV work was his finest, including "The Introduction of Tobacco to Civilization," wherein a telephone call from Sir Walter Raleigh prompts skeptical laughter in England:

"Are you saying 'snuff,' Walt? What's snuff? You take a pinch of tobacco (starts giggling) and you shove it up your nose! And it makes you sneeze, huh. I imagine it would, Walt, yeah. Goldenrod seems to do it pretty well over here. It has some other uses, though. You can chew it? Or put it in a pipe. Or you can shred it up and put it on a piece of paper, and roll it up—don't tell me, Walt, don't tell me—you stick it in your ear, right, Walt? Oh, between your lips! Then what do you do to it? (Giggling) You set fire to it! Then what do you do, Walt? You inhale the smoke! Walt, we've been a little worried about you . . . you're gonna have a tough time getting people to stick burning leaves in their mouth. . . ."

Said H. Allen Smith, "That thing about tobacco and cigarettes is possibly the greatest single comedy routine I've seen or heard in my entire life."

Newhart salved his TV ego bruises by playing Vegas at $35,000 a week. Reflecting the tastes of the Vegas crowd he did routines about nudist camps and topless clubs as well as sharp bits like "The Man Who Looked Like Hitler."

In 1964 Newhart and Carol Burnett starred in the ill-fated variety show "The Entertainers." Newhart returned to nightclubs, became a relaxed, amusing guest on talk shows and appeared in movies, as the bureaucratic Major Major in *Catch-22* and then as the Madison Avenue wiseguy of *Cold Turkey*.

Newhart's last album, appropriately titled "This Is It," might explain another reason for his gradual move away from stand-up. The liner notes report that "Newhart's slow-created tales come uncommonly hard-born . . . the routines in this album have been gestating around in Newhart's creativity for periods ranging from six months to six years." And for all that, the lp lasted 13 minutes on one side, just 10 on the other.

In 1972 Newhart starred in his own situation comedy. As psychologist Bob Hartley, Newhart once more portrayed an everyman type, but instead of a solo in stand-up, he played against a cast of overly extroverted morons. Deadpan, low-key, good-natured and only mildly caustic with his overweening wife, idiot neighbors and glum patients, Newhart reflected the 70's, when people were trying to be tolerant in life, using the pop-psychology formulas they were learning from the era's bestselling self-help books. A typical "I'm ok, you're ok" exchange with his wife went like this: "Bob, do you love me?" "Sure," "Why?" "Why not?"

The show was a minor gem, and like its powerful lead-in, "The Mary Tyler Moore Show," it lasted until its star felt it was going to wear out its welcome.

"I'd heard it's boring to play golf 365 days a year, but I'd like to find out for myself," he said after the series ended. Within a short time, he was appearing again on talk shows, at dinner theaters and in movie houses: "When I saw the script for the movie *First Family*, I was bowled over. It was hilarious. It couldn't miss. I don't think it ever showed in theaters. They put it on airplanes the first night. But if I were to see a script like that again, I'd do it."

Newhart resumed his chores in sit-com in 1982, scoring once again with a high rated series. He insisted on performing before a live audience to make sure the laughs were genuine, and coming in the expected places. Whether performing in sketches or stand-up, his point of view on the audience remains the same: "There's no drug in the world as depressing as a routine that doesn't work. The audience is saying they don't like you. On the other hand, I can't imagine a better feeling than when they're having a good time and it's because of me. Controlling an audience like that gives you a real feeling of power, and power is what this business is about."

He told Johnny Carson, after some 20 years in the business, "Singers come and go. But as long as people do stupid things, we comedians will always be around."

NICHOLS AND MAY

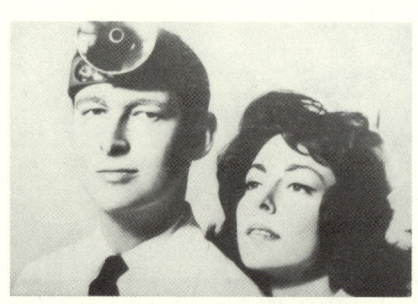

MIKE NICHOLS b. Michael Peschkowsky, November 6, 1931, Berlin, Germany
ELAINE MAY b. Elaine Berlin, April 21, 1932, Philadelphia, Pennsylvania

Records:
An Evening with Nichols and May (Mercury OCM 2200), Nichols and May Examine Doctors (Mercury MG 20680), Improvisations to Music (Mercury SR 60040), Best of Nichols and May (Mercury SR 60997), Retrospect (Mercury SRM 2 628).

When Mike Nichols, who studied acting under Lee Strasberg, and Elaine May, who learned the Stanislavsky method from Maria Ouspenskaya, joined forces, they created humor by acting out characters. They brought the actor's gut emotion to these comic creations, and there was a seriousness in their comedy that went beyond the dedication of two actors trying to portray, in all their intensity, the raw emotions and inner flaws that lead to moments of serio-comic truth. When Nichols and May zeroed in, they didn't satirize only the superficial voices and mannerisms of their targets, they tried to get at the motives and emotions at the core.

Nichols's father, Dr. Paul Peschkowsky, fled the harrowing Nazi death purges in Germany and migrated to New York. Nichols attended some of the better, neurosis-producing private schools in New York before going on to the University of Chicago to study medicine.

Elaine May's father, Yiddish actor Jack Berlin, took her with him on a bewildering series of road tours around the country. From an early age she was on the stage, neglecting her schooling to appear in plays.

She enjoyed the fantasy world of the theater and her own world of far-off fairy tales and fanciful legends discovered in books. At the University of Chicago she met Mike Nichols, and was often seen attending some of the more interesting classes, though few realized that she was not officially enrolled.

Nichols and May were part of an improvisational group, The Compass Players. They developed a talent for routines based more on an intimate understanding of character than on a desire to dazzle with gratuitous, ad-libbed jokes. In the cabaret environment, away from the more traditional nightclub settings and impatient audiences, they didn't go for the quick laugh. Instead they created mini-plays using a form of acidic satire that subtly burned and sizzled until, seven minutes later, both target and satirist were reduced to ashes. Funny? Not necessarily, but satire doesn't often produce belly laughs. Satire comes from behind gritted teeth or twisted lips, and the belly laugh is more often just a slightly painful twinge from deep in the gut.

"Mother and Son," one of their best-known routines, is nothing but a study of the psychic destruction of a guilty son by his manipulative mother. She doesn't stop until the grown man has literally regressed into infancy. The "Jewish Mother" theme has since become a cliche, but in the late 1950's this routine was innovative, a rare display of pathos on the comic stage, pathos at its most pathetic. The audience could ruefully recognize the devices the mother uses for manipulation, and giggle over each twist of the knife. The problems begin when the son fails to call home:

"I didn't have a second," the guilty man explains. "I could cut my throat. I was so busy."

"I sat by that phone all day Friday, all day Saturday, and all day Sunday," the mother mourns. "Your father said to me, 'Phyllis, eat something, you'll faint.' I said, 'No, Harry, no, I don't want my mouth to be full when my son calls me!'"

The mother reveals that she is sick, "you know what it is . . . it's my nerves. And I went to the doctor . . . I told him . . . I have this son . . . he's too busy to pick up a phone and call his mother. When I said that to him, that man turned pale!"

Mother and son continue to joust. The mother will go to the hospital ("they'll x-ray my nerves"). The son tries to be firm, to counter the outrageous hypochondria, the demands for attention. He keeps trying to explain that he's needed at his job—helping to launch the Vanguard missile. His mother will hear none of it: "Someday, someday, Arthur, you'll get married and you'll have children of your own, and honey, when you do, I only pray that they make you suffer! That's a mother's prayer . . . I'm sorry that I bothered you . . . I hope I didn't make you feel bad."

"Are you kidding? I feel awful!"

"Oh, honey, if I could believe that I'd be the happiest mother in the world!"

She gently, cloyingly breaks him down, eventually telling him, "You're my baby. You'll always be my baby . . . I worry . . . is it so hard to pick up a phone and call your mommy? Please baby. . . ."

The son, his voice taking on the numb, mechanical edge of a child repeating what the mother wants to hear, says, "I promise . . . I love you, Mommy."

"Goodbye, baby."

"Goodbye, Mommy!"

This kind of satiric psychodrama left some critics exhilarated, others reverential, but a few questioning the team's viciousness in ripping at some of the rawest nerves in man's psyche. "We're not bitter people," Nichols said in defense. "We're not working out our personal revenges. The problem is to draw the line between satire and nastiness." He insisted that the Nichols and May routines were not quite so premeditated, merely born of improvisation: "Neither of us knows what's going to happen. Somehow, just about the time in the development of a scene, we both sense which way we're going. . . ."

Although the duo favored improvisation, fans enjoyed some of their most famous, enduring routines, like "The Disc Jockey" (a satire of name-dropping and showbiz insincerity) and "The Telephone." The latter is a grinding seven-minute Kafkaesque study; a man discovers he has lost his last dime in a public telephone and is led through maddening, weakening conversations with a variety of telephone company authority figures, alternately cold-hearted and histrionically maternal.

Another well-known routine concerns a distraught man trying to arrange a funeral, only to be victimized by a conniving saleswoman who keeps finding "extras" to charge him for. To keep this particular black comedy bearable, the team overplay their parts, the woman too efficient, the man wavering tearfully. They even add funny names (Nichols is Charlie Maslow-Freen of Southeast Huguenot Walloon Drive) to underline the element of absurdity.

Most Nichols and May sketches score vividly despite the absence of quotable jokes, remaining memorable for the comic situation and the human emotions humorously, harrowingly portrayed. Some of their one-liners are almost non-jokes, like the memorable line in a dialogue between two empty, ennui-filled conversationalists, where one muses mightily, "I can never believe that Bartok died on Central Park West."

The team made a few studio albums which were mostly situational and devoid of jokes. One bit, "A Little More Gauze," is a tense study of a doctor and nurse trying to remain professional as they feud over the apparent end of their affair. In desperation, the doctor refuses to complete the operation, holding the patient's life at ransom. The nurse eventually capitulates and the doctor pointedly adds romance to his instructions: "Clamp . . . darling."

An Evening of Nichols and May ran over 300 performances on Broadway after opening on October 8, 1960. The duo also entertained radio audiences, appearing weekly on NBC's "Monitor" program.

Nichols and May weren't alone in developing "non-joke" humor. Lenny Bruce offered stream-of-consciousness ad-libbing, and Shelley Berman explored pathos. But they were among the first to carve out new concepts of satire for others to follow. And professionally, they took a serious artistic stance. They bypassed the 1960 Emmy Awards show when they were asked to abandon a sketch that lampooned a sponsor's product. They refused to overextend themselves on variety shows, and ceased guest appearances on one program because they felt the show had grown stale. They retained their integrity and their goals, and when these goals no longer included comedy, they broke up, eventually finding success in films, on stage and behind the scenes.

"We had to end it while we could still face each other," Nichols said. "We just got bored. We're both very restless types."

Nichols made a splash directing The Graduate in 1966. He has since directed many important and interesting movies, as well as establishing a name for himself as a director on Broadway. May's career as a writer and director began to take off with A New Leaf, and she, too, has an impressive list of credits since going solo.

Nichols and May have maintained contact with each other. Some years ago they performed together at New Haven's Long Wharf Theatre, playing George and Martha in Who's Afraid of Virginia Woolf. In the Spring of 1985 they signed to appear with Joan Rivers to appear in "Comedy Relief," a Broadway evening with profits going to raise funds for fighting Acquired Immune Deficiency Syndrome. Chances of more than sporadic reunions of the two remains slim. Their old records, two and a half decades later, still keep their names linked and still have a great appeal for many listeners who have found that the problems the duo satirized are still, for the most part, with us.

RICHARD PRYOR

In the late 1960's, a skinny, worried-looking black kid named Richard Pryor turned up on "The Ed Sullivan Show." He did standard bits like a routine about dating: "Ever try to check yourself out?" he asked, pantomiming a nervous date sniffing his own armpits and breathing into his hand to check for bad breath. With the audience giggling mildly he added,

"Deodorants are dangerous, man. Ever read on deodorant cans: 'Caution, contents highly inflammable. May explode.' I don't know about you people, but I don't want nothin' under my arm that's gonna explode!"

Funny, but not funky. A real situation, but not reality. Although he'd "made it," Pryor grew dissatisfied with being "just another young Ed

Sullivan Show comic," a junior Bill Cosby at best. He began passing up invitations to appear on the show. He began sprinkling his live act with obscenities and had run-ins with club management. As the 60's ended, so did Pryor's career as a standard stand-up. Fed up with agents, managers, show business people, corny audiences and safe humor, he walked offstage in mid-act at the Aladdin in Las Vegas.

Gone were the standard gags and the pat, acceptably broad race jokes: "Look! Up in the sky! It's a crow. It's a bat. It's Supernigger! Yes, friends, Supernigger. Faster than a bowl of chitlins . . . Supernigger's X-ray vision enables him to see through everything—except Whitey."

Pryor eventually turned up in small black clubs, trying out experimental, uninhibited comedy. He switched off the slick highway of shtick and returned to the trail of honest humor blazed by Lenny Bruce. "Lenny was alone," Pryor once said. "He was way ahead of his time. There is so much shit happening because of guys like Lenny." But he added, "it really doesn't make much sense to make another martyr."

He offered up a conversational style of monologue, a ramble that managed to hit all sorts of topics. On bodily functions: "We all fart. That's human. You don't fart, you blow your brains out!" On women: "You either fuck or fight, one or the other." On race:

"Niggers and white people fight. I'll always be rooting for the nigger, even if he bad. Please whup the white folks, I don't want the white folks to win. Even Jerry West—I wish that motherfucker couldn't play. I seen him make niggers look ridiculous."

Like Lenny, Pryor was sometimes funny, sometimes not. He could be obnoxious, pointlessly vulgar and rambling as easily as he could be raunchy, satiric or clownish with dozens of facial expressions and voices. His most telling characterizations were parodies of whites that often veered into deliberate racism and parodies of the winos, junkies and street people he had known since childhood.

Pryor doesn't discuss his early years often, and rarely does so with nostalgia. He grew up in a broken home, spending some time with his grandmother—in her brothel. He was a teenage father (Melissa, the first of four children, was born in 1957) and got into trouble in almost every way a street kid could. He showed some talent in school plays and performed at the Carver Community Center in Peoria. After Army service, he worked as an emcee and comedian at local clubs in Illinois and in Canada before heading for New York in the early 60's.

But it was the 70's version of Richard Pryor that won a huge following. He'd released one album and had some good earlier Vegas and TV credits, but it was only in the 70's that he became a major star with his truthful, sometimes painful raps about sex, drugs and social problems.

While he was perfecting his new style of monologues with diligent try-outs in small comedy shops, he was earning praise for his writing. He won a 1973 Emmy for his work on a Lily Tomlin special, and in 1974 worked with Mel Brooks on *Blazing Saddles.* That year he won a Grammy for his platinum album "That Nigger's Crazy," which was such a success it crossed over from the intended black audience to whites as well.

Whites found in Pryor a black man who could do devastating parodies of white mannerisms, who had a raw sense of satire on race that was shocking, intimidating, but intriguing. Younger whites were especially drawn to this new Lenny Bruce who was offering unsparing and exciting insights into the black experience, talking in a new way (not Lenny jazz, but Pryor black slang) and adding unbridled and uncensored humor.

Pryor ridiculed thin-lipped whites who were too stiff and hung up to

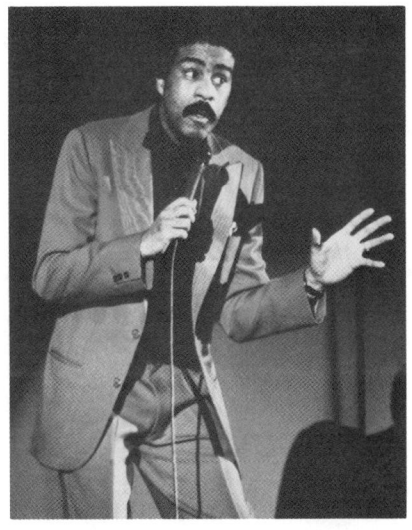

b. December 1, 1940, Peoria, Illinois

Records:
That Nigger's Crazy (Reprise MS 2241), Is It Something I Said (Reprise 2285), Bicentennial Nigger (Warner 3114), Wanted (Warner 2BSK3364), Live on Sunset Strip (Warner BSK3660), Here and Now (Warner 23981-1), Richard Pryor (Reprise 6325), Greatest Hits (Warner 3057).

TV:
The Richard Pryor Show (NBC 1977), Pryor's Place (CBS 1984).

Films:
Lady Sings the Blues, Silver Streak, The Wiz, Wholly Moses, Bustin' Loose, Wild in the Streets, Wattstax, The Bingo Long Traveling All-Star and Motor Kings, Car Wash, Stir Crazy, Superman III, Brewster's Millions.

Video:
Live and Smokin' (Vestron), Live on Sunset Strip (Columbia), Here and Now (RCA), Live in Concert (Vestron), Lily Tomlin Special (Karl), Saturday Night Live (Warner Video).

Bios:
This Cat's Got 9 Lives (Robbins and Ragan), Delilah, Black and Blue (Rovin), Richard Pryor (Nazel), A Man and His Madness (Haskins).

laugh loudly and enjoy life. He ridiculed the prissiness of a white man cursing, and imagined white people's amours: "Think we'll be having sexual intercourse this evening?" He compared "white folks [who] fuck quiet" to the black version: "Niggers make noise: Oh you motherfucker! God damn!"

Far from being suppressed, Pryor was lauded by critics, encouraged to be even wilder, more biting, blatantly racist, closer to the edge. His improvisations, facial contortions, sly imitations and rich slang lingo turned up on a steady stream of records. These included Grammy winners in 1974, 1975 and 1976, and a series of poorly recorded reissues from Laff Records, which Pryor hinted were not authorized.

People magazine called Pryor "the most imaginative and ferocious social critic in show business, the black ghost of Lenny Bruce." The suggestion was that Pryor might literally become a black ghost, that he was doomed to Lenny Brucian self-destruction.

Every comic has his influences, and Pryor's link to Bruce is obvious. Both were lone social satirists of their respective ages, both were undisciplined in their private lives, both took drugs and both favored truthful, free-form raps.

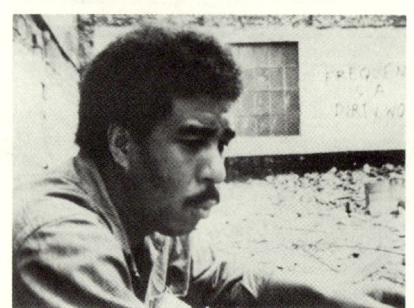

Lenny talked about stag movies being illegal, but the violent *Psycho* allowable. Pryor echoed, "You can't talk about fucking, but if you talk about killing, that's cool. I can't understand it myself. I'd rather come."

Bruce did a bit on the words "to come," saying "if those words offend you—you probably can't come." Pryor added, "I ain't never been mad cummin' . . . some people don't cum. I know President Nixon don't cum. If he does, he apologizes."

Bruce: "I'm going to piss on you . . . some of the ringsiders have objected to the bit. . . ." Pryor: "When the show don't be funny, I take out my dick and piss."

Just as Bruce became entangled in drugs and prosecution, Pryor tumbled into his own pit of drugs and perceived persecution. Each year saw new headlines: ten-day jail sentence for tax evasion, $100,000 lawsuit for beating up a motel clerk, furor over anti-gay slurs (he claimed gays were cruising for sex on Sunset Boulevard while Watts burned), a domestic melee ending with bullets being fired into his Buick while his fifth wife ducked for cover.

Pryor was tacitly encouraged in much of this. As the angry black comic, he was expected to be offensive on talk shows and didn't disappoint. Some interviewers condescended to him, which only fueled his rage the way indulgent parents inflame a tantrum-prone child. Thrown interview questions guaranteed to provoke an outburst, he exploded. Once he intimated the need to "kill some white people" in South Africa, and he regularly dished out racist comments for the public prints.

In 1977, NBC brought Pryor to TV for a proposed series of ten shows. His outrageousness was too much for them. Their censorship was too much for *him*. In one sketch he fought back, putting on a sexless body suit designed to show that he'd "given up absolutely nothing" to NBC— except his balls. NBC clipped that segment out, and it ended up broadcast as a news item all over the country. After five shows, NBC and Pryor called it quits.

The ghost of Lenny, the demons inside Pryor, a comic mind sizzling in the midst of red-hot fame, psychic pain, confusion, drugs . . . something had to happen.

On June 9, 1980, it did. Pryor's spree of rage, outrage, box office success, high comedy and wild living nearly came to a fiery end forever. Attempting to "freebase"cocaine, Pryor set off a sudden inferno that engulfed him in flames. He raced out into the street a human torch, his upper body afire.

At the hospital he was given a 30% chance of survival. Newspapers headlined "Richard Pryor Near Death." But Pryor held on. The grim ordeal lasted for months, but during that time he saw, perhaps for the first time, that people cared. He was deluged with fan letters, celebrities like Jim Brown lent their time and support, and critics, no longer wanting him to flirt at the edge of destruction, were now talking about his great comic genius.

In the wake of the accident, Pryor's movie *Stir Crazy* became the third highest grossing film of the year. It was an important cross-over film for him. But for stand-up, his "performance" movies remain milestones. For the first time, a filmed one-man show became a box office smash. And each of his performance movies since has been a success.

Before Pryor, it was unheard of to give a stand-up comic an entire movie or TV show in which to demonstrate his art. After Pryor, cable and TV network hours of solo comics became common. Although Lenny Bruce's "Performance Film" was there first, it was hardly big box office. It was Pryor who gave this final measure of respect to stand-up as an art form.

On stage Pryor's humor was as sharp as ever after the accident, but more philosophical and tolerant. "White people didn't come to see me till I burnt up," he joked. But his racially mixed audience and new acceptance led him toward new directions in comedy. He could wring laughter from tears, from the literal pain of the fire. He did bits on his hospitalization, even frisky ribaldry:

"Strange people say God was punishing me. If God wanted to punish my ass, he would've burnt my dick. When the fire hit, my dick went to work: Emergency! Piss! Come! Do something! Don't let the fire get to the balls!"

There was more vulnerability in Pryor, and it showed in his routines on understanding women, sharing the fright and insecurity behind macho behavior. He handled racial humor with more tact. Yet he remained outrageous. On drugs: "They call it an epidemic—because white people are doin' it." On Ronald Reagan: "The motherfucker looked at me like I owed him money. He look like a dick. Not a hardon, just a dick with clothes on."

"There's been a whole lie that comics can't be funny unless they're unhappy," Pryor has said. "It's a shame to think that way because it's not true. You don't have to be miserable to be successful. You don't have to take drugs and drink yourself to death or act irrational or be different on purpose to be anything. It's a shame to think of all the wonderful artists who acted their lives away. They never stopped to get hold of themselves."

He's been thrown lows, highs, and now more consistent highs. He received six consecutive Grammy nominations. His box office hits have vindicated Columbia's $40 million contract with him, once considered reckless.

"I don't have the energy anymore to act angry," he told journalist Tony Brown. "I don't want to play a game with my life anymore." The fire incident gave him a new life, but "I got scared. I didn't know I had a problem. I tried the drug again. Back in the same thing. Better get some help. And I did. Everything was fine except real life. It was nobody's fault—*mine*." Evaluating himself, he added, "A 44-year-old burn-up—literally burnt up black uneducated man living in so-called racist America—how's it possible to be where I am unless there's a God?"

REINER AND BROOKS

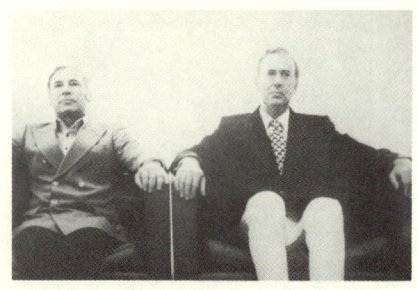

CARL REINER b. March 20, 1922, New York, New York
MEL BROOKS b. Melvin Kaminsky, June 28, 1926, Brooklyn, New York

Records:
Best of the 2000 Year Old Man (Capitol ST 2981), 2000 Years with Carl Reiner and Mel Brooks (Capitol SW 1529), 2000 and One Years (Capitol SW 1618), Reiner and Brooks at the Cannes Film Festival (Capitol SW 1815), The Incomplete Works of Reiner and Brooks (Warner Brothers 3XX 2744), 2013 Year Old Man (Warner Brothers BS 2741).

Video:
The 2000 Year Old Man Cartoon (Media Video), Timex All Star Comedy Show 1962 (Video Yesteryear).

"The funniest record ever made. People used to listen to that record and laugh their guts out. They used to get lockjaw from laughing so much . . . hernias . . . appendicitis . . . cardiac arrest . . . killed a whole family in Iowa, nine people actually died from laughing so much. The relatives tried to sue but they threw it out of court. Couldn't get a judge or a jury to stop laughing once they heard the evidence."

This is Mel Brooks talking about "The 2000 Year Old Man," naturally. Recorded in 1960, the dialogue between an interviewer and a comically blunt old (make that *very* old) Jewish man became an instant classic. And it briefly made a comedy team out of Brooks and Carl Reiner.

They had first worked together a decade earlier when they wrote material for Sid Caesar. At private parties, Reiner and Brooks would often entertain, ad-libbing impromptu interviews.

"During the fifties," Reiner told *The New Yorker*, "we spent our days inventing characters for Caesar, but Mel was really using Caesar as a vehicle. What he secretly wanted was to perform himself. So in the evening we'd go to a party and I'd pick a character for him to play. I never told him what it was going to be, but I always tried for something that would force him to go into panic, because a brilliant mind in panic is a wonderful thing to see . . . there was no end to what he could be—a U-boat commander, a deaf songwriter, an entire convention of antique dealers."

With so many famous comics and producers at these parties, it was only logical that the team be "discovered." And at the insistence of George Burns and Steve Allen, the latter having considerable contacts in the record world, the duo went into a studio, ad-libbed for two hours, and from that produced a hit. For Brooks, a hit was sorely needed:

"The record came out. Saved me. Sold maybe a million copies. And we did two others, 2001 and The Cannes Film Festival." Before the records, Brooks was floundering, unable to find work after the Caesar show folded, unable to save his first marriage. But the 1960–62 Reiner and Brooks albums, and the TV appearances, gave him renewed confidence. "That was a turning point for Mel," Reiner recalled. "It gave him an identity as a performer for the first time."

The popularity of the 2000 Year Old Man character even led to commercials, where Brooks became the 2500 Year Old Brewmaster. But for the two men who grew up in Brooklyn and the Bronx, there were new worlds to conquer, and no way they could stay together as a team after the TV appearances promoting the records.

Brooks won an Oscar for his cartoon short *The Critic*, and began work on *The Producers*. Reiner was busy with "The Dick Van Dyke Show," patterned loosely after his family's experiences in suburbia while he was writing for Sid Caesar.

Over the years, the Reiner and Brooks albums continued to sell, with new fans discovering the "2000 Year Old Man" and his sharp wit and wisdom.

"The more serious the situation the funnier the comedy can be," says Brooks. "Comedy is a red rubber ball and if you throw it against a soft, funny wall, it will not come back. But if you throw it against the hard wall of ultimate reality it will bounce back and be very lively."

The 2000 Year Old Man laughed in the face of the ultimate reality, mortality. He endured. And that's better than his creator Brooks can hope for: "If Shaw and Einstein couldn't beat death, what chance have I got? Practically none."

Brooks played hardball with fear.

"Everything we do is based on fear." Singing began as screaming for help. Getting married helped two people look out for each other with dangerous animals lurking about. And the handshake? "Also stems from fear—to see if a fella had a rock or a dagger in his hand. You held that hand, you looked, opened it up, shook it a little—make sure he didn't have a small stone or a marble he'll stick in your eye."

Of course much of the routine simply revelled in the amusing character of the old Jewish man, his problems with fatherhood ("I have over forty two thousand children—and not *one* comes to visit me") and his "peppy ways."

"The 2000 Year Old Man is a pastiche of everyone around me," Brooks admits, "my mother, my uncle Joe, my grandmother. When I became him, I could hear 5,000 years of Jews pouring through me. Look at Jewish history. Unrelieved lamenting would be intolerable. So, for every ten Jews beating their breasts, God designated one to be crazy and amuse the breast-beaters. By the time I was 5 I knew I was that one."

The 2000 Year Old Man joked about historical figures and religion and reduced 2,000 years of human achievement to a commercial for Saran Wrap: "You can see right through it! You can put a peach in it, and another peach—" "But sir, you equate this with . . . the discovery of space?" (After a pause) "That was a good thing."

The old man delineated tragedy and comedy:

"Tragedy is if I cut my finger. Comedy is if you walk into an open sewer and die."

Often the Reiner and Brooks routines were joys to observe just for the sight of two comedy geniuses flexing their muscles. Take this quick, ad-libbed exchange that shows two minds having fun:

"Fruit cured diarrhea, sir?"
"Peaches!"
"Oh? What kind? Alberta—"
"No . . . cling."

You can almost hear the smile in Brooks's voice as that line came to him, with Reiner the omniscient straight man leading the way.

And along the way, the 2000 Year Old Man had some serious points to make. Being old: "We mock the thing we are to be. Yes, yes, we make fun of the old then we become them. Look at that man bent over and spitting. In a few years we're bent over and spitting . . . oh, we shouldn't have laughed." But then again, there's laughter. Even laughter in knowing when someone is dead: "Simple, you put a finger in his nose. If he doesn't say, 'Hey, take your finger out of my nose,' he's dead."

The worldly wise old man could say of life, "As long as the world is spinning we'll be dizzy and make mistakes." But for an opposite view, the team tried a routine about a two-hour-old talking baby who can describe early life in grim detail. Take morning sickness: "The moment [mothers] realize that there's a living creature inside, then they puke."

The 2000 Year Old Man routines were made into a cartoon special and a book. The "incomplete" works of Reiner and Brooks were gathered into a boxed set. In 1973 the team found time to record a fine sequel on the 2013 Year Old Man.

From there Brooks went on to direct and co-star in one of the most successful movies of all time, *Blazing Saddles*, and create other highly successful films. His finest work can be seen in the films previously mentioned and the experimental *Silent Movie*, the clever *High Anxiety*, and a neglected gem, *The Twelve Chairs*.

Carl Reiner has directed many comedies over the years, including *The Comic, Oh God* and the skillful comedy exercise *Dead Men Don't Wear Plaid*. In 1984 he directed one of the best constructed, most beautifully timed and comically acted comedies of recent years, *All of Me,* which (like "The Dick Van Dyke Show") is almost a primer in how to execute comedy with a blend of broad and subtle jokes, wit and pantomime, plot and pace, and the discipline not to overplay any comic situation.

Reiner and Brooks are both married, both have three children, and are still talking to each other. Brooks's wife, actress Anne Bancroft, has taken a hand in managing singer Estelle Reiner, who made her New York debut at Michael's Pub in 1984.

DON RICKLES

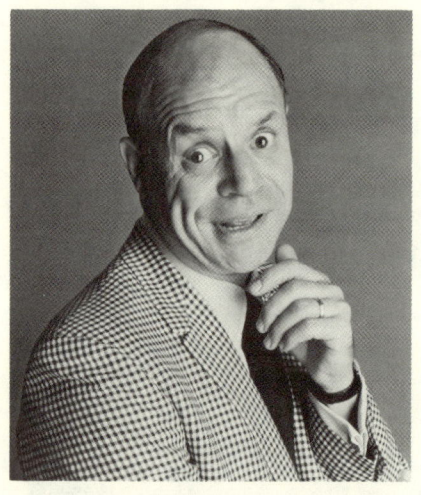

b. May 8, 1926, Queens, New York

Records:
Hello Dummy (Warner Brothers 1745), Don Rickles Speaks (Warner Brothers 1779), Magic Moments from The Tonight Show (Casablanca SPNB 1296).

TV:
The Don Rickles Show (ABC 1968–69), The Don Rickles Show (CBS 1972), C.P.O. Sharkey (NBC 1976–78), Foul-ups, Bleeps and Blunders (ABC 1983–   ).

Outrageous or just tasteless? A champion fighting bigotry or someone using bigotry to give people vicarious thrills? "People either love me or hate me," says Don Rickles.

Dubbed "Mr. Warmth," Rickles in concert blends ad-libs with his prepared material for a show that appears to be a spontaneous free-for-all. He involves the audience by cleverly seizing on one person at a time, doing some jokes on whatever physical or ethnic trait offends him, and then continuing with prepared jokes on the same subject. Then someone else in the audience gets on his nerves, and the cycle is repeated.

"Look at this front row!" he starts off. To a staring fan, "Are you on the toilet? You wanna magazine?" The person looks Italian. "Are you Italian? You, the one with the flies all around." Then, after a spate of general Italian jokes, it's on to a new ethnic group: "You're Chinese? You're not Chinese? Then get your eyes fixed!" To a black man: "We need the blacks—so we can have cotton at the drugstore." To a Puerto Rican: "We need the Puerto Ricans! (A pained expression) For what?" To a fat man: "You get any heavier we're gonna put cords on your can and put ya in the Macy Parade." After asking if a particular person is married, he goes into prepared wife material with the Rickles flavor: "Got any kids? How many? One kid? Don't you fool around at all? . . . Get yourself in heat. My wife lays in the room goin' 'Go, Geronimo, Go.' Last night I was Cochise. I had to stand on top of the sink in the nude, and she was in the living room with a bell on her tochus. She was goin' 'Wagon Train, coming through the pass!' And I had to ring the bell."

The shock humor puts the crowd off-balance, as do the constant darts thrown out at random: "That was a good one, right, queer?" "Look—the Italian guy—oil all over the table." "The Jew's laughing and the black guy just picked his pocket!" No one knows what will come next from the short, profusely sweating man on stage who twists his face into a ceaseless set of grimaces registering irritation, boredom, outrage and chagrin. But the face never really shows anger.

"My style is to rib people I like," Rickles says. "If there's anger in it, it isn't funny. Audiences always know what I am saying is, beneath it all, being done with a certain kind of love and respect. I think there's an element of catharsis in what I do. People laugh because they can see that ultimately it's all a satire of our attitudes and prejudices."

There's no doubt that people understand that Rickles is neither a bigot nor seriously antagonistic. He insists he's never had a serious run-in with an insulted fan. In fact, "People try to get seats up front where the odds are better that I'll get to them," he says. "I think most people understand that I'm not speaking with venom. You gotta remember, I'm trying to create a character out there . . . there's a fine line between being nasty and ribbing a guy in a way that he knows is in fun.

"I guess insult comedy is the best way to describe what I do but I'm very much aware of the thin line that exists between this kind of comedy and outright cruelty. I have had years of experience in this business and it has given me an inner control panel that tells me what's funny and what isn't. I don't go in for sick humor about really bad personal problems."

Rickles, even though he deliberately includes in his act such serious lines as "I live for the day when every bigot will rot in hell," has still been doubted by critics, and even Buddy Hackett says, "He's the furthest thing from the truth."

Actually, it *is* truth that makes audiences laugh. When Rickles calls a woman in an ostentatious fur coat "an old beaver in heat," they laugh out of shock and agreement. Rickles often says what people are really thinking. To a fat ringsider: "6'6" and 240 pounds? What do you eat for dinner? Furniture?" Often there needn't be a big joke attached. To Howard Cosell he said, "From the bottom of my heart . . . I say you're annoying and you should go away!" Not a pearl, but it was greeted with approving laughter. To Ricky Schroder, the cute child actor: "You were great in 'The Champ'—snivelling and whining. . . ." And to Joe Piscopo, "I hope Eddie Murphy robs your house!" No wit, but solid shocks and a release of hostile aggression.

"My main problem is that my humor depends on my face," says Rickles. "If you take a quote from me—in print it's different. I read it and say ouch! Seeing it in cold print bothers me. It's what's not in print that's important, my honesty and my love for people."

Rickles's love of people was evidently not reciprocated when he was growing up. "I wasn't a great student and I could never get a date," he recalls. "When you're short and shy and not good-looking, the only way you get any notice is by telling jokes and getting a lot of laughs. This doesn't mean I got the girls. I didn't, but I did get a lot of laughs." He grew up in a strictly orthodox Jewish household: "I'm still very pious, very conscious of being Jewish. I'm a serious man, serious about my work, my family."

After Navy service during World War II, Rickles attended the American Academy of Dramatic Art in New York, a classmate of Jason Robards, Jr., and others. "I was going to conquer the world as an actor," he thought. At 5'8" and 220 pounds, he was often cast as a heavy. On the side he "worked up a little $10 a night act for burlesque clubs. I was a straight stand-up comic in those days and I really stunk." He worked terrible joints, ending up "cancelled out of the worst strip joint in Boston." The hecklers wanted two things: the girls and Rickles's blood. "You got such a low class of people in those joints. I gave it right back to them. Believe me, it took guts to yell back at a bunch of guys bigger than you."

Jack E. Leonard had built a career out of insult humor, and Rickles too found it lucrative. But it took time. His father, an insurance salesman, told him, "Anything that's tough pays great dividends." He also felt his son had something unusual to offer: "If you're different, if you work in a different way, you have a chance."

Rickles's big break came in 1956 at the Slate Brothers Club in Los Angeles. Frank Sinatra was in the audience and Don was hot: "I'll never forget it and at the time I had never met the man. I said, 'Frank, I've seen you in nightclubs, I've watched you in movies, I've listened to you on records, and I say this from my heart—Frank, your voice is gone. It's all over for you, you're making a fool of yourself. You've got to find some other work.'"

Fortunately, Sinatra enjoyed the brash young comic and so did other entertainers who found themselves deflated by his bullying bombasts. In 1958, Rickles was getting $100 a night to play the Concord. Ten years later, the pay was $5,000, but those were ten tough years, with Rickles working clubs and pursuing an up-and-down movie career during which he received some good notices (*The Rat Race*) but nothing consistent.

Into the 60's the climate was right for Rickles and his unsparing brand of mayhem. To a black: "You look like you fell into a bucket of M & M's." To an elderly woman: "Hi ya, Mom, I spoke to the home—you go in Friday!" Sniffing with annoyance he announced, "There's a definite odor in this section—the old guy is starting to go bad." Pausing to kiss the hand of a female ringsider he said, "What'd you make for dinner? Fish?"

Russell Baker, writing in 1968, complained that Rickles was indulging in "mere billingsgate. An hour of Rickles contains less true insult than one line of Groucho Marx." But Groucho was a different type of insult comic. He close-ended his insults so there was rarely a chance of getting topped ("Were you fat when you left Vassar or did you leave Vassar-lean?"). He was usually insulting in a mild way, loosening up his target rather than destroying it. And for Groucho insult was just another way of attacking with ad-libbed wit, not waiting for a straight line.

Rickles is actually a comic character: he looks like the typical middle-aged salesman who, sweaty and red-faced from daily frustration, ends up blurting out the kind of malformed insults he has kept to himself for years. The remarks aren't usually witty, but part of the humor is their inane hyperbole. "You hockey puck!" he'll scream at someone, his eyes bulging and mouth distended. Rickles is Everyman on a rampage, and what frightens critics and minority groups is seeing this average man's hostility and rage exposed, even comedically. This isn't Groucho playing word games, or a wounded Lenny Bruce or Richard Pryor fighting fire with fire. It's Joe Salesman, playing before middle America on "The Tonight Show" or in Vegas.

It's no wonder that so many average members of his audience go away imitating him. In everyday life, many people's insults sound a bit like Rickles's. "I keep hearing about amateurs who see me in action then try the same technique on their wife or their boss or their best friend. If you're lucky, you'll get away with only a thick lip," says Rickles. The reason lies partly in what Rickles has said all along: *he* delivers the insults with comic outrage and he spares no one.

There will always be debate over whether Rickles mocks prejudice or tacitly reinforces it. It's undeniable that some people enjoy racial humor as a safety valve for their frustrations or anger, but it's also true that Rickles presents the jokes in the most absurd way possible. There is also the dual nature of the man himself: he came upon insult humor as revenge against a rejecting, hostile audience (and possesses a certain kind of hostility found in many comics) yet he is a pious, devoted family man with his own very evident sensitivity that goes beyond the mawkish disclaimers he enunciates at the end of his show.

Meanwhile, "Mr. Warmth" continues to perform before enthusiastic crowds and, unlike some other insult comics, leaves himself vulnerable to barbs from others. Milton Berle cracked in his presence, "What can you say about Rickles that hasn't been said about hemorrhoids?" On a dais Joan Collins added, "Last night he came down with food poisoning—he bit his tongue." And Pat McCormick offered the classic line, "Rickles will be a little late, he's out walking his rat."

In addition to his stand-up work, Rickles has always kept busy with acting projects. In recent years he's done summer stock, notably *The Odd Couple* opposite Ernest Borgnine. And he's withstood his mother's urging that he should "tell nice stories like Bob Newhart."

JOAN RIVERS

"Can we talk?"

A two million dollar contract for a year at Caesars Palace. A quarter of a million dollars for nine weeks of guest-host chores on "The Tonight Show." A million dollars for a new comedy album. Plus commercials, a line of greeting cards ("Happy Birthday to the meanest queen since Marie Antoinette"; "Happy Birthday, tramp—you've turned more tricks than Houdini"), t-shirts with her "Can we talk" catch-phrase on them. . . .

On paper, Joan Rivers is the most successful woman in the history of stand-up comedy. On stage, it's easy to see why. Oddly enough, Rivers's ambition was not humor at all. "I was on the literary magazine in school," she recalls, "the yearbook, the college newspaper. I was a literary major and I won the prizes, but I always thought I was going to grow up to be Sarah Bernhardt and be a great dramatic actress."

Growing up in the middle-class surroundings of Larchmont, New York, Rivers may have had dreams of glory, but she was inhibited by her own perception of reality. She believed she was fat and unattractive. She insisted her sister was smarter. But like many shy and insecure people, she also had the drive to change her situation in the most public way possible.

In 1951, a young Joan Molinsky managed to get a bit part in a Jack Carson movie, *Mr. Universe*. She had hopes that this would be the start of something, but it would be 17 years before she got another bit (a role in 1968's *The Swimmer*). She attended Barnard College and, after graduation in 1954, worked as a fashion coordinator at a clothing store and married the store's heir. The marriage ended after six months. The end of the marriage marked the beginning of a six-year struggle to make it in show business.

An office temporary, she was typing by day, trying out her routines at night. At one point she was "Pepper January," strip-club comic. "I was crossing back and forth," she recalls, "a revue performer, a writer, doing my own act in the Village, and also Second City improvised theater. It was a very exciting time. Bobby Dylan was on the same bill with me—$6 a night. He passed the hat same as me. Barbra Streisand. You were just so happy and grateful to be working. You never thought in terms of making it."

She made it to Broadway in *Talent '60*, appeared in more revues including *From the Second City* in 1962, and after some work for the USO was temporarily mired in the comedy team of "Jim, Jake and Joan."

"Lenny Bruce saved my life," she says. "I was doing miserably. Finally, I watched Lenny's act every night for three weeks. I learned from Lenny that you could tell the truth on stage." Actually, her style grew to be closer to that of her friend Woody Allen.

Joan injected gut humor into her act, releasing her hostilities and

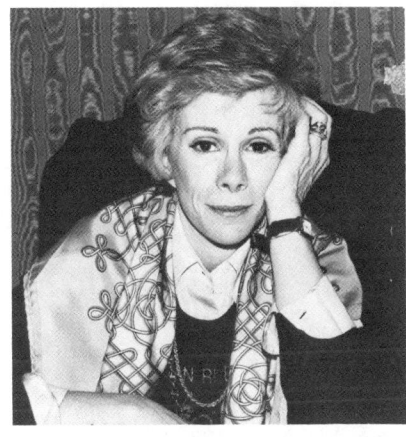

b. Joan Molinsky, June 8, 1933, Brooklyn, New York

Records:
Mr. Phyllis and Other Funny Stories (Warner W 1610), The Next to Last Joan Rivers Album (Buddah BDS 5048, rereleased as Arista BL58096), What Becomes a Semi-Legend Most (Geffen GHS 4007).

TV:
The Girl Most Likely To.

Film:
Rabbit Test.

Books:
Having a Baby Is a Scream, The Life and Hard Times of Heidi Abromowitz.

insecurities in ceaseless jokes about herself. Although nobody seemed to notice back in the 60's, Woody Allen and Joan Rivers were Mr. and Ms. Neurosis, two nervous, unattractive losers driven by lethal wit and enough inner toughness to twist their problems into a new, forceful brand of humor.

Allen took off quickly, leaving his job as a writer for Garry Moore. Rivers still had to lean on writing jobs, from work for "Candid Camera" to gags for such unlikely subjects as Phil Foster and the rubbery puppet "Topo Gigio." At the time, critics ignored Rivers, apparently because her material was based on "trivial" women's problems. Her most popular routine was about her hairdresser, "Mr. Phyllis." Supporters like Bill Cosby said, "She will not pretend to be the dumbest girl in the world . . . she is intelligent . . . a funny woman that you can love." She had some off-beat bits in her repertoire, like a Woody Allenesque routine about a wig she bought. She befriended it like a pet, picked it out at a "wigpen," taught it tricks ("Curl!") and had some good times till the moppy thing slipped away and was run over on the highway. And in another surreal bit she noted, "I have bad luck with plants. I bought me a philodendron. I started small. And I put it in the kitchen and it drank my soup."

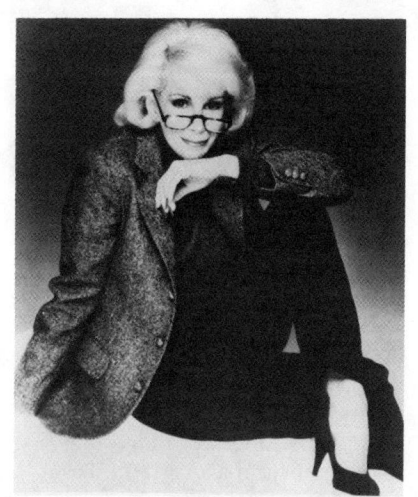

In 1965 she got a shot on Johnny Carson's "Tonight Show." At that time she also met producer Edgar Rosenberg. He was interested in having her work on a proposed Peter Sellers movie script. Instead, four days later, he proposed marriage. Her daughter, Melissa, was born in 1968.

Rivers became a favorite on TV in the late 60's, expanding her truth in comedy to cover the problems of married life, from the honeymoon to pregnancy to flagging sexual interest ("If my husband didn't toss and turn in his sleep, we'd never have had a kid"). She had a never-ending supply of gags about nasty stewardesses and vicious nurses (like the one who short-sheeted her bed in the maternity ward and said during the delivery, "Still think blondes have more fun?").

She had a syndicated TV series, "That Show," and became established with her character of the flat-chested, desperate deb who couldn't get a date, the one now mired in the life of an unfulfilled housewife: "Every woman walks out of my show feeling it's not so bad that her body isn't perfect, that she's aging . . . that she's not the best there is in bed. We all have the same problems, the same pain, and if you lay it all out on the table it doesn't seem so scary." Her humor, she said, "is based on the philosophy of ha ha, I said it first. I mean, you don't have to tell me my slip is showing. Oh no, I said it first." But gradually Joan Rivers turned the anger outward.

She wrote a TV movie, "The Girl Most Likely To," which she describes in her urgent and triumphing way as "The absolutely true story. I had a *terrible* blind date in college. As I came down the stairs he said to a friend, 'You must be kidding.' I met him 18 years later at a cocktail party. He didn't remember me. He was a Beverly Hills doctor literally on the make and carrying on. I thought, wouldn't it be wonderful to scream, 'Don't you remember Joan Molinsky!,' take a gun and shoot him. My husband said, there's a screenplay in that.

"In the movie the girl kills off everybody who was mean to her and it struck a chord 'cause everybody's been hurt and everybody has revenge daydreams." When the movie aired in November of 1973, it won a 42 share of the audience which made it the most popular TV movie yet shown. Yet, she adds, "it was rewritten seven times and the first time I saw it I literally went out and threw up! How's that for liking yourself?"

Rivers got the attention, at last, of the Hollywood elite. But she chose to ignore them and finance her next movie herself. This was *Rabbit Test*, a rather undisciplined assortment of gags stitched around the premise of the first pregnant man. Rivers mortgaged her home to finance the film. It was a terrifying gamble and the strain she felt was evident to anyone who saw her promoting the film in city after city. Fortunately, the film was a success.

In stand-up, Rivers continued to use self put-down ("My body is falling so fast my gynecologist wears a hard hat") but also began to turn the humor onto others, most notably the stars she was now meeting socially and as a talk show hostess. For these people, she was as unsparingly, comically truthful as she had been about her own shortcomings.

At 5'2", 107 pounds, the constantly dieting Rivers was appalled at the way glamorous Elizabeth Taylor let herself go: "This woman has more chins than a Chinese phone book!" She attacked homely royalty, laughed at the "child bearing lips" of Mick Jagger, and insisted Bo Derek was so stupid "she saw a sign saying 'Wet Floor' so she did!" Unpredictable, fun to watch, Rivers emerged as a superstar, a constant guest on "The Tonight Show" and now "the female Don Rickles."

Actually Rickles attacks face to face and Rivers takes the "town gossip" approach behind the back. Rickles is blunt; he might tell Elizabeth Taylor, "you need *two* chairs—make yourself at home, Liz, eat the seat cushion," while Rivers uses gags and visual pictures, like the image of Taylor lodged between the arches of McDonald's after a burger binge, coaxed out by the promise of a Twinkie and someone greasing her thighs.

Like Rickles, Rivers insists, "If I thought I hurt anybody, I'd go crazy." The point was made when, in an elaborate practical joke, Johnny Carson hired a Queen of England look-alike to meet Joan accidentally at an airport and feign distress at her jibes. The result, aired on TV, showed a genuinely embarrassed, humble Joan Rivers offering apologies, and looking to her husband, Edgar, for moral support.

The incident showed the sensitivity of Joan Rivers, the fact that she, like most comics, cares about the subjects she attacks and still feels a certain insecurity and need to be liked. In Rivers's case, her reaction when a joke bombs also betrays her sensitivities. She flashes a wearily disappointed smile, and in a conciliatory voice says, "That was a *good* joke" the way one would say to someone "those were my *best shoes* you accidentally stepped on." She is always more prone to a sigh of exasperation than a put-down when a joke fails.

Rivers works hard on her jokes. "A monologue grows," she says, "it evolves from inspiration and adrenalin on stage. I work at night in a small club that holds 80 people. I bring my notes of the jokes I think might be funny up on stage. Then I improvise from them. The next day I sit and listen to a tape recording of the show and pull off the jokes I like. Then I bring those on stage the next night and improvise from there until the thing begins to form.... I've never sat down ever and written a monologue. It's always trial and error on stage, with lots of notes. I'm always writing notes to myself." She holds out her purse filled with, among other things, a small blizzard of scrap paper.

As for being a female comic, she admits, "it's a very difficult life for a woman getting started. You have to hang out in clubs till three, four o'clock in the morning for no money. You have to take yourself there, get back, and when you go out on the road it's even worse for a woman, terribly lonely." But, she adds, "I'm so tired of hearing that because you're a woman you can't get a break in comedy. If Hitler came back with 10 good minutes you'd be talking to him next week. In comedy it doesn't matter—if you make somebody laugh it's golden."

And Joan Rivers has reached a golden plateau after her first splash in

1965, the big TV movie in 1973, and her emergence as a superstar a decade later.

Rivers's life and work were in the headlines constantly in 1984. She made the cover of *People* magazine the traumatic way: in a report on the nearly fatal heart attack of her husband, Edgar. She triumphed later in the year, achieving a writer's dream, a place on the *New York Times* Best Seller List for her book, *The Life and Hard Times of Heidi Abromowitz*. It was a meditation on one of her popular stand-up characters, the town slut. On Heidi's infant precociousness: "She did things with her pacifier that most women still haven't done with their husbands."

Sensing backlash from her celebrity insults, Rivers wisely began to back off slightly from the Elizabeth Taylor put-downs and superstar send-ups and resumed telling more jokes about herself: "I'm having hot flashes—I went to my gynecologist. He didn't use rubber gloves he used an oven mitt!" And "I'm Jewish—if God had wanted me to exercise he would've put diamonds on the floor."

Offstage she has the reputation for being a warm, caring and supportive wife, mother and friend. An interview with Joan Rivers is a relaxed, one-to-one experience far different from the fast and frantic style she uses guesting on "The Tonight Show." On happiness, she says, "I don't think you have to be miserable to produce comedy. I think you have to be aware of misery. How's that for one of the great all time nonpithy answers? I'm not miserable, but you have to go outside of yourself and be aware of other people's unhappiness and what's going on around you. But you yourself don't have to be sad. You don't have to lose an ear to paint great."

WILL ROGERS

"His humor and his comments were always kind. His was no biting sarcasm that hurt the highest or the lowest of his fellow citizens. When he wanted people to laugh out loud, he used the methods of pure fun. And when he wanted to make a point for the good of mankind, he used the kind of gentle irony that left no scars behind it. He loved and was loved by the American people."

President Franklin Roosevelt's remarks about Will Rogers still stand, and so does the legend of the cowboy philosopher, the man who offered up satirical observations that made people laugh—and think.

Part Cherokee, with "just enough white blood to make my honesty questionable," Rogers grew up in what was simply known as Indian country. Eventually he called the town of Claremore home. "My mother died when I was ten years old," he recalled on a Mother's Day radio broadcast. "Folks have told me that what little humor I have comes from her. I can't remember her humor but I can remember her love and understanding of me."

He attended a one-room school and then spent two years at the Kemper Military School in Boonville, Missouri: "I could have gotten to West Point but I was too proud to talk to a congressman." Rogers didn't last in school, joking "I went to Kemper one year in the fourth grade, one year in the guard house. Then one night I just up and left. I don't want any enterprising youth in this audience to think I did the right thing. . . . I'll always regret that I didn't take a chance on fifth grade."

Rogers traveled the world as a cowboy and rancher, appearing in

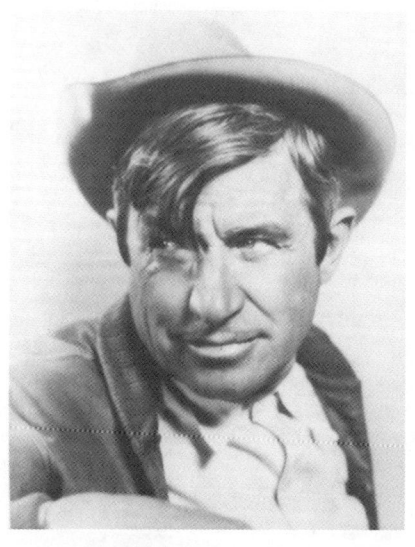

b. November 4, 1879, Oolagah, Oklahoma; d. August 16, 1935

Wild West shows where he became known as "The Roping Fool." His amazing dexterity with rope tricks brought him to vaudeville stages, and even the newsreels wanted footage of the roper in action: swinging two lariats and roping both a horse and rider as they rode past.

Once, filling in time between his tricks, he said, "Swingin' a rope's all right—if your neck ain't in it." It got a big laugh, but the shy cowpoke was shocked. He decided not to speak on stage again and risk another outburst in the midst of his roping. Fortunately, his vaudeville friends told him it was a great idea to spice up the act with some humor.

Chewing gum to counter his nervousness, studying the newspaper for interesting, topical things to joke about, Rogers evolved into a full-time humorist, with ties to Mark Twain and a long tradition of slyly witty rustic philosophers. He became a star of the Ziegfeld Follies beginning in 1907, and topped bills along with such stars as W.C. Fields and Fanny Brice. Appraising the beautiful Follies chorus line, he remarked, "Isn't it sad to think that in 20 years these gals will be 5 years older?"

Rogers moved to California, making dozens of silent films including *A Connecticut Yankee in King Arthur's Court*. He began a newspaper column that was syndicated to over 500 papers and was a frequent guest on radio. He even found time to experiment with comedy monologues on records. Here is his opening for one rare 78 rpm disc:

"You know these talking machines are great. When you come to a theater or movies to see some of us and you don't like our act, just outta courtesy you have to stick and see us through. On one of these if you don't like us you just stop the machine, take the record off and accidentally drop it on the floor. Then the only annoyance is sweepin' up.

"Now, folks, all I know is what little news I read every day in the paper. I see where another wife out on Long Island in New York shot her husband. Season opened a month earlier this year. Prohibition caused all this. There's just as many husbands shot at in the old days, but women were missin'. Prohibition has improved their marksmanship 90%. Never a day passes in New York without some innocent bystander being shot. You just stand around this town long enough and be innocent and somebody's gonna shoot ya. One day there was four shots. That was the best shootin' ever done in this town. It's hard to find four innocent people in New York. That's why the policeman never has to aim here. He just shoots up the street, no matter who he hits it's the right one."

It was a straight line that brought Rogers to the attention of President Woodrow Wilson: "The Germans wonder how we can train our boys so quick. Well, they only know one word: forward." He became a favorite of Wilson's successors, too, even though he showed them all his brand of good-natured irreverence.

In front of Roosevelt he said, "Now, Franklin, I can call you Franklin . . . you used to come to the Follies as a boy to see our show! You used to come as an old man to see the show, too! Here tonight, you aren't allowed to refer to politics because this stadium was dedicated to art, sports, and any *useful* enterprises."

At the opening of the Coolidge Dam in Arizona, he remarked in front of the guest of honor, "Mr. Coolidge is the best Democrat we ever had in the White House—he didn't do nothin' but that's what we wanted done."

The *New York Times* remarked, "while it's easy to call a spade a spade, he did so and yet made the spade like it." He also broke some rules in comedy. He had probably the worst delivery of any star comic:

Records:
The Wit and Wisdom of Will Rogers (Caedmon TC 2046), The Voice of Will Rogers (American Heritage P 11794), Will Rogers' U.S.A. (Columbia SG 30546), Will Rogers Radio Broadcasts (Mark 56 # 569), Will Rogers (Murray Hill M 51220; 3 lps), Will Rogers Says (Columbia ML 4604).

Films:
Two Wagons Both Covered, Doubling for Romeo, Going to Congress, They Had to See Paris, Ambassador Bill, Will Rogers: Champion of the People.

Books:
Rogerisms, The Cowboy Philosopher on Prohibition, The Cowboy Philosopher on the Peace Conference, What We Laugh At, Illiterate Digest, Will Rogers' Autobiography, Letters of a Self-Made Diplomat, Will Rogers' Political Follies.

he would pause, mumble, drawl out a punchline and sometimes step over it with a few added words. Part of this was his rambling, ad-libbing style, and a little his natural shyness and humility.

Yet Rogers had definite ideas about humor: "A gag to be any good has to be fashioned about some truth. The rest you get by your slant on it and perhaps by a wee bit of exaggeration so people won't miss the point."

A tireless fundraiser for charity, Rogers regularly flew around the nation to appear at benefits, lending aid to victims of floods and natural disasters. He loved to experience new places and see new people. He planned an extensive tour for the summer of 1935. In his last radio broadcast of the season, June 9, he said,

"Everybody is trying to save the country. Only they are trying to do it in different ways, and it is too big, the country is too big for all of them put together to spoil anyhow. So goodbye, and I'll see you in the fall. Thank you very much."

Two months later, Will Rogers and his pilot, Wiley Post, were dead. Their plane developed engine trouble and plunged into a river bank near Point Barrow, Alaska.

The nation mourned as for a war hero or a President. The mourning may have lasted a short time, but the remembrance has never faded. Forty years after his death, Rogers's wit and wisdom were brought together in the stage show *Will Rogers' U.S.A.* starring James Whitmore, which collected many of the comedian's most famous lines and demonstrated just how timely they were. Here, Korea and Vietnam come to mind as Rogers notes:

"Youth For Peace March. I've been readin' alot about that lately. The kids don't want us in the Japanese War. They're marchin' to keep us from war. Seems they're gettin' the same training as they would in the military. But folks, if you're gonna travel 7,000 miles to find a war, you really have to be looking. 'Course the thing we do worst in this country is mind other folks' business. But the joke's on the kids anyway. We say we ain't got no war, and the other side says we ain't got no war. Of course the guys gettin' shot say it's the best imitation they've seen yet. But don't worry, we got the best politicians in this country that money can buy."

Although he will forever be known as the man who said, "I joked about every prominent man in my lifetime, but I never met a man I didn't like," there is a large, complex and often biting collection of observations waiting to be discovered in Rogers's books and recordings. Unfortunately, many of the existing records of him are in poor condition and culled from ad-libbed radio appearances. Those looking for a place to start might, in this case, do better with the reenactments performed by James Whitmore. Of Whitmore, Will Rogers, Jr. said, "A vigorous and strong personality, he somehow transforms into Will Rogers. Listening to him I can see my father."

ROWAN AND MARTIN

The two super comedy teams of the 1950's were wildly funny: Abbott & Costello, Martin and Lewis. They were also wildly unreal, utilizing crazy routines and broad slapstick. Waiting in the wings, Dan Rowan and Dick Martin decided to innovate, not imitate.

"We looked at all the other acts and decided to stay away from imitations, song and dance routines and slapstick," says Dick Martin. "No funny clothes or funny faces to get laughs either." They developed real humor that was closer to the audience: "In every family there's one person you can't stand. That's me, with Dan as my brother-in-law. The audience identifies with us." If anyone influenced them, it was Phil Ford and Mimi Hines: "They're always themselves, the same as we try to be."

Of course, their success was not so easily calculated, and their first taste of it did not come for many, many years. Their first year together, 1952, saw them pull in just $6,000.

Dan and Dick had both been writers before embarking on their nightclub career. Rowan's parents were carnival performers. His father died when Dan was very young, and when he was 11, his mother passed away, too. Left in an orphanage, Rowan ran away, taking odd jobs as a trash collector and furnace stoker. He toiled at a gas station to work his way through high school in Pueblo, Colorado. He was encouraged in his writing, and confident enough to head to California where he hoped to find work. He did, first in the mail room at Paramount, and then behind a desk as a junior writer. He joined the Air Force in World War II, enduring flying highs and one low: a crash landing in a dry riverbed.

Dick Martin had a more stable up-bringing, but a dim future working in a factory helping to assemble Fords. He too had writing talent, which he proved by selling jokes to nightclub comedians when he moved out to Hollywood. He also sold gags to such radio shows as "Duffy's Tavern," but to make a living he worked in a tavern tending bar. During the war he was classified 4F.

In the years after the war, Rowan went to college and then sold cars for a living. Martin, as a straight man, had failed to make a dent in show business with two different partners. There was little to suggest, when they were introduced to each other, that they would become better acquainted, partners or famous. But after collaborating on comedy routines for other teams, including Noonan and Marshall, Rowan and Martin took a chance as stand-up partners, starting with a $300 a week gig in a club in Albuquerque, New Mexico.

"On the same program with us was Dreamy Darnell, a stripteaser," Rowan recalled. "Indians and cowboys came in and dared us to do our stuff. But they accepted us."

From 1952, Rowan and Martin polished their act and their characters, developing a few sketches that they could call their own. There was the Shakespeare routine (which Noonan and Marshall had turned down), wherein Dan, the serious actor, is heckled by good-time drunk Dick. And there was the subtle spy bit, where Dick would parrot, a split second later, the detailed instructions of tight-lipped Dan, with an occasional comic misunderstanding.

They signed a contract with NBC in 1957 but little came of it. In 1958, with Martin and Lewis and Abbott & Costello finished, the movie world wanted a new duo. Universal had a film script called *Once Upon a Horse* ready. As Hal Kanter, its writer-producer, put it, in hunting for stars he discovered "two young men, who were unknown to millions, battling

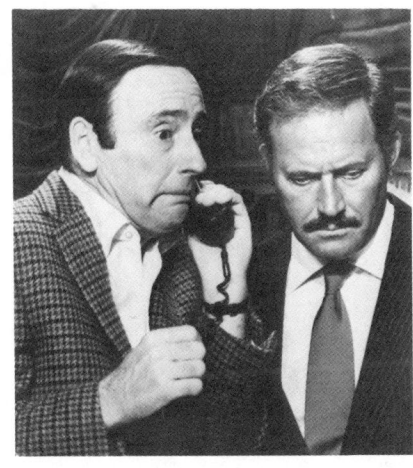

DAN ROWAN b. July 2, 1922, Beggs, Oklahoma
DICK MARTIN b. January 30, 1923, Battle Creek, Michigan

Records:
Rowan and Martin at Work (Trey 901; reissued Atco SD 33-257), The World of Rowan and Martin (Epic FLM 13109), Rowan and Martin's Laugh-In (Epic FLM 15109 and Harmony KH 30976).

TV:
The Rowan and Martin Show (NBC 1966), Rowan and Martin's Laugh-In (NBC 1968–73).

Films:
Once Upon a Horse, The Maltese Bippy.

obscurity in a half-filled nightclub." The low-key western left the team's obscurity level intact.

Rowan and Martin continued to work nightclubs and TV, performing reliable routines wherein the detached, tolerant Rowan would go through his paces with the often corny, deliberately dumb and flighty Martin. In their routine about doctors, Rowan begins:

"You are a doctor."
"A DM."
"An MD!"
"MD. MD."
"Doctor, in medicine today it seems to me most men are specializing."
"Well, what's happened a lot today in medicine is that we have found that, in medicine, many of the people, particularly doctors, are specializing."
"Yes. Well, I'm certainly glad you cleared that up."
"We were talking about that just last Thursday at the doctor place."
"The hospital!"
"The hospital."
"And how about you, doctor, what's yours?"
"Bourbon if you have it."
"No, in what field do you operate, sir?"
"We don't operate in a field, we have a new building. . . . I'm a surgeon. C-E-R-G-O-N."
"You're a general surgeon?"
"Yes I do."
"You do general surgery?"
"Yes I am."
"Whichever is correct, we realize you don't operate alone."
"No, we like to have a patient there. . . ."

In 1966 the team did a summer show as a replacement for "The Dean Martin Show," a program they'd appeared on often. They did well enough to spark NBC into giving them a series.

"We started to sense that the day of the long comedy sketch was coming to an end," says Martin. "The attention span of the public started to shorten. You couldn't sit at a bar and tell a four-minute joke anymore. The people were getting bored with long stories."

Long gone were their situation comedy routines (these can be heard on their 1960 "At Work" album) and even faster ones where flippant Dick would irritate dour Dan with his carefree comedy on drinking and dating. Instead, Rowan and Martin produced "Laugh-In." At the time, bracing for trouble, Rowan said, "We waited a long time to do the kind of TV show we wanted to do, and whether the Bible Belt likes us or not, we're going to do 13 shows."

Of course, they were on for years. Their show was a springboard for such talents as Goldie Hawn, Ruth Buzzi and Lily Tomlin. The show's catch-phrases included "Sock It to Me" (once spoken on the program by Richard Nixon), "You bet your bippy" and "Look that up in your Funk & Wagnalls." With their conservative dress, the duo may have been a reassuring presence to mid-America. Generally the team let others perform the more outlandish character sketches while they did stand-up and emcee work.

The two were very professional with each other on the show. Off camera, they steered clear of each other, so as not to strain the partnership. This wasn't difficult, since the men had completely opposite interests. Martin, true to his character, was a lively single. Rowan called him "Charley Night Life. He never misses a party . . . he's one of the most popular guys in Hollywood and one of the easiest to get along with . . . smiling, cheerful, apparently free from worry. It's uncanny."

Martin characterized Rowan as "Mr. Worry Wart . . . he sweats over getting every line down pat." Rowan, quite serious offstage, was the one who encouraged "Laugh-In's" anti-war humor and social satire. Not surprisingly, he also enjoyed getting away from it all through sailboating, his favorite form of relaxation.

Gradually "Laugh-In" lost popularity, and the team felt the show also lost taste. They became less and less involved with it. In 1976 they worked on "The Rowan and Martin Report" for ABC, but the show didn't make it. The team retained their steady nightclub clientele, and in 1981 appeared on TV in "The First Annual Ultra Quiz." But after so many years, and so many triumphs, Dan Rowan announced his retirement. He took his wife and his love of the good life to France.

Dick Martin turned up on game shows, both as guest and host. A producer ("The Waverly Wonders") he's been involved behind the camera for "Newhart." "Laugh-In" has returned in packaged reruns, once more amusing audiences with its fast-paced gags.

ANNA RUSSELL

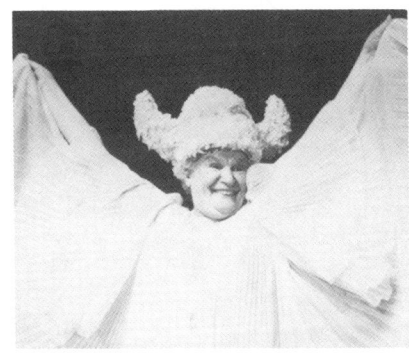

b. Claudia Russell-Brown, December 27, 1911, London, Ontario, Canada

Records:
Anna Russell Sings? (Columbia ML 5494), Anna Russell Sings Again? (Columbia ML 4733), Square Talk on Popular Music (Columbia ML 5036), Guide to Concert Audiences (Columbia ML 4928), In Darkest Africa (Columbia ML 5195), Practical Banana Promotion (Columbia ML 5295), The Anna Russell Album (a double-record reissue of her first two albums, Columbia MG 31199).

Book:
I'm Not Making This Up.

Anna Russell's career as a serious opera singer was so horrid it was funny: "I started off as a lumpy, silly sort of person," she recalls. "I was spotty, pimply, fat, and for some preposterous reason, I wanted to sing. I enrolled at the Royal College of Music in London, mainly because nobody told me not to. I was a bit of a mongrel, part British, part Canadian, part Australian. I had no sense of humor at all, and probably no talent, either."

There was, to be fair, quite a glimmer of talent, at least enough for composer Sir Ralph Vaughan Williams to take an interest in Russell. But as though to seal her fate, the unfortunate girl took part in a hockey game at school and "I got smashed in the face with a hockey stick. That ruined my acoustic. The sinus cavities and all that. I had no range, no color. But I could sing loud. And it grew louder and louder and awfuller and awfuller."

Thinking positively, the 16-year-old opera student, who came from a family that included several classical performers, toured in a road show version of *Cavalleria Rusticana*. But again, the results were not quite encouraging:

"A tenor half my size was supposed to hurl me to the ground during a duet. I turned on my ankle, went spinning across the stage and into the prop church which came tumbling down. The audience roared, the orchestra dried up they laughed so hard, and the performance was over. So was my career. My life's work was shattered, after five years of hard preparation. I went into a snit, but I got over it."

There was a change from opera to light comedy, a divorce from her first husband, and a move to Canada. There Anna became popular with short comic numbers like "I Wish I Were a Dicky Bird," and she began to develop clever introductions for her songs. Eventually she created a longer program suitable for a one-woman show. Her charm, eccentricity and good-natured opera lampoons earned her a devoted following.

From the stage she noted, "What one needs to be a big-time opera star is a glorious voice, lots of money, sex appeal, political motivation and back-stabbing bitchiness." Disdaining the joys of playing such roles as Wagner's Brunhilde, she added, "Who would want to do all that bo-jo-to-ho-ing anyway, prancing around in a brass bra?"

For the classical music audience, so generally polite and often eagerly forcing appreciative laughter to signal recognition of a modest "musical joke," it would have been easy for Anna Russell to play for giggles. Indeed, before such an audience she made the most of mild asides like: "The story opens in the River Rhine . . . *in* it!" which drew broad laughter. But she went further than that, contrasting the drily sophisticated lines with outlandish outfits, eccentric facial expressions and a boundless zest in performance.

She satirized Gilbert and Sullivan and bagpipes ("It's a very unsanitary instrument—it works on the blow-suck-push-twiddle system") and urged the audience to take part in whimsical sing-alongs of fractured folk pieces and lieder. Of course, her most-requested routines involved a retelling of Verdi's *Nabucco* and Wagner's Ring cycle.

In the latter, she introduced the characters, from Wotan ("The head god and a perfectly crashing bore") to the Valkyries ("They're all virgins and I'm not the least bit surprised"). And, with the audience tittering and clapping gleefully, she would say in all candor, "I'm not making this up!"

Time magazine called her "the crown princess of musical parody," while the *Times* of London simply considered her "the world's funniest woman." For decades she toured the world, delighting audiences who came to hear live the classic routines they'd played over and over again on disc. Many would laugh wildly at lines they had memorized already, like Russell's one-liner on lieder singers: "They are judged like cheese: the older and rottener they are, the better."

It was part of her artistry that Russell *could* coax fresh laughter from material the audience already knew. With Russell, audiences left wanting more, even though they knew what the "more" would be: perhaps an encore song like "I'd Be a Red Hot Mama—If I Didn't Have These Varicose Veins."

The delirious diva retired to Australia in 1955, but after all the farewell performances, she was urged to come back. "What I didn't realize," she said in 1983, "is that people enjoying a bit of nonsense is not predicated on me being 18 and sexy. So long as I've got a loud enough voice, it doesn't matter how antique I've become."

A pattern of farewells and comebacks culminated in a series of concerts in the spring of 1984 that she vowed would indeed be her last.

Her final tour was a roaring success, audiences loving her sassy lines ("Most singers have resonance where their brains ought to be"), her bizarre costumes (her "drag" as she called it) and her dynamic presence. It was the legs, not the voice or heart, that were tired after the show.

Russell lives in a retirement community in Canada on a street called Anna Russell Way. She enjoys gardening and was delighted to have won first prize for the best garden in Heritage Village. She donated her income from her last tour to the lovely area, which is green, lush and peaceful. Except, of course, when she practices her singing and piano playing.

MARK RUSSELL

As far as Mark Russell is concerned, politicians are laughably ephemeral. After all, they come to Washington and stay two, four, maybe six years on the average. Yet he's been in Washington for over two decades. It's no wonder he treats them all with such irreverence.

It's probably not surprising that, like most iconoclasts, Russell had a strict and straight upbringing. He attended parochial schools including the all-male Canisius High School and, after some brief university time, enlisted in the Marines.

When he got out of the service, Russell found work as a cocktail pianist. Realizing quickly that his talents were not strong enough musically to vault him much higher, he decided to find a more distinctive identity.

An admirer of risque pianist Charlie Drew and the gleeful sicknik Tom Lehrer, Russell began to write parody songs. He tried them out at Washington's Carroll Arms Hotel, and they went over very well.

In the tense nation's capitol, Russell found politicians and those working for the government eager to laugh at his brand of kidding. "Welcome to Washington," he'd say. "This is where your laws are made. And broken. By the same people, in many cases."

Russell's technique was to scan the newspapers and write quickie spoofs on the latest scandals. Usually these were rather obvious, and set to such mundane tunes as "Old MacDonald Had a Farm" or "Won't You Come Home, Bill Bailey," but his audiences didn't mind. With light piano accompaniment filling in, he'd offer gags on all topics, including one-liners like these:

"Here's a definition. Definition of a sadist. A sadist is a guy who does nice things to a masochist . . . (piano interlude) . . . the story of a rabbi on the West Coast. Very discouraged. Half of his congregation had turned Quaker. Or as he put it, 'Some of my best Jews are friends' . . . (music) . . . (using a put-on tough voice) All right, you men are here to become Marines. It won't be easy, some of you will make it, others will crack. Those who make it will go on to grand and glorious things. Those who crack—will be Marines! Ohh, it was a rough outfit. I'll never forget the day the Chaplain went over the hill. . . ."

By 1961 Russell had moved to a new hotel, the Shoreham-Americana, and by concentrating more and more on social and political humor had developed a solid following. Changing events kept him constantly supplied with material. He toured clubs like The Blue Angel, Mr. Kelly's and The Village Vanguard, but remained something of a Washington legend, a sight worth seeing when in town. He even had a local television show for a while, giving forth with fresh observations that often drew approving laughter:

"The FCC came along and it said no more cigarette commercials on television. That might be overdoing it a little. I'd much rather watch a pretty girl offer me a cigarette than an old lady ask if I'm constipated."

Although he recorded his first album during the Kennedy years, it was during the Nixon administration that he (and many other political humorists) reached a peak. He did some fairly straight one-liners ("The other day Nixon sent the crime bill to Capitol Hill—somebody stole it") but as usual scored with jokes that were really more like statements of disapproval, getting applause if not all-out belly laughs: "There's a dance called The Spiro Agnew. You take two steps forward, two steps back, put

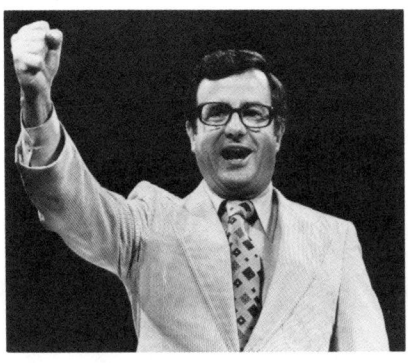

b. Mark Ruslander, August 23, 1932, Buffalo, New York

Records:

Up the Potomac Without a Canoe (Columbia CS 8572), Face on the Senate Floor (WEET 001), Wild Weird Wired World of Watergate (Deep Six).

Book:

Presenting Mark Russell.

your foot in your mouth and fall on your nose." When Watergate broke, Russell was ready, hoping to bang out the chords to a new tune: "Bail to the Chief."

Unfortunately Nixon's fall coincided with hard times for Russell as well. Domestic problems plagued him, and a divorce in 1975 led to a traumatic breakdown. He was not seen at the Shoreham for four months.

A TV deal with the PBS network gave Russell a much needed boost. He was discovered by a national audience, and also found he was earning as much money from five yearly specials as he did from a whole season at the Shoreham. His PBS specials rarely display needle-sharp wit, but there's a good deal of bludgeoning parody. As he says, he's "a political cartoonist for the blind."

With his wide, crooked smile, insinuating smugness and the overpowering verve of a carnival barker, Russell enunciates the jokes and then hammers them home with quick parodies on the piano. Taking on the famous "subway vigilante" case in New York, where Bernhard Goetz shot four blacks who he claimed were about to mug and rob him, Russell sang a new version of "Ghost Riders in the Sky."

The last stanza of it is typical of Russell's technique: boiling down issues into caricatured laugh lines:

"The liberals want the maximum of punishment to bear. Conservatives will probably run Bernhard Goetz for mayor. 'No Subway Vigilantes' goes one angry refrain, of those who in the city ride in taxis and complain.

"See the people arming up, the situation's worse. There's an old lady with a cannon and it's hidden in her purse. See the kindergarten where they practice with their guns. See the quick draw Avon Ladies, see the pistol packin' nuns!"

For his non-musical jokes, Russell is again very simplified. On Yuppies he rants,

"They want tax credits for a membership in Club Med. They wouldn't even be in the same room with anyone not wearing a real fiber—they wouldn't be in the same room with an artificial fiber. They wouldn't salute the flag if it wasn't 100% cotton."

Reporting on the festivities at the second Reagan inaugural, he held up a souvenir decanter of the event, which contained red, white and blue jelly beans. He said, "The theme of the inaugural was 'We the people.' So these are the 'We the People' jelly beans. Unfortunately, the black ones are on the bottom."

At one point the comic was deemed sarcastic yet inoffensive enough to become a co-host on "Real People," introducing various oddball stunts and personalities. At the moment he is a firm fixture on educational TV, and in concert. With such lasting appeal, a politician desiring a longer stay in office might think seriously about Mark Russell as a running mate.

NIPSEY RUSSELL

This smiling comic, noted for his ready quips and ad-libbed comedy rhymes, was a performer from childhood, when he tap-danced on the streets of Atlanta. Displaying talents both intellectual and physical, the prodigy was a whiz in high school, graduating at an early age and then enrolling at the University of Cincinnati where he received his M.A. degree in Old English literature. His unfailing ability to concoct quick, witty rhymes on any subject probably comes from his continued mastery of the classics, particularly Shelley, Chaucer and Keats. He is also fluent in French.

A captain during World War II, Russell worked in Montreal after the war, and was featured on the Robert Q. Lewis series "The Show Goes On" in 1949. He worked with Billy Eckstine on the road and was a regular at Harlem's Baby Grand in the 50's. Through the 60's, Russell saw his salary rise in proportion to his fame, moving up to $4,500 a week. Through it all, he remained modest and studious, and even today maintains a quiet apartment in New York.

When black comedians made a breakthrough in the 60's, Russell was already a veteran, his style influenced by such comics as Bob Hope. He didn't want to jump on the Dick Gregory bandwagon and limit himself to racial humor. He told interviewers that he hoped black comedians could achieve the same status as black ballplayers in the years after Jackie Robinson. Just as a Dave Winfield or Rod Carew is considered a "great player," not a "great black player," Russell wanted people to consider him as simply a "comedian."

"It's only natural that, at first, we should rely on jokes about race relations and civil rights," Russell allowed. "Humor is based on the way a man looks at life's ironies, and being a member of a minority group can certainly be ironic . . . but when you keep harping on one issue, you neglect other subjects worth poking fun at."

Early on, at the Apollo, Nipsey used lines like: "We've always had integration in the South . . . we just want it now in the daytime." But he did political humor as well: "I was just listening to a high government official on TV. I don't know whether he was drinking or smoking, but he was high." He claimed to have tried to interview a delegate to a Democratic Convention: " 'Do you think there's too much ignorance and too much apathy,' I asked him. He said, 'I don't know and I don't give a damn.' "

"I have no political convictions," he privately admits. "I'm a party line crosser. If I'm booked to play a political party's affair, I'll use jokes about the group I'm not working for that evening."

Early on, Russell's stand-up style recalled that of Will Rogers. He favored short, Rogersesque lines ("New York is a funny town. You can drown in whiskey and starve to death . . . everybody says have a drink, nobody says have something to eat"). In the nightclub setting, though, he had to pepper these observations with more standard jokes and his crowd-pleasing party rhymes: "I went to see my girl the other night. She came to the door in her nightie. She stood between me and the light. And Good God, Almighty!"

Russell's early discs contain this unusual blend of risque story and carefully worded and delivered satire. According to his manager, these "party" albums are now something of an embarrassment to him.

In 1959 Russell was featured at a Carnegie Hall benefit to raise funds for Martin Luther King, Jr. This appearance was a major break, leading to

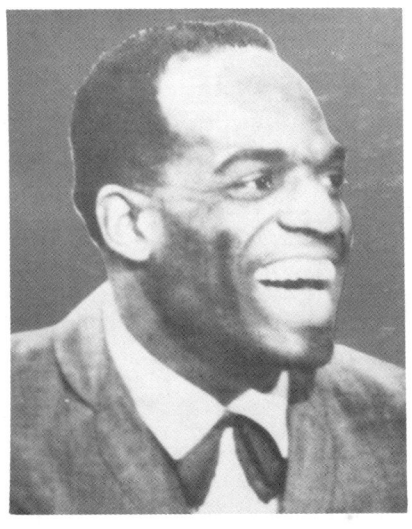

b. October 13, 1925, Atlanta, Georgia

Records:
Star of the Jack Paar Show (Surprise SUR 99), Laff Lectures (Humorsonic 702), Birds and the Bees (Humorsonic 703), Sing Along (Humorsonic 706), Harlem's Son of Fun (Borderline).

TV:
Car 54, Where Are You? (NBC 1961–62), Barefoot in the Park (ABC 1970), Dean Martin Show/Comedy World (1972–75), Juvenile Jury (1982–   ).

Broadway:
Tambourines to Glory.

Film:
The Wiz.

an appearance on "The Jack Paar Show" at the request of guest host Orson Bean.

"During all the years I entertained at the Baby Grand," Russell recalled, "90 percent of the audience was white. But when I tried to break into television, I was told that white folks wouldn't understand what I was talking about."

Russell did make great strides after his first variety show appearances. In 1961 he became one of the first blacks to have a co-starring role in a series when he played a police officer on "Car 54, Where Are You?" In 1965 he turned up on the talk show "Night Life" and was a regular for years on "To Tell the Truth."

In 1970 he was a co-star of TV's "Barefoot in the Park," and over the years appeared regularly on the various Dean Martin shows. He's made movies (*The Wiz*) and in the 80's he's starred in the cable TV revival of the quiz series "Juvenile Jury."

MORT SAHL

A stand-up comic is supposed to tell jokes with punchlines. The comic is supposed to dress in a suit. The comic is supposed to keep things light and inoffensive.

These rules were the norm for the nightclub—until the arrival of Mort Sahl. Mort paved the way for an entire generation of new and experimental comedians.

He wasn't comfortable in a suit, so he wore slacks and a sweater. He contrasted Will Rogers's "I never met a man I didn't like" with "Is there any group I haven't offended?" He dared to joke about a variety of social and political taboos. And he even satirized the old notion of the stand-up comic: "It's great to be a clown," he'd say sarcastically, "and make the corners of people's mouths turn up." Then free-association: "I'm just here to take your minds off the fact that we're trapped in this mine shaft. . . ."

Most of all there was the free-association, an unheard-of style of nervous digression, stops and starts, one-word allusions and the hip jargon of the jazz fan, the student, the intellectual and the psych major. Sahl's delivery remains a compelling part of his art. Many simply love to hear him talk. He offers a seemingly ad-libbed, slippery stream-of-consciousness monologue with jokes mixed with hostile observation, sly wit and sharp shards of broken gags that he lets the audience piece together for themselves, marking time with a cynical laugh before it sinks home. His hip, assured delivery and cadence lend importance and irony to many lines that may not in fact be that pithy.

"It wasn't smart not to laugh at Mort Sahl," Enrico Banducci, owner of the Hungry i recalls, "and you would hear certain people say, 'What'd he say? What'd he say?' And someone would say, 'Hey, dummy, don't you understand what he said?' and laugh—but they didn't understand either. But they were laughing." Lenny Bruce watched Sahl work and he told Banducci, "Boy he's great. You know, I could be a Mort Sahl, I could be a social satirist just like Mort."

Mordant, salty Mort Sahl wasn't always the lean and hungry intellectual. The satirist was once, in his own words, "a Martinet." His father was a government worker who, in a brief period of rebellion, quit to run a tobacco shop in Montreal. Later the family settled in Los Angeles where Mort developed a fascination for the military. The gung-ho Sahl teen was

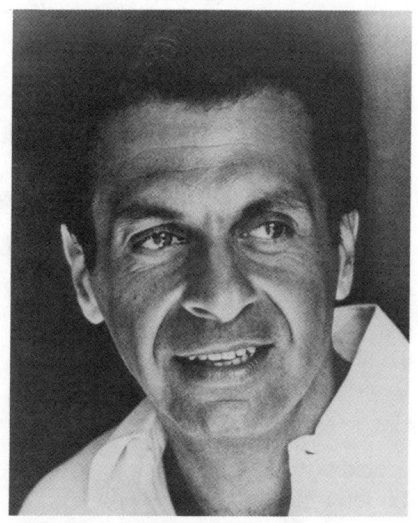

b. May 11, 1927, Montreal, Canada

Records:
The Future Lies Ahead (Verve MGV 150002), Mort Sahl 1960 (Verve MGV 15004), A Way of Life (Verve MGV 150006), At the Hungry i (Verve MGV 15012), The Next President (Verve MGV 15021), At Sunset (Fantasy 7005), Great Moments (Verve MGV 15049), The New Frontier (Reprise R 5002), On Relationships (Reprise R 5003), Anyway Onward (Mercury MG/SR6 61112), Sing a Song of Watergate (GNP Crescendo GNPS 2070).

Video:
Hungry i Reunion (Pacific Arts).

Book:
Heartland.

in the ROTC, and loved to wear his uniform to school. He won an American Legion Americanism Award and ran away once to join the Army. He dreamt of attending West Point but before he could do much about it, he was drafted and sent to an Air Force base in Alaska. This cooled his enthusiasm for military life.

"A few months under the heel of authority killed it for me," Sahl recalls. He ran a post newspaper called "Poop from the Group" and his satiric comments got him 83 consecutive days of KP. Still establishment-bound after the service, Sahl majored in city management and traffic engineering, graduating from the University of Southern California in 1950.

A period of odd jobs and magazine writing followed. Sahl became involved in the bohemian lifestyle of the area's students. His girlfriend Sue encouraged his attempts at stand-up comedy and impressions. From Berkeley they moved to San Francisco, where the free-thinking beat underground was waiting for something different in comedy. "The audiences are all intellects," Sue told Mort, "which means if they understand you, great, and if they don't, they will never admit it."

Sahl's "bravery and bravado" caught on. Fantasy Records recorded a 1955 concert at the Sunset Auditorium in Carmel (and released it after Sahl's Hungry i recordings for Verve in 1959). Already the Sahl style is evident. He talks about jazz, about a hi-fi nut who used his house as a speaker and put his family in the garage, and did bits on cars: "I want to assert my masculinity—shift my own gears." He reported on intellectuals and neurotics, and a bank hold-up in which a robber's note, "act normal," was returned by the teller marked "define your terms."

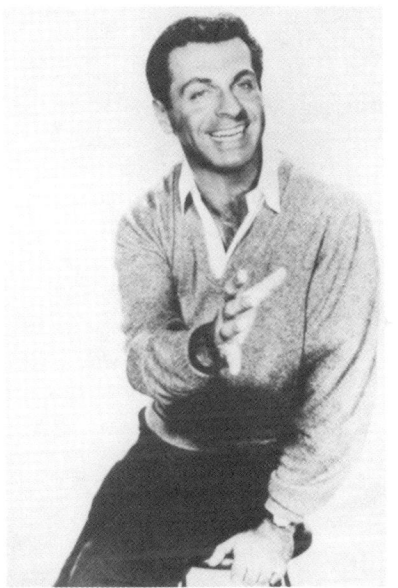

At the Hungry i, where he first attained fame, Sahl brought a newspaper on stage and his work became more topical and political: "Joe McCarthy doesn't question what you say so much as he questions your right to say it." The newspaper served a very basic purpose initially: "I wrote my key lines on paper and stapled them in the newspaper because the silence would make me forget my lines . . . I would digress because I had no discipline. And when I digressed I got my first laugh."

Early on Sahl developed a nervous giggle which helped cue the crowd and underline that no matter how hostile or truthful, there was humor in there, and something to laugh about. The giggle eventually gave way to an even more pronounced barking laugh. The *New York Times* called it "his he-heh black gurgle, as though he were laughing himself to death at all he knew." *The New Yorker* reported that "he erupts into a staccato two-syllable bark" which logically had to come from someone with "big white teeth . . . and a wolfish grin." It's no wonder he became known as "Will Rogers with fangs."

Sahl attacked everything and everyone, using lines that not only hadn't been heard on a stage before, but the kind of thing people barely dared to say in the privacy of their own homes. "I'm not so much interested in politics as I am in overthrowing the government," he'd say. Then he'd talk about a McCarthy jacket with an extra zipper to go over the mouth. He'd note that "Nixon's been on the cover of every magazine except True," or toss off a stream-of-consciousness pun like "A woman's place is in the stove."

The Eisenhower years saw the "Ike-conoclast" (as he was sometimes called) rise to fame. A 1959 Grammy nominee, Sahl was the first comic to have a best-seller with a spoken word comedy lp. Verve seemed to issue fresh records every other month as Sahl covered the U-2 incident, the Eisenhower era's end and the Kennedy-Nixon campaign: "Nixon's trying to sell the country. Kennedy's trying to buy it."

Sahl appeared on the cover of *Time* magazine, a titanic accomplishment for a mere stand-up comic. Magazines regularly quoted his latest jokes. On the missile gap: "Maybe the Russians will steal all our secrets—then they'll be two years behind." On Nixon's visiting Russia: "He can't call anyone a Communist over there and hurt their career." On capital punishment: "I'm for capital punishment. You've got to execute people. How else are they going to learn?"

Mort attacked unfashionable targets, too: "I went to my dressing room between shows and an attorney for the NAACP was waiting for me. He wanted to know why I don't have any Negroes in my act."

Mort asserted during election years, "whoever wins, I will attack him," but with all his Eisenhower jokes, he was perceived as a liberal Democrat, especially by the liberal Democrats of the media. Having written some of the "Kennedy wit" for Senator John Kennedy, few believed Sahl would attack him. Naturally, he did. His album "New Frontiers" was loaded with quips, and they weren't the mild kind that turned up on "The First Family."

The intellectuals and liberals Sahl thought were his undying fans turned against him. TV variety shows closed their doors to him—if he insisted on doing Kennedy jokes. Sahl's income began to shrivel. And, ironically, the Kennedy supporters didn't want to hear from Sahl when he began to talk about the assassination conspiracy. His income dropped from $400,000 a year to $19,000.

As Lenny Bruce was obsessed with the law, Mort became obsessed with the lawlessness in Dallas. When he managed to get a gig on "The Steve Allen Show" or a club date, he'd talk mostly about the Warren Report. For this he was criticized, and it was reported that he'd lost his sense of humor.

"According to Gallup, 88 percent of the American people don't believe in the Warren Report. I certainly wouldn't want it on my conscience that I disturbed the faith of the remaining 12 percent," Sahl remarked sourly.

The blacklist intensified. In Lenny Bruce's case, it ended with a suspicious death. For Mort Sahl, there was a suspicious auto accident, the result, a broken back.

During the Johnson era, Sahl slowly regained his momentum. He worked college campuses, and when LBJ became a monster in the eyes of the media, Sahl was brought back to help slay him. "Whenever there's a political bloat, Mort sticks a pin in it," Hubert Humphrey once said. Now Johnson and Humphrey were ripe targets. Sahl noted Humphrey's subservience to LBJ, mock-quoting him as saying, "It's a beautiful day today, just as President Johnson promised."

Sahl enjoyed renewed success in the Johnson and Nixon years, and found unexpected fortune in Las Vegas, learning that the town "has become populated with busloads of middle Americans, and I found I appeal to them. I guess I appeal to anybody in pain." He had a classic line, which he has since updated: "Two hundred years ago, we had Jefferson, Washington, Ben Franklin and Tom Paine, and there were four million people. Today we have 200 million, and the top guys are Carter and Nixon . . . Darwin was wrong."

Sahl wrote a combination autobiography/essay called *Heartland*, the title reflecting Sahl's new respect for mid-America. He took deadly aim at the liberal press: "Hitler said that he always knew you could buy the press. What he didn't know was that you could get them cheap."

Sahl's book was attacked in the press as bitter and self-serving. It was bristling, challenging and as compelling as his monologues. The one-liners were stronger than ever: "The Christians confuse you with mercy. The Jews want to bring you justice." He attacked former supporters

Hugh Hefner and Woody Allen. When Woody dared suggest during Mort's blacklisting that he could always write a book about JFK's assassination, Mort was furious: "I should have beat the hell out of him, but it looks like somebody did already."

It's hardly surprising that an iconoclast would attack both friends and enemies. But over the years Sahl's barbs on liberals, conservatives, Democrats, Republicans, homosexual cliques in the arts, un-intellectual actresses, students, blacks, the press, talk show hosts and anything else that came to mind bewildered those who never got the message that "is there any group I haven't offended" might include *their* group. From time to time, Sahl would insult the audience as a whole. "Keep paying attention like that," he said after a remark was greeted with silence, "and maybe someday you can talk to your children." On another occasion, when Sahl's view was unpopular enough to get a hissing response, he said, "I like that hissing. I wish you could articulate your position." Sometimes reckless and opinionated as well as satirical and incisive, Sahl never stopped throwing grenades, even if some seemed to self-destruct in his hands.

Sahl hosted local TV and radio shows in Washington, D.C., and Los Angeles during the late 70's, and began a new career as a screen writer, working with Paul Newman, Robert Redford and Clint Eastwood on a variety of projects. As with most movie scripts in Hollywood, they've remained on the shelf, unproduced.

There is still a very strong following for Mort when he goes on tour, delivering his analysis of what he's seen in the papers, on TV, and in person at Hollywood gatherings and White House parties. Reporting on liberals amazed that their children ended up conservative, voting for Reagan, he said, "If anybody comes up to you and says 'My kid is a conservative—why is that?' you say, 'Remember in the 60's when we told you if you kept using drugs your kids would be mutants?'"

"I beg you," Sahl wrote once, "join the battle for your own sake. Give our existence meaning. Lack of purpose is the worst: it's the insanity with no meaning."

After over 30 years, Sahl continues as a relentless, vibrant satirist. In fact, at peak confidence, blending attacks on liberals and conservatives, new moralities and old values, Sahl is currently on an upswing, appealing to anyone who wants to knife through the news and share Sahl's satiric insights.

SOUPY SALES

"Soupy says: don't bite your nails—your nails don't bite you . . . be careful crossing streets—you might get that run down feeling. . . . Keep your chin up. It'll keep the milk from spilling on your clothes!"

The star of one of the most popular kid shows of all time, Soupy was probably the first stand-up comic children paid attention to. He loved to tell classic gags, new corny one-liners and silly jokes that got him laughs—and a pie in the face. He performed with such a spirit of good-natured fun and easy-going hipness that adults began to pay attention, too.

Growing up in Huntington, West Virginia, Soupy appeared in amateur shows in school and was impressed by Ritz Brothers movies. Harry Ritz remains his favorite comic. For years the story was told that his real

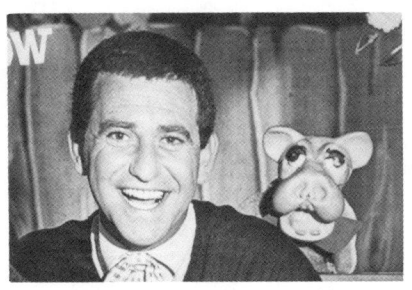

b. Milton Supman, January 8, 1926, Franklinton, North Carolina

Records:
The Soupy Sales Show (Reprise R 6010), Up in the Air (Reprise R 6052), Spy with a Pie (ABC Paramount 503), Do the Mouse (ABC Paramount 517), Bag of Soup (Motown S-686), Still Soupy After All These Years (MCA 5274).

TV:
The Soupy Sales Show (local and ABC network versions 1953–66; syndicated 1979), Sha Na Na (syndicated 1978–80), Donkey Kong (voice on the cartoon series, 1982–   ).

Films:
Two Little Bears, Critic's Choice, Birds Do It, Don't Push, I'll Charge When I'm Ready.

Broadway:
Come Live with Me.

Video:
Video Bloopers (includes the uncut "nude" blooper scene; Video Dimensions).

name, "Milton Hines," led kids to call him "Soupy Heinz." The truth, contrary to many published reference works, is that his name was Supman, not Hines. The nickname came logically enough: "In the South they just naturally called Supman Soupy," he says. He adds with a placid shrug, "It got confused because I used the name Hines when I was on television in Cleveland and people picked up on it ever since." People also moved his birthplace to Franklin County, or Wake Forest, but the affable comic isn't too distressed about such biographical misinformation.

A journalism major at Marshall University, Sales received his B.A. degree and became a script writer for a Huntington radio station. On the side, he did stand-up: "I can recall driving 80 miles to appear at these clubs for $15 a night. The money wasn't much but the experience was invaluable."

In World War II he served on the U.S.S. *Randall* in the Pacific. Afterwards, it was back to stand-up work and a job as a radio station disk jockey. His mix of comedy, music and patter led to a television job in 1950, as host of "Soupy's Soda Shop" for a Cincinnati station. After a stint in Cleveland, he moved to Detroit in 1953 to star in his own children's show. He was the summer replacement for "Kukla, Fran and Ollie" in 1955, and in 1957 he added a Saturday morning network show to his local Detroit program.

"The Soupy Sales Show" moved to Los Angeles in 1960. His blend of one-liners, stand-up gags and slapstick comedy became so popular that he often defeated network shows in the ratings. Many celebrities dropped by to get hit by a pie. In the tradition of the early "Ernie Kovacs Show" and "Carson's Cellar" Soupy kept things loose and lively. The laughter of the camera crew could be heard quite clearly. In 1961 Frank Sinatra took a pie in the face; that episode outdrew even "Rawhide" in the L.A. ratings.

Soupy's first album, on Sinatra's Reprise label, sold 25,000 copies in the first four days of release in Los Angeles. The fad was on. Soupy moved to New York, and the mania spread across the nation with him. There were Soupy Sales cards, books and toys, and in 1965 Soupy's 10-day stint at New York's Paramount Theater recalled the frenzied days of Martin and Lewis. Young fans mobbed the place.

Soupy appeared on "The Ed Sullivan Show" with his routines, and demonstrated his comic abilities on many sit-coms, playing a wide variety of characters in guest roles. Bringing back the fast-paced humor and silliness of vaudeville, Soupy revelled in running gags like a visit from some irate and unseen next-door neighbor (a hand gesticulating in the doorway was all that accompanied the voice), an old Spike Jones record mouthed by Pooky (a hand-puppet lion) or an eccentric dance like "The Soupy Shuffle," a kind of sideways version of Curly Howard's backward skip. Children especially loved the growling and cooing "White Fang" and "Black Tooth," two dogs seen only as hairy paws. Adults especially loved an occasional double-entendre along the way.

Although most of the stories are exaggerated or apocryphal, Soupy did have some overboard moments doing his kiddie show. The most famous was the time he was suspended for jokingly telling kids to mail him some "green pieces of paper" from their parents' wallets. Sometimes the joke was really on Soupy. Once he opened the front door of his stage home to be confronted by a jiggling nude dancer. Home viewers saw only the usual empty doorway, but the practical joke worked on a smiling, weakened Soupy who was speechless and delighted for ten seconds before shutting the door and trying to keep the live show going.

The pies flew fast and furious until 1966 when Soupy left the show to appear on Broadway in *Come Live with Me*. The show didn't make it, but Sales rebounded via the comedian's best friend, the quiz show. He brought his ad-libs and patter to "What's My Line" as a panelist from 1968 to 1975, and also did summer stock, TV specials and stand-up gigs.

Into the 70's he briefly hosted "The New Soupy Sales Show," and later spent three years on the nostalgia show "Sha Na Na." He soon discovered that his young fans, now grown up, never outgrew their penchant for a good, silly gag. In fact, one old fan was on TV with "The Uncle Floyd Show," a fulfillment of every amateur's desire to pretend to be Soupy.

Snobbism in comedy has only recently been dealt the poke in the eye it deserves. For years acts like Laurel and Hardy or The Three Stooges were denigrated for using slapstick. Now, being silly has been recognized as a very special talent. Into the 80's, Soupy Sales has emerged as perhaps the greatest proponent of the fun, corny gag. Corn *is* fun. "You show me a sculptor who works in the basement," Soupy says, "and I'll show you a low-down chiseler!"

Instead of a mechanical delivery of rote oldies, a la Henny Youngman, Sales delights in retelling the classics, and in sharing shaggy dog stories and wacky jests with his unpretentious, equally loose audience. Of course, for grown-up kids, there are jokes that are silly but adult. He tells one about a woman who is attempting to buy a hair remover at a drugstore. She needs it to remove ingrown hairs from her dog's ear:

"The druggist says, you want the cream or the oil? If you're using it under your arms you want the cream. Rub it in really good, but take my advice, don't use any deodorant for two days, it could irritate your arms. She says, 'It's not for my arms.' So he says, 'If you're gonna use it on your legs, you need the oil . . . but don't wear stockings for three days, it could irritate your legs.' And she says, 'It's not for my legs.' She says, 'I want to put it on my Schnauzer.' And the druggist says, 'In that case, don't ride a bicycle for a week!'"

The title of his latest record says it all: "Still Soupy After All These Years." With an open-mouthed chuckle, twinkling eyes and deceptive skill in making it look easy, Soupy has an unrivaled future as the saver and savior of good old gags—and sappy, soupy, silly new ones.

JEAN SHEPHERD

Confidential and conversational, Jean Shepherd's style of monology was unique. It gained him a large cult following on radio, and assured him of packed auditoriums and nightclubs when he chose to tour. He recorded four albums: two studio discs of his quiet monologues, one live, and one that (in a technique pioneered by Murray Roman) collaged live material, sound effects and musical interludes.

In the late 50's *Cue* magazine described him as "a philosopher without portfolio, a wit who never tells a joke, a man who makes you laugh but would never be described as a comic."

Shepherd was a "big brother," telling, in exaggeratedly hushed, intimate and conspiratorial tones, little truths and long, shaggy reminiscences. He rambled on with tales of his Chicago boyhood, his army days, his love for the mediocre Chicago White Sox, and these anecdotes

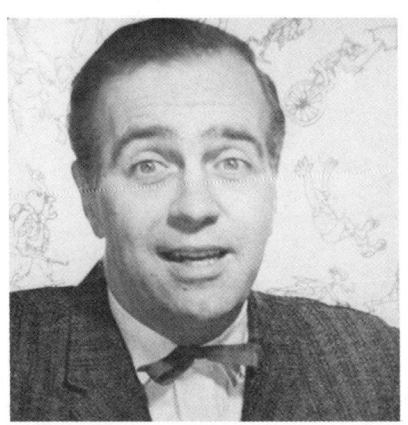

b. July 26, 1923, Chicago, Illinois

Records:
Jean Shepherd and Other Foibles (Elektra EKS 172), Will Failure Spoil Jean Shepherd (Elektra 195), Live at the Limelight (Quote Q-4), The Declassified Jean Shepherd (Mercury SRM 1615).

Books:
In God We Trust All Others Pay Cash, Wanda Hickey's Night of Golden Memories and Other Disasters, Fistful of Fig Newtons.

became little semi-precious gems of Americana. Years later, Hal Holbrook would tour the country in a Mark Twain review, recounting some of Twain's tall tales and anecdotes, doing essentially what Shepherd was doing in the 50's and 60's, turning the misadventures of "Banana Nose" ballplayer Zeke Bonura into the stuff of epic myth, vividly portraying mid-American characters like his own father, who drank beer first thing in the morning ("to get the guts working") and who always believed a pill to turn water into gasoline existed, but was being suppressed by the government.

"Comedy deals with situations," Shepherd once said, "humor looks at the conditions that create them."

Shepherd could muse about almost anything, including this bit of childhood universality:

"The fear of discovery. Yes, how many times had your mother said to you, when you were on your way to the Warren G. Harding School (or your equivalent), 'Did you change your underwear! If you get hit by a car, I don't want them to think. . . .'

"Can you imagine a Mack truck hitting this little squirt. . . . Five minutes later, the surgeon says: 'Look at that underwear!'"

Shepherd could also endear himself to audiences by sharing a one-liner like this: "Ever look at the people around you and say, 'How the hell did I ever wind up with these idiots?'"

"Jean Shepherd is merely a vehicle for communicating to us not only that the emperor has no clothes on, but also that we are *all* naked emperors," Paul Krassner wrote. Of course, other satirists were communicating, too. Guys like Mort Sahl. They got much more press coverage than Shepherd.

"They don't have followers, they have acolytes," he said, in a bitter parody of "bitter" comics. He describes a guy very much like Mort Sahl ("he dresses very casual—an old sweater. And he carries a prop . . . maybe a newspaper") who, in a cave-like club, comes out every hour to deliver "the word."

When the comic says "Adlai Stevenson," the crowd roars. "Now he's beginning to swing," Shepherd whispers mockingly, "he's really giving us the truth." The comic says "Ike!" and the crowd goes wild. Then he offers the topper: "Golf balls!"

Sahl indeed seemed to get envied giggles simply for one-word free-association at times, something that didn't happen often with Shepherd. Twenty years later, when the New York Times reviewed Sahl's autobiography, they ironically chose Jean Shepherd to deliver the knife. It was not a positive review.

At his best, Shepherd animatedly portrayed, with awe and wonder and satiric detachment, the idiocies and dangers of modern living. One of his most popular bits describes an unusual form of addiction:

"Am I chicken? Am I chicken? Just look me in the eye and ask me if I'm chicken," the young Shepherd says to a boy's schoolyard dare. "Five minutes later I got my mouth full of this sticky stuff, and at first it tasted sweet and made me kind of sick, kind of funny and sick. . . ."

Shepherd wonders about this odd substance the boy has given him, dared him to try. His mother notices a strange smell on his breath. But worse, Shepherd discovers that he's hooked on this stuff. And instead of getting more free, that schoolyard boy makes him *buy* some.

He notices a prophetic sentence printed on a box of the stuff:

"The more you eat the more you want." And it's true. Before long, the boy is cadging nickels and dimes from his relatives so he can secretly buy more. It doesn't taste bad anymore. It tastes *good*. And there are even odd little prizes buried in among the bits of gooey popcorn and peanuts.

"The more you eat the more you want. They are not kidding, man. I'm on this stuff for four years. When you first start, you think you're just doing it to get the magic fit-all finger ring. But it's just a come on, like all the rest of life. The more you eat the more you want...."

In his quiet, chillingly satiric way, Shepherd's "Crackerjack" parody typifies his ability to blow up a part of everyday life and find something pathetic, painfully foolish and human about it.

Shepherd, who began making records in the early 60's, has shifted almost completely to magazine articles, books of comic prose, and television specials. Of his 1984–85 edition of "Jean Shepherd's America" (the first premiered in 1971 on PBS) he described the 13-part show as "about a funny man doing crazy fun and games on a little screen that nobody would remember 10 days later." The shows should endure a bit longer, and so should the old albums which are now high-priced collector's items. There are some interesting things to be found on the discs, especially the unique performance: quietly effective and conversational in the studio, animated, celebratory and ironic live.

ALLAN SHERMAN

It was an unlikely hit, but in August of 1963, "Hello Muddah, Hello Faddah" by Allan Sherman reached #2 on the Billboard charts. "God, I'm a lousy singer. Sour notes. High notes I reached for but couldn't make. Not enough breath." Sherman was appalled by his voice. But it was appallingly funny. And people loved the nightmarish "letter from summer camp" he sang to his parents:

"... Now I don't want this to scare ya, but my bunkmate has Malaria. You remember Jeffrey Hardy? They're about to organize a searching party...."

Sherman's own childhood was far worse, scarred by conflict and insecurity. When he was six, his mother and father were divorced. His mother announced that he had to choose whom he wanted to live with. This was not new for Mrs. Sherman, who had been married and divorced at 16, but it was bewildering news for the young boy. Since his mother had been the one to ask, he decided to stay with her. He did not see his father again for ten years.

The boy's guilt and confusion blossomed into misery and insecurity as Sherman struggled through school, attending 21 different institutions. His mother, whom he characterized as a swinger, had more boyfriends than he could count and, along the way, a few more husbands. With all the traffic, Sherman was often dumped with relatives. One was his lively grandfather who took him to Yiddish theater and sang funny tunes around the house.

Sherman grew up chubby and self-conscious about his large hooked nose. But at the University of Illinois in 1941 he was able to enjoy himself, writing humor for the student paper and discovering his ability to create musical parody. After enlisting in the Army, and withdrawing a few months later due to asthma, Sherman returned to school where he gained some attention for writing a patriotic musical (lyrics by Sherman,

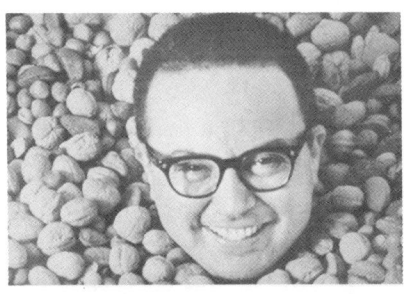

b. Allan Copelon, November 30, 1924, Chicago, Illinois; d. November 21, 1973

Records:
My Son the Folksinger (Warner 1475), My Son the Celebrity (Warner 1487), My Son the Nut (Warner 1501), Allan in Wonderland (Warner 1539), My Name Is Allan (Warner 1604), For Swinging Livers (Warner 1569), Live (Warner 1649), Togetherness (Warner 1684), More Folk Songs with Friends (a reissue of old material: Jubilee 5019), Best of Allan Sherman (Rhino 005).

Play:
The Fig Leaves Are Falling.

Books:
A Gift of Laughter, The Rape of the APE.

music borrowed from *Oklahoma!*). He starred in another show, a musical satire of Adolf Hitler.

The same year, 1943, he met Dolores Chackes, who first helped him get over his sensitivity about his physique, and then helped him get thrown out of school (he was expelled for entering a sorority house with her). Later they married.

Sherman dreamed of a career in show business, but his was not to be an easy, magical trip to the top. In his debut performance, at Danny Thomas's Chicago nightclub, he forgot his lines and was met with catcalls. His humiliation was not complete until he stumbled through the crowd and saw his own mother, drunk, at one of the tables.

Disappearing behind the scenes, he switched to writing comedy. He managed to sell his work to Jackie Gleason, Lew Parker, Joe E. Lewis, Jack E. Leonard and Frances Faye. He regained his confidence and moved to New York in 1945, but was disappointed when his periodic attempts to find a market for his comedy songs failed.

In 1951 he recorded a 78, changing "A Bushel and a Peck" to "A Satchel and a Seck." Jewish novelty tunes were popular—when sung by Mickey Katz. Sherman's entry never made a dent.

The struggling writer developed the idea for a new game show, "I've Got a Secret," and finally made a name for himself. But he didn't make much money. He was so desperate to get a contract with Goodson and Todman Productions that he practically gave away all royalties to the program. But at least he latched on as producer.

Sherman produced "I've Got a Secret" for several years, and then went on to produce Steve Allen's talk show for Westinghouse. Once again, Sherman walked into disaster: he simply didn't work out in this complex role, and was out. Down and out and on unemployment. In his autobiography, he wrote, "I had reached the bottom of the bottom of the bottom." All he had was his family: "That made it even worse. Because there they were and they loved me and I loved them, and there was nothing I could do for them. Nothing."

He tried to sell his parodies again. He created a Jewish version of "My Fair Lady," with songs like "With a Little Bit of Lox," "The Chrain (horseradish) in Spain Tastes Good with 2¢ Plain," and "I Got The Customers to Face." For "On The Street Where You Live" he noted "lanes are curving there . . . names are Irving there." He forgot about two things. They were named Lerner & Loew. They refused to grant permission for parody. Sherman began using public domain material, like folk songs. Capitol Records said "We don't think there's a market for this type of thing," but Warner Brothers thought differently. They decided not to press Allan's dirty version of "Big Bad John," "Big Bad Jim" (written for Warner exec James Conkling) but instead gave him the go-ahead for a folk parody album.

Frantically inspired, Sherman knocked off song after song, and on August 6, 1962, recorded "My Son the Folksinger" in 45 minutes at an informal studio session in front of 100 celebrities and friends. Stars like Steve Allen, Jerry Lewis and Harpo Marx wrote liner notes to help the unknown singer along. And the album was a startling success. Like "The First Family," it took off so quickly that printing plants couldn't keep up with demand. Over a million copies were eventually pressed.

The comic counterpoint between Sherman's plain and humble voice and elegant musical arrangement was funny in itself, classic violins deflated by an ill New York wind. More than that, though, listeners were treated to excellent parody delivered with deft puns and wordplay.

Most Sherman fans have a favorite example. "Glory Glory Hallelujah" became "Glory Glory Harry Lewis," the stirring story of a garment worker who spent his time "trampling through the warehouse where the drapes of Roth are stored."

He turned "Greensleeves" into a homely madrigal about Greenbaum, a knight who could smite dragons, though he privately wished he "could kick the habit—and give up smoting for good."

Often the title alone is enough, like the rousing "Won't You Come Home Disraeli." If there wasn't enough material for a complete parody, Sherman offered quickies, like this version of "Aura Lee": "Every time you take vaccine, take it Aura Lee. As you know the other way is more painful-ly." As unassuming as some of his gentle jests, Sherman was an unlikely star, but managed to rise to the challenge.

Sherman found himself playing Carnegie Hall on New Year's Eve, 1962. "Before I begin," he told the crowd, "I'd better explain why I look different tonight from the way I really look. You see . . . I look exactly like Cary Grant . . . anyway, with the kind of material I do, looking like Cary Grant is not the proper image. So I hired these publicity people—they work on your image—they decided I ought to look short and fat and wear glasses . . . if it works I'll keep it in the act."

Sherman fought against "psychological tension" that he felt played a part in his developing laryngitis, and he fought against throat problems caused by his lack of training as a singer. He continued his tour across the country, winning over audiences with topical parodies he injected, and a piece, "Overweight People," that satirized the intimate style of singers like Judy Garland. Instead of perching at the edge of the stage to sing "Over the Rainbow," Sherman plotzed down and sang of the day "where every little thing I taste won't wind up showing on my waist, or worse—behind me."

Eventually Sherman became smooth enough to host "The Tonight Show," and his live shows co-billed with Harpo Marx (Harpo's last appearances) are legend. In July 1963, the Grammy-winning comic was singing before 18,000 people at the Hollywood Bowl. In July 1964, he was playing before the largest audience ever seen at the Berkshire Music Festival at Tanglewood. But by July 1966 Sherman was in the process of a divorce. Sales of his albums were down, and his autobiography was no longer hot in the bookstores. He tried a new image, doffing his glasses and taking 30 pounds off his 5'7", 225-pound frame. He had some fine songs on his "Togetherness" album, but the public was evidently saturated with the Sherman formula for parody.

In 1969 he wrote *The Fig Leaves Are Falling*, a Broadway musical that closed after one performance. He wrote a book about sex and morality in America, *The Rape of the APE: American Puritan Ethic*, but it wasn't the success he hoped it would be. Sherman's dietary problems and asthma weakened him, and he died of respiratory failure at 48.

Along with *My Fair Lady* and Tijuana Brass albums, Allan Sherman records were a glut in thrift shops at a dollar a copy. But slowly the public began to reassess Sherman's work. His records began to rise in price, the last few becoming $20 collector's items due to their small press runs.

Today there is a new-found, genuine appreciation for his effortless parodies. While the songs that simply "kosherize" a well-known tune with Jewish names or terms may still mystify gentiles, his best material remains deeply witty, warmly humorous and easy to love. The new respect for Sherman has happily extended to a reappraisal of *Rape of the APE*, which remains a very complete, often very funny social study. The man who made one of the biggest splashes in the history of novelty records and stand-up comedy has at last won the right to be thought of as an enduring comedian.

RED SKELTON

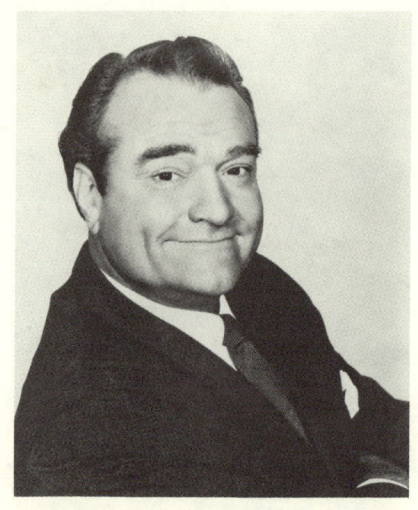

b. Richard Skelton, July 18, 1913, Vincennes, Indiana

Records:
Red Skelton (Mark 56 #699), Red's Rogues Gallery (Radiola MR 1108), Golden Age of Comedy (Evolution 3013), My Favorite Story (20th Century Fox TFM 3106), Red Skelton Conducts (Liberty LST 7425), Music from the Heart (Liberty LST 7477).

TV:
The Red Skelton Hour (CBS 1951–70; NBC 1970–71).

Films:
Having a Wonderful Time, Whistling in the Dark, I Dood It, Whistling in Brooklyn, The Fuller Brush Man, Southern Yankee, The Yellow Cab Man, Three Little Words, The Clown.

Video:
Hollywood Goes to War (includes "Guzzler's Gin"; Video Yesteryear).

Books:
I'll Tell All, Red Skelton in Your Closet, Red Skelton's Gertrude and Heathcliff, Clown Alley.

Bio:
Red Skelton (Arthur Marx).

Red Skelton's beginnings in show business are the stuff of romantic legend. His father was a circus clown who died two months before Red was born. As a youth, Skelton was drawn to comedians. He saw one on stage: "The people around me were laughing their heads off." He thought, "What a lucky buzzard that comedian is. People like him."

Red kept coming back to see the show, "studying the mannerisms and facial expressions, memorizing each word. I began to imitate his act around Smith and Kramer's poolroom. When I started to get laughs and applause, I felt like jumping over the moon."

As a newsboy, he couldn't see shows as often as he would've liked. One day a customer bought all his papers and got him a front row seat for the show. The man was Ed Wynn, and his performance inspired Red even further toward his goal of entering show business.

When the "Doc Lewis Medicine Show" came to town, Red joined the charlatan who sold "elixir" at a dollar a bottle. The redhead was good at drawing crowds for Dr. Lewis, especially when he began entertaining them with slapstick. He recalls, "I fell off the stage once. When I got up, the audience laughed. I decided to fall again to see if I could get another laugh. But that time I jumped up real quick to let them know I wasn't hurt, and the laugh was louder. Now, when I fall, I have to get up even quicker. At my age the audience is really afraid I might be hurt."

From the medicine show, the teenager worked as a blackface singer and dancer on a Mississippi riverboat. He worked in a flea circus, burlesque, and at carnivals all across mid-America. He told jokes, too, and discovered that if one failed, he could rescue it with a pratfall or a bit of visual humor. Before varied audiences he learned the common denominators of laughter.

When the Depression hit, Skelton learned a new way of making a few dollars: the Walkathons. Walkathons and dance marathons were a peculiar and grueling phenomenon of the era, later chronicled in *They Shoot Horses Don't They*. Skelton emceed many of these interminable endurance contests and at one of them met his first wife, Edna, who had been an usherette at the Pantages Theater in Kansas City.

Skelton did anything and everything to keep audiences entertained. In vaudeville he performed spectacular falls into the orchestra pit. With Edna managing him, he found more bookings, but business was still slow. Stalled in Canada in 1936, Skelton idly observed a man eating donuts in a local coffee shop. He became fascinated with the unintentional comedy of the scene, and developed what was to become his ticket to the bigtime, his "Donut Dunking" routine.

In what he calls a "verbamime" (a pantomime where the artist tells the audience exactly what he's going to do), Skelton acted out the sneaky dunker, the fussy dunker, the slosher, and every other type, downing donut after donut, pausing for raucous facial expressions. Like Abbott & Costello, Skelton conquered Broadway with his seemingly effortless style, honed before vaudeville crowds. Nobody but Bud & Lou could make "Who's on First" work, and nobody but Red could get an audience roaring over "Donut Dunking" or the standard gags he dusted off and used in his monologues.

Red began appearing on Rudy Vallee's radio show and in top theaters, and even entertained before Franklin Roosevelt. In 1938 he brought his donut dunking to a short film for Vitaphone (*Broadway Buckaroo*) and featured it in his first full-length film, *Having a Wonderful Time*, in which he was the comic relief.

With the same quickness as Abbott & Costello, Red was upped to star billing and thrown into dozens of movies. He also had his own radio show starting in 1941, where he popularized his catch-phrase ("I dood it!") and characters like the "Mean Widdle Kid," a male Baby Snooks. He wrote his autobiography, I'll Tell All, which some insist told very little. To this day some of the colorful anecdotes about his early years remain unsubstantiated, and some insist that Red has doctored his birthdate from 1910 or even 1906.

Back in the 40's, newspapers began to report on some of the comic's eccentricities. The strangest was the "triangle." Red divorced Edna and married again, yet Edna remained on the scene for years as friend and business manager, the woman he often called "Mommy."

Over the years Skelton's quirks have been well documented: he won't get into a bathtub full of water (the water must be added after he's in), he hates talking on the telephone, he chews up but doesn't smoke 20 cigars a day, he's a perfectionist who is often physically sick before going on stage and then physically exhausted after the show. Then there are the paradoxes. He's been characterized as deeply conservative and inoffensive, yet he enjoys raucous "R-rated" rehearsals and once stopped traffic by projecting a stag film from his window onto a blank billboard. He's warm and friendly, yet bewilders employees with his suspicions and sudden firings. He has the dedication of an artist, yet once threatened to destroy his old TV shows to prevent syndication. "I'm even an enigma to myself," he says. Probably his most famous comment was to a TV Guide interviewer: "I'm nuts and I know it, but as long as I make them laugh they ain't gonna lock me up."

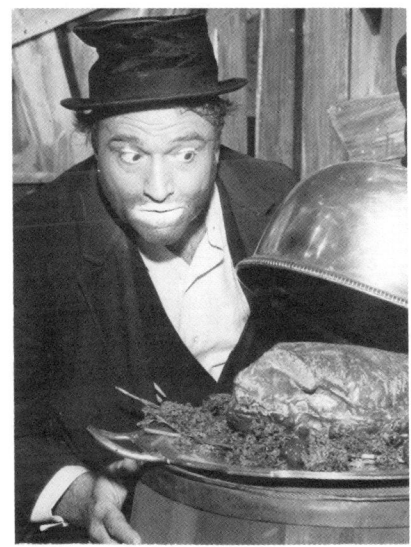

One of Skelton's most popular routines began on radio—but not on Red's show. It was "Guzzler's Gin," which Edna found while going through old radio scripts for possible material. Although not original with him, it's become one of his standards. The premise is simple: while extolling the virtues of his sponsor's gin, an announcer takes a shot too many and becomes the ultimate comic drunk. With outrageous faces, slurred diction and energetic pantomime, Skelton flipped and flopped his way to a boffo, blotto finale. It was yet another example of a bit that could not be performed as well by anyone else.

In 1951 Red shifted his radio show to television and was an immediate Top Ten hit. A few years later, Skelton was weighed down with problems; he was using up all his best visual comedy and working under the increased technical demands of live TV. The same things had spelled disaster for another Red, Red Buttons. Skelton's heavy drinking didn't help matters. But Red managed to hold himself together, only to face even more trauma. In 1958 his son died of leukemia. For years Red kept the boy's room just as it was the day he died, and he would go in there and sit in silence.

Into the 60's, Red put much of the sorrow behind him. He changed houses, gave up drinking, stopped competing with himself by continuing to make movies, and concentrated on his TV show, which soared into the Top Ten again and remained one of the hottest programs through the decade.

Fans couldn't get enough of his cast of characters, including San Fernando Red, George Appleby, Cauliflower McPugg, Clem Kadiddlehopper and Freddie the Freeloader. Every show opened with a monologue and ended with a "silent spot" of pantomime. Some of these were laced with pathos, like his legendary "Old Man Watching a Parade."

Emerson College gave him an honorary degree, and he earned praise of the highest order: "You have a sensitivity and concern for the burdens and suffering of your fellow man."

Skelton's sensitivity was displayed in his eulogy to his late friend Ed Wynn. He talked of laughter, and its arch enemy, silence: "A clown is a warrior who fights gloom. When deafening silence greets his gestures, the agony comes—the loneliness of a lover saying goodbye, a prelude to death. The tears in the eyes dry to a dull glisten. Every nerve reaches out. There is no medication to relieve the pain, no understanding to wrap the wound in. He stands there and bleeds."

Red's show went off the air in 1971, not from low ratings, but from improper demographics. His show was appealing mainly to kids, old folks and rurals—not the affluent, urban, upwardly mobile 30 year olds most sponsors wanted to reach. It was a cruel slap in the face, an insult Red still hasn't forgotten.

Now Red spends time writing, composing songs and symphonies, and painting. His works have sold for $20,000 each, and he does a lively business selling lithographs. And he still tours. At first he played mostly State Fairs, but then he conquered Carnegie Hall, and has since given many Royal Command Performances in Europe. After years of criticism for his sentimentality (his "Pledge of Allegiance" was read into the Congressional Record) and his "low" pantomimes, critics have begun to see the genius of his stand-up work, and the brilliance of his miming, which has been praised by experts including Red's friend Marcel Marceau.

Skelton is one of the very few who can command the stage with verbal humor *and* pantomime. Verbally or visually Red is exhilarating from the start, coming out dimpled and smiling, clapping his hands at the audience, a devilish twinkle in his eyes:

"I feel good tonight!" he begins, perhaps to allay his own backstage nerves.

"I feel good! People tell me 'Gee, you look good.' There are three ages of man—youth, middle age, and 'gee, you look good.' They say, 'Gee, you must exercise a lot.' The only exercise I do is acting as pall bearer for my friends who exercise a lot. But I don't let old age bother me. There are three signs of old age. Loss of memory . . . I forget the other two. . . . My doctor said I look like a million dollars—green and wrinkled."

In cold type, the jokes aren't much, dusty classics at best. But they aren't simply spoken by Red. He acts them out, he revels in each one, and he laughs as heartily as the audience, slinging his arms from side to side, his eyes moist with glee, his tongue sticking forward in his open mouth.

Stan Laurel once said, "I love his talent, but I hate the thing he does with it when he does that deliberate and undeliberate breaking up. In my opinion this is the worst possible thing any comedian can do—the worst." But Skelton isn't just *any* comedian. The free-wheeling giddiness in Red fuels the audience, and it's presented with such sincerity, warmth and good nature that the crowd rolls along with it.

It's magical when he flips his old felt hat up, sideways or down to crown his portraits of old ladies, little kids or cowboys. A hair-fluttering sneeze from Red is a beautiful little comic vignette. He wrings huge laughs from the simplest pantomimes: a woman putting on a girdle, a man eating popcorn, a tailor sewing on a button. As the two seagulls, Gertrude and Heathcliff, he notes: "Red Skelton's for us." "Yeah—he's for the birds." Actually he's for everyone who likes to laugh from the belly and cry from the heart.

And at show's end, both he and the audience exhausted, he gives his benediction:

"I want to thank you for allowing me to be a part of your evening. I sincerely hope I haven't said or done anything to offend anyone. If I have, I didn't mean it. I hope you have had as much fun as I have. It is a lot of fun to try and make people laugh. Regardless of what your heartache might be, while laughing, for a few seconds you have forgotten your troubles. Perhaps in a moment of sorrow, you'll remember something I've said or done, and it will bring a smile again. Thanks for coming, good night, and may God Bless."

SMITH AND DALE

The comedy team of Smith and Dale met as a comedy team should: with a bang. "It was on Delancey Street in New York's Lower East Side when I ran into Charlie," Joe Smith recalled, "and I really mean ran into him. We each had hired a bicycle and were having a Sunday afternoon ride. I came scorching around the corner and smashed right into Charlie."

A fight broke out and when the owner of the bicycle shop came out, he said, "You fellows remind me of Weber and Fields, the way you argue. Take an hour off from this fight and go and talk, because you seem to have a lot in common."

After this historic collision in 1898, Joe and Charlie decided to try their luck in the plentiful cafes, saloons and theaters around town. They danced, sang and told jokes, getting three dollars for their first job as party entertainers.

The team of Sultzer and Marks was not destined to last long: "We got a job at the Palace Garden, a small club," Smith said. "We go to the place, we see a poster. At the bottom we see the name Smith and Dale, no Sultzer and Marks. I go to my brother, who is sort of manager of the place. I ask him who is Smith and Dale. 'That's you,' he says. My brother tells me he went to a printing place to print some cards for us. The printer tells him he has 100 cards. The name on the cards is Smith and Dale, comedians. He says he'll sell the cards for a quarter because the fellows who ordered them cancelled."

Smith and Dale experimented with blackface comedy, all kinds of accents and types of routines. In 1901 they were part of the "Avon Comedy Four," but became a duo again later. They evolved their classic "Dr. Kronkheit and His Only Living Patient" routine around 1906, and toured Europe as stars in 1909. In 1915 the "Kronkheit" routine appeared in *A Hungarian Rhapsody*. Over the years, they developed three-minute, six-minute, fifteen-minute and other length versions of that sketch, to suit the circumstances of the show they were in. Here is an abridged sample from this vaudeville standard. Smith speaks first.

"Are you a doctor?"
"I'm a doctor."
"I'm dubious!"
"I'm glad to know you, Mr. Dubious."
"I'm still dubious."
"Mr. Dubious, are you a married man?"
"Yes and no."

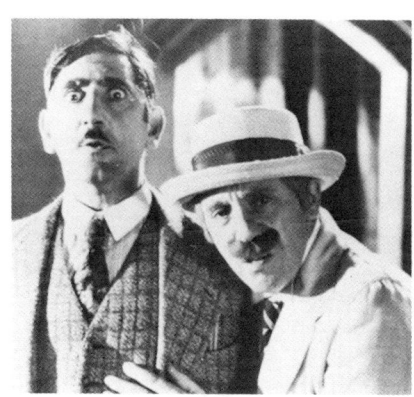

JOE SMITH   b. Joe Sultzer, February 16, 1884, New York, New York; d. February 22, 1981
CHARLIE DALE   b. Charlie Marks, September 6, 1882, New York, New York; d. November 16, 1971

Record:
At the Palace with Smith and Dale (Jubilee 2035).

Compilations:
Golden Age of Comedy (Evolution 3013), Smith & Dale and Moran & Mack (Timestu TS 81600, rereleased as Bramal 59), The Great Radio Comedians (Murray Hill compilation set).

Films:
The Heart of New York, Two Tickets to Broadway.

Broadway:
Mendel Inc., Crazy Quilt, The Sky's the Limit.

"What do you mean, yes and no?"
"I am but I wish I wasn't!"
"Have you any children?"
"I got three beautiful children, a boy and a girl."
"Well, what's the other one?"
"So young who can tell."
"Mr. Dubious, what's your complaint?"
"Before you I saw another doctor. He said I had snoo in my blood."
"Snoo? What's snoo?"
"Nothing, what's snoo with you! But doctor, I'm sick, every time I eat a heavy meal I don't feel so hungry after."
"Maybe you don't eat the right type of vitaminees! What type of dishes are you eating?"
"I should eat dishes? What am I, a crock-odile?"
"No, no, you don't seem to grapse me, what I speak."
"I don't grapse you? Well, if I don't grapse you, you don't grapse me! Besides, you've been eating radishes."
"Don't you like radishes?"
"I love radishes, but not when *you* eat them!"
"So when you drink, vat kind of drinks, liquids—"
"Doctor, (wiping face) don't speak so fluidly!"
"Please, my time is liniment."
"Don't rub it in."
"I have no patience!"
"I shouldn't be here either."
"Now, mister, I'm trying to help you."
"Look, doctor, look at my hand, look how it's moving."
"Did you ever have that before?"
"Yes."
"Well, you got it again."
"And I got rheumatism on the back of my neck. That's a bad place for rheumatism, the back of my neck."
"No, where would you want a better place than on the back of your neck?"
"On the back of *your* neck."
"You should go to Mount Clements for rheumatism, that's the best place."
"The best place?"
"That's where I got mine. Now look me in the face."
"I got my own troubles."
"The whole trouble with you is you need eyeglasses."
"My eyes are all right!"
"You owe me $10."
"For what?"
"For my advice."
"Well, Doctor, here's $2, take it that's my advice!"
"You cheapskate, you come in here, you cockamamie—"
"One more word and you only get a dollar."
"Why—"
"That's a word! Here's the dollar!"

Smith and Dale starred in *The Passing Show of 1919* and were regulars in reviews thereafter, touring Europe, headlining London's Palladium in 1929. Their routines, told in comic Jewish dialect, were timeless. As Joe Smith said, "An old joke is a new joke if you haven't heard it before."

They were still stars through the passing decades, appearing in *Bombshells of 1943* among other revues. In 1946 they met President Harry S.

Truman, who shook hands saying, "Are you a doctor? I'm dubious!" Joe Smith answered, "How do you do, Mr. Dubious."

In 1951 they were still going strong, headlining with Judy Garland at The Palace. And in 1962, the ageless team took over the Mayfair Theater on Broadway for *Old Bucks and New Wings.* They regularly appeared on television variety shows, resurrecting the sketches about doctors, tax consultants and other occupations that had always won them laughter.

Asked once if Smith and Dale had many fights over the years, Smith answered, "We do so much arguing on stage that we don't have anything left to argue about offstage."

More than six decades after that bicycle smash-up on Delancey Street, Smith and Dale were still actively performing. After the death of his wife, Dale moved to the Actors Fund Home in Englewood, New Jersey. When Smith's second wife died, he too found the place to his liking: "We'd rather be here because we know people here." They staged shows and entertained the many visitors who came out to see them.

Smith, who was still giving interviews at age 96, was very much alive when Neil Simon's *The Sunshine Boys* opened on Broadway. "I like it very much," he told *The New Yorker.* "Of course, it's a paraphrase, but it's very well done . . . the trouble with the show is that people think I have something to do with it. I'm even getting letters asking for seats. . . ."

Smith insisted that, unlike what occurs in the play, "I never did poke Charlie hard. I'd point my finger at him, and, if necessary, give him a little jab when I said 'You're making a mountain out of a mothball' but I never hurt him. . . . And as for all that about my spitting in his face during the act when I pronounced my 't's, why, it was *he* who spit in *my* face when he pronounced his 'p's."

The veteran comic could look back on all those years and say, "We were about as close as two men could be. . . . Charlie's buried in Woodlawn Cemetery and I'll be laying alongside of him. We have a headstone and it says 'Smith and Dale.' I wanted to add: 'Booked Solid.'"

THE SMOTHERS BROTHERS

The changes in the 1960's were personified, in comedy, by the Smothers Brothers. They began their career in 1960, saw it ebb by 1969, and along the way changed from innocent, crew-cutted young folk singers to long-haired (well, as long as they could manage) political and social satirists. During the decade they issued ten comedy albums.

Born in New York, the brothers (plus sister Sherry) grew up in California, where the family had moved following the death of their father, Major Thomas Smothers, in a prisoner of war camp. Although part of their comedy routine involved the idea that "Mom liked Dick best," the boys did everything together and equally, attending Southwestern Military Academy, Redondo Beach High School and San Jose State College where they put together their music and comedy act.

There was a lot of opportunity for folk acts back then. The "folk boom" was on, begun by Harry Belafonte, The Kingston Trio and others. With Tom providing the leadership and optimism, the boys performed more and more. An engagement at San Francisco's Purple Onion was a breakthrough.

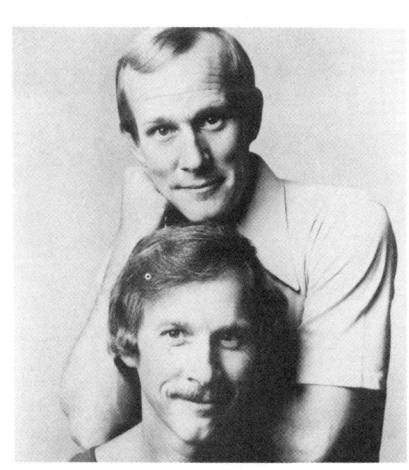

TOM SMOTHERS   b. February 2, 1937, New York, New York
DICK SMOTHERS   b. November 20, 1939, New York, New York

Records:
Purple Onion (Mercury SR60611), Two Sides (Mercury SR60675), Think Ethnic (Mercury SR60777), Curb Your Tongue, Knave (Mercury SR60862), It Must Have Been Something I Said (Mercury SR60904), Tour de Farce (Mercury SR60948), Aesop's Fables (Mercury SR60989), Mom Always Liked You Best (Mercury SR601051), Golden Hits Volume 2 (Mercury SR601089), The Smothers Brothers Comedy Hour (Mercury SR61193).

TV:
The Smothers Brothers Show (CBS 1965–66), The Smothers Brothers Comedy Hour (CBS 1967–69), The Smothers Summer Show (ABC 1970), The Smothers Brothers Show (NBC 1975).

Broadway:
I Love My Wife.

Video:
Bing Crosby Show 1963 (Video Yesteryear).

Of an appearance on his TV show, Jack Benny recalled, "When they first bounced onstage in their bright red blazers, shoe button eyes shining and faces freshly scrubbed, I was sure they had mistaken the studio for an eighth grade dancing class. But the minute they opened their mouths it was clear that I had hired the funniest comedy team around."

At first they sang standards like "Tom Dooley" or "Tzena Tzena" with the humor coming from comical introductions, false starts and fighting by-play. During a duet, Dick would shout, "Take it, Tom!" and the obstinate brother would say, "No," starting an ad-libbed argument.

1962's "Two Sides of the Smothers Brothers" showed the duo divided between their folk past and comic future. On their Grammy-nominated third album, Tom and Dick's characters were etched. Tom, in reality the older brother, was the childlike fool, playful and undisciplined, stuttering and inarticulate, prone to comic temper tantrums when frustrated. Dick behaved like the prissy older brother, trying to keep his sibling in line while the parents were out.

"You know why I'm mad most of the time?" Dick would say to Tom. "Because it's difficult being an only child."

The sibling rivalry theme progressed through the years, giving them their identity and the catch-phrase "Mom always liked you best." They also specialized in cute novelty songs from such writers as Mason Williams, Jerry Bock and Sheldon Harnick, and Oscar Brand. They not only picked excellent material, they gave it sparkle in performance. The comedy is virtually nonexistent in such songs as "Church Bells" and "Jenny Brown," for example, when heard performed by the original composer.

Gradually the brothers experimented with bits of irreverent humor, even if it started with parodies of folk songs ("When John Henry was a little baby, sittin' on his daddy's knee . . . his daddy picked him up, threw him on the floor and said 'This baby's done wet on me'") or mock-ups of pop standards ("You better not cry, you better not shout, you better not pout I'm tellin' you why: Santa Claus is Dead"). Eventually they were performing things like Pat Paulsen's "Mediocre Fred," about a dullard who led an uninteresting life—except for the nights he'd "climb over the moat, find some people sleeping and he'd bite their throats!"

The boys were still pure Americana. Many of their satires were on classic American and folk figures like Paul Bunyan and Hiawatha, their humor very good natured, mildly sassing teachers' history lessons. With their crew-cuts and neat red blazers, they marked a return to naive, innocent comedy after the late-50's "sickniks" like Sahl, Bruce and Berman.

Their first TV show was a mild sitcom: "There's miracles to start but they always come apart," was the show's theme song. Tom as a ghostly "apprentice angel" tried to help Dick out in his everyday existence on earth. The short-lived show gave Tom a look at the production end of the business. It also gave him an ulcer.

Their second show, a variety series, was a huge success in 1967. By this point in the decade, folk singers like Bob Dylan had turned to protest, and so did the brothers. From guests like Glen Campbell and Nancy Sinatra, the boys turned to Mort Sahl, Joan Baez, Elaine May and The Beatles. They satirized President Lyndon Johnson, included drug humor (a continuing character was "Goldie O'Keefe"), and gave David Steinberg the chance to do religious comedy.

The brothers waged a constant war against CBS censors, who often ripped entire segments out of the show, from Pete Seeger songs (it was the brothers who courageously ended his long TV blacklist) to the words

"Please talk peace." "We stand out because nothing is being said," Tom remarked. "We would be moderates anywhere else. We stand out as rebels or anarchists only because of the great lack of anything pertinent on television." Indeed, by today's standards, their humor is milk mild.

Typical of their political satire was the time Tommy told his brother he had discovered a clue to how the government was being run. "There's a theory of clothes and politics. There's a definite corrolation. You can tell who's running the country by how much clothes people wear." Dickie is intrigued. "You mean some people can afford more clothes on, and others less on?" Tommy nods. "The ordinary people are the less ons." "Then who's running the country?" "The more-ons!"

CBS, looking for a reason to drop the show (although it was the only series to dent the ratings of NBC's "Bonanza"), claimed they weren't getting previews on time. The brothers were cancelled. Four years later, in 1973, they won a breach-of-contract suit against CBS, but it was too late.

The Smothers Brothers had been replaced by "Hee Haw" and other variety shows. A mild new show in 1975 (using Carol Burnett's producer) was unsuccessful. Getting a bit too old to complain about who mom liked better, wised up after the 60's, and with folk music dead, the brothers found themselves adrift, viewed as icons of a past decade along with other 60's figures. The Beatles broke up before the 70's began: it seemed that the brothers were finished, too. "Tom's more interested in show business than I am," Dick commented. "I could be happy out of it."

On December 30, 1976, the Smothers Brothers made their farewell appearance at the Aladdin Hotel in Las Vegas. That same year they started a winery, which today produces gold medal-winning products. Tom appeared without Dick in a few movies, but couldn't establish a new character to replace his cute and boisterous "dummy buffoon."

In 1978 the brothers re-teamed, appearing on Broadway in the musical comedy *I Love My Wife*. After a year, they took the show on the road. They began making a few concert appearances as well, timing them so they wouldn't interfere with their wine business schedule.

A tour with Joan Rivers in 1983 re-established them, and they developed some new routines, including a nostalgia act revolving around such childhood pastimes as yo-yo tricks (which Tom would perform ineptly and sometimes rather eptly). And they continued their comic arguments. After a prissy put-down from Dick, Tom might turn and say:

"Why are you beating this with a dead stick?"
"When you talk like this you act like a stupid fool, Tom!"
"That's my job!"

Both divorced and in their mid-40's, the brothers now have several tongue-in-cheek lines parodying their old sibling rivalry. And in the interest of nostalgia they're not only back doing their old bits, they're back in their red suits. "I don't like doing it to tell the truth," says Dick. "Tommy wants us to do it because it's traditional with the act. It lets people know who we are—when they see red jackets they don't confuse us with other people."

In 1984 the duo appeared as humorous on-screen narrators for several HBO specials that took a look at the bizarre, funny and often perverse TV commercials politicians have utilized during election years. Their work on these specials demonstrated that the Smothers Brothers have not abandoned their interest in political satire, and that they could be effective in a low-key setting, sans references to childhood.

DAVID STEINBERG

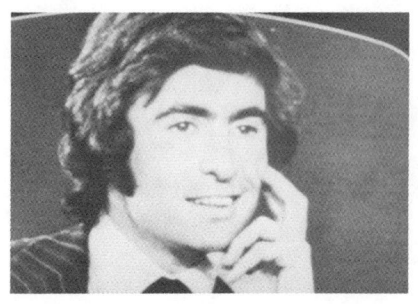

b. August 9, 1941, Winnipeg, Canada

Records:
The Incredible Shrinking God (Uni 73013), Disguised as a Normal Person (Elektra EKS-74065), Booga Booga (Columbia KC 32563), Goodby to the 70's (Columbia PC 33399).

Video:
Comedy Tonight (Vestron), In Concert (RKO), Showbiz Ballyhoo (USA).

Religious humor of any kind was a firm taboo on TV—until David Steinberg began delivering comical "sermons" on "The Smothers Brothers Comedy Hour" in the late 60's. Like the biblical David, little David Steinberg stood alone as he delivered the barbs. The Goliath TV network shuddered a bit, and the letters from outraged viewers poured in, but Steinberg stood his ground. At last, it was the right time and the right place for such material.

Steinberg did bits that reflected a young generation's religious cynicism:

". . . And God looked down and saw that the land and the people were bad. If He didn't look down so much maybe things would pick up." When God tells Moses, "I am that I am," Moses coughs politely and says, "Thanks for clearing that up."

His humor, in retrospect, was mild. In a new version of the story of Lot, Lot's wife turns out to be such a nagging nuisance that, as they leave Sodom and Gomorrah, Lot says, "Dear—God told me to tell you to look back." Pausing in the midst of fables on Jezebel and Solomon, he acknowledged that he had missed Onan: "I can't do Onan tonight—I suggest you go home tonight and do it yourself."

His first album of religious satire, released when he was only 27, had liner notes by Nelson Algren. It was Algren who correctly established Steinberg's place among the other comics who had dabbled with religious material in nightclubs: "Lord Buckley's God looked upon Man with the golden eyes of love. Lenny Bruce's stayed in a towering rage. David Steinberg's God won't answer unless you call Him Mike. . . . That's the nice thing about Mike—there's nothing formidable about him."

Steinberg was able to kid about biblical incongruities, and God's tendency to put the "anthropomorphic ZAP!" on people. He could even touch upon that most delicate of problems: God's seeming playfulness with mortal men's lives.

The son of a rabbi, Steinberg says, "I was the only one in my family who *wasn't* funny. They all shared this vicious, Russian-Yiddish sense of humor, and because I was the youngest, I was usually the victim. One of the recurring jokes was how quickly I cried. Now, when you cry quickly, that's not funny."

Steinberg enrolled for religious training and at 18 was sent for a year to Israel. "In Israel I studied theology and ran after girls. I went to Chicago and studied some more theology and ran after some more girls. By this time I'm sounding like Harpo Marx. I saw Lenny Bruce and something happened to me."

At the University of Chicago, he began performing comedy. He was impressed by Nichols and May's work, and was shocked when the director of their Second City troupe invited him to join, based on Steinberg's performance in a school production of *Candide*.

Steinberg earned a Masters Degree in English literature and in 1964 was one of the improvisational stars of The Second City. Although he had the ability to perform manically (as seen in his Groucho-influenced audience participation routine pretending to be an insane psychiatrist), Steinberg never lost the intellectual style of delivery, and an intimate, conversational approach to monology.

After his Second City appearances he landed a job in the off-Broadway *Mad Magazine* revue, *The Mad Show*. This encouraged him to try serious dramatics, but short runs on Broadway in 1967's *Little Murders* and 1968's *Carry Me Back to Morningside Heights* lessened his enthusiasm.

Steinberg pursued comedy at The Bitter End, and in 1969 appeared for ABC in a TV series called "The Music Scene" where his catch-phrase "Booga Booga!" first turned heads.

Steinberg's big break came on "The Smothers Brothers Comedy Hour," where he performed his religious satires. Lines like "The Gentiles grabbed the Jews by the Old Testament" irritated the CBS censors. But so did almost any religious joke. Much to Steinberg's delight, he was propelled into the midst of publicity and controversy. He wasn't too delighted, though, when he received some of the blame for the cancellation of the series.

As it turned out, Steinberg appeared on CBS with his own variety show the summer after the brothers left the air. He soon became a comfortable enough figure in American living rooms to host "The Tonight Show" often.

Steinberg's humor was no longer religiously oriented. He did more diverse material, including an occasional fey one-liner ("The reason I feel guilty about masturbation—is I'm so bad at it"). He was still known as one of the "intellectual" comics, along with Dick Cavett. He used long words, cerebral metaphors and contrived wit that required a carefully enunciated, quiet, slow delivery to be understood.

In this bit, talking about a sexual encounter with an air-head, he delivers lines that would, for most other comedians, be too unwieldy to be appreciated. In measured tones, he begins:

"Imagine. You have attained undreamed of horizons of virtuosity. You have devised and executed maneuvers that would mystify even Masters and Johnson. You have become to sex what Julia Child is to a chicken. And as you're lying there in the afterglow of a moment that poets devote their whole lifetimes to describe, she turns to you and says, 'Hey . . . that was cute.'"

And David Steinberg was (and is) cute, utilizing his contrast between the intellectual and the passionately real. Over the years his audience has remained attentive to his humorous literary similes ("President Nixon has a face that looks like a foot," an old man's wrinkled neck "looks like the escalator at Bloomingdale's," someone trembles "like David Eisenhower at an orgy"). His answer to hecklers is appropriately impatient and intellectual: "Unless it's gonna be a witty exchange—it's a pain in the ass."

In 1973 Steinberg starred in the ABC TV-movie "Night Train to Terror," and developed into both a film actor and director. His credits include *Something Short of Paradise* in 1979. The following year he and Burt Reynolds formed a production company and signed with ABC. He has also continued duties as a talk show host, and in 1984 starred in a series of talk specials featuring famous guests. Even in this role, Steinberg retained his individuality. When asked why he avoided sensational questions (like asking Burt Reynolds about Sally Field) he replied, "I don't have any feeling that I have to give the audience what they want . . . only what interests me. That makes it a better interview."

As a guest on "The Tonight Show" in February of 1985, Steinberg was still displaying a sly, dry wit. In the presence of Johnny Carson, who had recently been in the headlines when his ex-wife demanded an additional $6,000 to her weekly $44,000, he mused about a TV movie, "Hollywood Wives": "Imagine the premise of 'The Hollywood Wives' . . . they're trying to convince us that there are wives of celebrities who do *nothing* but shop and have lunch! And just wait till they can divorce the celebrity . . . and just take everything that that celebrity's got." The audience roared as Carson broke up with embarrassed, gleeful chuckling.

Using the cerebral approach, Steinberg set up a premise. Having watched a TV actor do a commercial, he noted, "He says in the ad, I'm not a real doctor—but I play one on TV. And then he sells cough medicine! Well, I take that a step further. How about the President? He was an actor. How about him saying, 'I'm not a president, I just play one on television' . . . I feel like I'm in Reagan's mini series, and we're all gonna get cancelled."

Of his monologues, he says, "I really don't think about what the audience wants when I am preparing my material. Nor do I condescend to what a TV audience is supposed to be. To do so is to drop to the lowest common denominator."

When asked what his ultimate goal was, he once said, "To sexually satisfy the entire King Family, right before their big Thanksgiving Special." These days, he continues to fulfill his ambitions as a comedian in nightclubs, and as an actor and director. His place in comedy is assured by his thoughtful, literate humor, and by his being the first comic to successfully present religious satire on national television.

STILLER AND MEARA

When Jerry Stiller and Anne Meara met, it was a scream. Literally. Both were struggling actors, auditioning for practically every play in town. Waiting for an interview, Jerry heard a scream. Suddenly he saw a tall, pretty young redhead race out of the agent's office. She told him that the agent had chased her around the room.

When Stiller confronted the agent, the man chased *him* around the room, too! "In the end neither of us got a job," he recalls, "so we went out together to drink coffee and console each other. That was the start of our relationship."

It wasn't the start of a comedy team, though. Both were still intent on careers on the legitimate stage. Stiller had majored in drama at Syracuse University and worked in summer stock. Meara appeared in small productions on Long Island before studying acting at the Herbert Berghof Studio. She appeared with Zero Mostel in *Ulysses in Nighttown* and in Michael Redgrave's production of *A Month in the Country*.

Together, they joined the fledgling Shakespeare company run by Joseph Papp. The idea was to stage the Bard's work in Central Park: "In those days we didn't have a stage in Central Park. People just sat around us informally. So in the middle of a play you'd have a guy yelling from the grass, 'Ay, Romeo, give it to her! Give it to her!'"

Anne was often the leading lady and Jerry the fool or comic foil. When they discovered the ushers were making more money, they realized something had to give. They experimented with different styles they could use in a duo act for benefits, cabarets and clubs. Their experience in theater gave them the skill to develop two-character comedy sketches.

They were compared to Nichols and May, who also used character sketches, but this team was much warmer. They specialized in the natural humor of everyday people, especially opposites who have attracted but ironically remained opposite in some irritating ways. They slightly exaggerated moments of truth in a relationship:

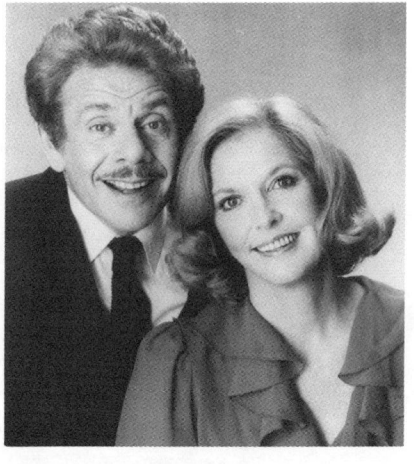

JERRY STILLER   b. June 8, 1928, Brooklyn, New York
ANNE MEARA   b. September 20, 1929, Rockville Centre, New York

Records:
Presenting Stiller and Meara (Verve V-15038), The Last Two People in the World (Columbia CS 9542), Laugh When You Like (Atlantic SD 7249).

"I hate you," Jerry mutters.

"You hate me? I hate you!"

"You don't know what hate is, the kind of hate I have for you."

"Listen," says Anne, warming up, "my hate for you is such a hot hate, I hate you with hot heaping hunks of hate!"

Jerry doggedly persists: "The heat of your hot hate could not begin to approximate the hateful hatredness with which I'm hatefully hating you right now."

Anne burns: "If it was possible to write the word 'Hate' on each grain of sand in the Sahara desert . . . all that hate on each of those hateful grains wouldn't equal one one-millionth of the hate that I'm hating you with right now!"

"You know how much you hate me? Double it! That's my hate for you!"

There is a pause in the fight. "I'd like to ask one question," Jerry deadpans. "Do you think this marriage can be saved?"

The battle rages on, until it becomes a brawl. "You matzo head!" Anne jeers. "You shillelagh shiksa," Jerry growls. "I'll give you shiksa. You don't know shiksa from Shinola." "You meshugenah Mother Machree!" "You Tel-Aviv Tummeler!" "You tooraloora tushy, you!" "You cockamamie knish!" "Let's stop this before it reaches the name-calling stage."

At last Jerry vows to leave, but not before he takes his Batman toothbrush, a gift from Anne. Anne is touched. They make up. And . . . yet another trifle brings them back to a final barrage of ludicrous argument.

The duo appeared in clubs like the Crystal Palace in St. Louis, New York's Bon Soir and London's The Establishment. Known soon as the funniest husband and wife team since Burns and Allen, they won a spot on a Merv Griffin afternoon talent showcase and became regulars on "The Ed Sullivan Show," appearing every two months. Many of the sketches they used on the show were variations on the theme of bumpy relationships, whether it was a young dating couple, or a husband and wife feuding about starch in the collar:

"Why would I want starch in a collar that says 'do not starch'?"

"To keep your chin up," Anne says sweetly. "You have a weak chin . . . so does your mother. . . ."

"Look dammit—"

"Don't you swear at me, you cretin!"

The battle royal begins, but this time they both have an idea. They'll follow a marriage counselor's advice and see things "from the other's point of view." Jerry apologizes: "You were *right* in putting starch in my collar," he says. Anne demands the same right of apology. "Don't tell me I was right when I was wrong." Jerry is conciliatory: "You're wrong in saying you're not right in putting starch in the collar." Anne: "You're wrong in saying that I'm wrong in saying I'm not right in putting starch in the collar." Jerry stops. "You're wrong . . . in saying what you just said. . . ."

They find the argument so stupid, they begin to laugh. Until Jerry notices something else: "There's no button on this shirt—" and off they go again.

What Stiller and Meara brought to these sketches, aside from the timing to make the escalation funny and the tangled rage sound true, were identifiable characters. Jerry's husband was comically deadpan, limited in vision, capable of anger but clearly a bit of the lost child, and vulnerable. Anne's comic wife had a variety of perfectly enunciated New York accents (depending on the sketch's setting) and was by turns pleading, caustic, tough and fragile.

The duo *did* perform standard shtick, but not in their domestic sketches. They saved the broad gags for things like the inevitable doctor-newswoman interview:

"You're just coming from the operating room?"
"No, I just came from the men's room. Are we on the air?"
"What is the first step on admitting a patient?"
"We get a check . . . as soon as the check clears, they're admitted. Otherwise we have to keep the baby."
"That's shocking, doctor."
"It is—when you consider the number of kids we have on the third and fourth floor."

Over the years Stiller and Meara found their way back to the theater, Jerry in shows like *Unexpected Guests, The Ritz* and *Hurlyburly,* the latter directed by Mike Nichols, Anne in *The House of Blue Leaves* and *Spookhouse.* Jerry has done a number of movies, many TV dramas and sit-coms, and was a regular on the series "Joe and Sons." Anne was a regular on sit-coms ("Rhoda" and "Archie Bunker's Place") and starred in the series "Kate McShane." She and Jerry appeared together in the film *Nasty Habits* and the TV movie "The Other Woman," which Anne co-wrote.

The most ubiquitous man-woman team on radio, Stiller and Meara have created and starred in dozens and dozens of commercials, most of them with a gentle comic edge. They've won practically every advertising award possible on behalf of their company, Stiller and Meara Enterprises. They are also well known for their charity work and their concern for causes big (the nuclear freeze) and small (their local New York block association).

They are also still very much in demand as a stand-up team, and many avidly request their old, poignant routine about Hershey Horowitz and Mary Elizabeth Doyle, the Jewish man and Irish woman who, after many a comic confrontation, would wistfully wish that "maybe someday, two people like us who wanna get married can just get married." Of course, they are living proof of that happy, harmonious possibility.

LILY TOMLIN

In December of 1969, a new young comedienne joined the cast of TV's "Laugh-In." She brought with her a wealth of exotic characters, like the stuffy-nosed, snorting terror of the telephone company, Ernestine:

"One ringy-dingy, two ringy-dingy," she'd enunciate. Reaching her party, Mr. Vidal, she offered the following:

"Mr. Veedle? You owe us a balance of $23.64. When may we expect payment? Pardon? When what freezes over? Mr. Veedle, you are not dealing with just anyone's fool. I am a high school graduate. . . . I think you'd prefer to pay up rather than lose your service and possibly the use of one eye."

With Ernestine, Lily Tomlin became a sensation. She won a Grammy for her first album, "This Is a Recording," and it sold thousands of copies.

Her fame as the nutty telephone operator was such that "When I was in Las Vegas, I went into a luncheonette and ordered a hamburger. The guy behind the counter went into a telephone booth, ripped out the dial, put it in a hamburger bun and gave it to me."

But there was much more to Lily Tomlin than Ernestine, a character that was essentially based on the callous telephone company woman created by Elaine May. There was the sticky brat Edith Ann, bag ladies, chic wretches, "Sister Boogie Woman" and even the quadriplegic Crystal. Lily developed into America's most critically acclaimed female stand-up, earning the kind of praise once heard for her early influences, Elaine May and Ruth Draper.

Tomlin's dedication to her comedy characterizations comes across in interviews. Even the essentially one-dimensional Ernestine has an unusual creative process: "Doing Ernestine is really a very sexual experience. I just squeeze myself very tight from the face down. The bottom line with Ernestine is that she is a very sensual person."

Born in Detroit, Tomlin's parents were from Kentucky. "They were just working people," she recalls. "My father was a job setter in a factory, my mother a nurse's aide in a hospital. They were funny, terribly funny, but then, everyone is, really."

Her father gave her some advice: "Babe, pay your own way. Don't owe anybody anything." It stuck with her. Early on Lily earned her own money by doing chores and odd jobs for neighbors. She skipped school when she felt like it, and grew up to be a member of "The Scarlet Angels," a clique of high school girls who "wore ballet shoes, pegged skirts and lots of black."

She was intrigued by the comediennes she saw on TV—stand-up Jean Carroll, satirist Bea Lillie and comic actresses Imogene Coca and Lucille Ball—but it wasn't until she went to Wayne State University that she seriously pursued dramatics.

She'd enrolled in pre-med: "I'm a Virgo, and most of them are hypochondriacs. Like I read up on leprosy when I was a kid and found out it had an incubation period of eleven years, so I spent a lot of time thinking I might have it."

A variety show needed material, and she managed to assert herself, breaking in despite some initial fears. Soon her interest in medicine flagged, and she was taking dance and mime lessons instead. She had a feeling she could make it in show business, but that meant leaving Detroit: "When I arrived in New York, I had $15 in my pocket but I didn't have the good sense to be scared."

One of the odd jobs Tomlin took was as a waitress at a Howard Johnson's at Broadway and 49th Street. She did her best with the sleazy customers, hum-drum hurry and depressing co-workers. For a time she even found amusement in trying to get applause from the diners for being named "Waitress of the Week." One day, with customers barking out orders and other waitresses whisking away her silverwear and trays before she could get to them, she brought the place to a halt:

"I rapped on the counter and I shouted, 'All right, this is the last time anybody takes my silver! I'm not serving another thing!' And I quit right there in the middle of the lunch rush. I've heard that most mental breakdowns occur in the restaurant business and I believe it."

Lily lived in an East Village apartment atop the B&H Dairy Luncheonette in a noisy, dirty area on Second Avenue. She lived there with her brother, visiting thrift shops, collecting items of movie memorabilia like Ruby Keeler's tap shoes, Harriet Hilliard's (later Harriet Nelson) gowns and Alexis Smith's clutch bag.

A 1965 appearance at Cafe Au Go Go helped her advance, and she gained some attention in *Below the Belt*, a Julius Monk–styled cabaret

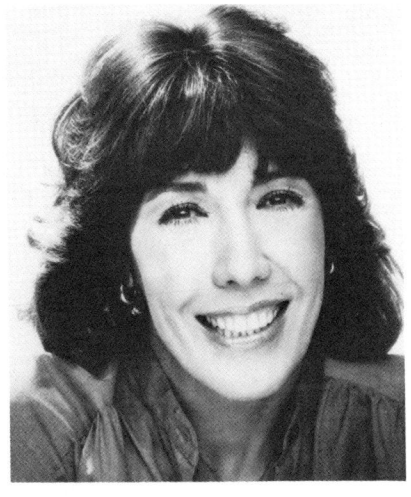

b. Mary Jean Tomlin, September 1, 1939, Detroit, Michigan

Records:
This Is a Recording (Polydor PD 24405; material from this album is included on "Comedy Classics" [ERA BU 3890]), And That's the Truth (Polydor PD 5023), Modern Scream (Polydor PD 6051), On Stage (Arista AB 4142).

TV:
Rowan and Martin's Laugh-In (NBC 1969–73).

Video and Films:
Nashville, The Late Show (Warner Video), Moment by Moment, The Incredible Shrinking Woman (MCA), Nine to Five, All of Me, Lily Tomlin Special (Karl Video), Saturday Night Live 1975 (Warner).

revue at Upstairs at the Downstairs. Meanwhile she worked as an office temporary, and was buoyed by landing a commercial for Vapo-Rub. She also did some brief work on "The Garry Moore Show," where Carol Burnett first achieved fame.

Her ability to interpret a variety of unusual, real women made some think of her as a young Carol Burnett. Her talent for unusual characters came from "the kinfolks . . . Lud, Pud, Odie Mae, Ermadee" and other relatives she encountered.

She impressed critics with her work in another review, 1968's *Photo Finish*, which led to a spot on "The Merv Griffin Show." She scored with a monologue about an unfortunate girl who couldn't understand, as she lit up her cigar, why she was having trouble with blind dates.

Tomlin found favor with many unusual monologues, including an early piece about a "rubber freak" housewife who loves to eat rubber bands and is finally rehabilitated—into an alcoholic.

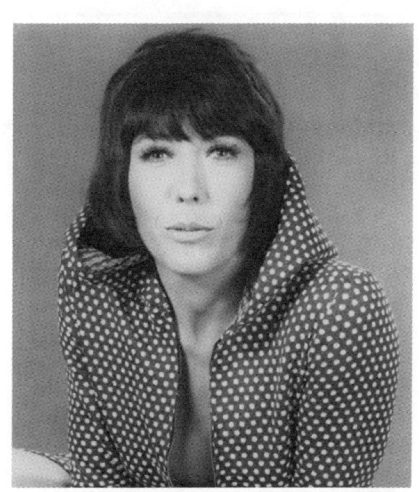

She did "How to Entertain Your Friends at a Wake," which included such suggestions as using the corpse as a ventriloquist's dummy, or shouting "Last one to the cemetery is a rotten egg." She did Nichols and May black humor; a guest at the funeral tells the widow, "It's a shame you didn't have any of his children. Everybody else did."

The short-lived "Music Scene" TV show was her next exposure, and that led to "Laugh-In." Her Ernestine bit was so popular the telephone company offered her a half million dollars to do ads. Tomlin was furious: "I was insulted because they wanted to turn my creation to their use. I was so horrified and insulted that they had the audacity to think I would do it."

She followed the Grammy-winning album of Ernestine humor with "And That's the Truth," featuring her new creation, bratty Edith Ann. Again critics noted the artistry behind the creation, and the serious intent mixed into the comedy. Edith Ann describes anger:

"You know what happens when you get angry? First your face gets just like a fist, and then your heart gets like a bunch of bees and flies up and stings your brain, and then your two eyes is like dark clouds looking for trouble and your blood is like a tornado and then you have bad weather inside your body."

The comedienne says the character evolved from a niece: "She'd sit down telling embarrassing truths about the family and friends. She'd be sticking out her tongue and blowing spit as she talked, always ending up with 'and that's the truth.' She was a wonderful little monster."

Tomlin brought her characters to Broadway in *Appearing Nitely*, and received a special Tony award. She won acclaim for a series of television specials, and achieved the rare honor (for a comic) of being given the cover of *Time* magazine.

Critics applauded the chances she took, some of her material bordering on pain. There was Crystal, the wheelchair-bound girl who, at an amusement park, is mistaken for a ride. There were the one-liners that recalled vintage Woody Allen:

"There will be sex after death, we just won't be able to feel it. . . . Things are going to get a lot worse before they get worse. . . . I worry about kids today—because of the sexual revolution they're going to grow up and never know what dirty means."

Because she lived with comedy writer Jane Wagner, much was made of Tomlin's unisexual image, as well as her highly visible support of women's liberation. She dodged questions on her sex life with "It's like most people's—inadequate." And she could also kid feminists, asking rhetorically, "What would your position be if you were a passenger on the *Titanic*?"

Like many comics, Tomlin switched from stand-up to the movies, only to find difficulty in getting suitable roles. At first she scored in such films as *Nashville* and *The Late Show* with Art Carney, but just when she seemed on her way to solidifying her box office power, she was roasted for *The Incredible Shrinking Woman* and *Moment by Moment*. For the latter, critics took the opportunity to jeer at the look-alike androgyny of both her and leading man John Travolta.

Now Lily divides her time between stand-up and movie roles, and has won praise both for her latest stage work, and for such recent films as *All of Me*.

"I've tried to keep a balance," she says. "Coming from television you get a certain audience which follows you. From the stage, you get a hipper, smarter crowd. The movies bring in another element. Combined, you don't know what you've got. Every night during my concerts, I know there are at least 1,000 people sitting there who really wouldn't be caught dead in the same room with each other. Trying to make them all laugh, all understand is the fun of it."

JACKIE VERNON

"I once owned a pair of love birds that hated me . . . just yesterday my Charlie horse bit me . . . we were so poor, we used a substitute for margarine."

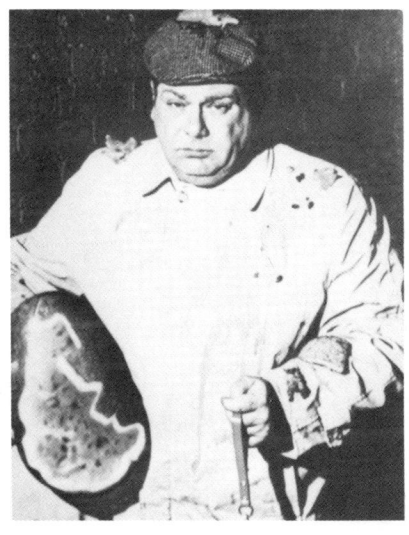

b. Ralph Verrone, 1928, New York, New York

Records:
A Wet Bird Never Flies at Night (Jubilee JGM 2052), A Man and His Watermelon (United Artists UAL 3577), The Day My Rocking Horse Died (United Artists UAS 6679), Sex Is Not Hazardous to Your Health (Beverly Hills BH 1133).

Video:
Hungry i Reunion Concert (Pacific Arts).

Baleful eyes, a high deadpan voice, lips pursed into a pout, pudgy body limp and motionless, Jackie Vernon is the personification of the loser. He was stand-up's first successful failure. Facetiously introduced as "Mr. Excitement," Vernon got instant laughs just by walking center stage. Audiences could instantly feel superior to the 5'8", 240 pounder, a comic who looked like an egg but was even more pathetically defenseless against the world.

Vernon came by his sad-sack stance naturally enough. He grew up in tough neighborhoods, attending Theodore Roosevelt High School in the Bronx. To the neighborhood kids, he was the fat boy nicknamed "Curly Joe." His father had been a welterweight in the 1920's, fighting as Gus Vernon, but after a little sparring, it became evident that Jackie would never follow in his footsteps.

Following service in the Air Force, Vernon and some spirited friends became "The Looney Lunatics," a comedy band with Vernon on trumpet. Little by little, the band gained enough momentum to peter out entirely. In 1955 Vernon stepped out as a comic. One of his first bookings was at the Red Rock Inn, in Lodi, New Jersey:

"I bombed so badly the owners said they wanted me to take a ride with them after the club closed. Up pulled a black sedan and I knew I was in for it. I sat in the back . . . sweating, wondering what was going to happen next. Finally, we crossed the George Washington Bridge. . . . One of the owners said to me, 'Do you know what that is?' 'Ye-yeah,' I stuttered. 'Well, don't ever cross it back into New Jersey again, fat boy. Ya hear?'"

For Jackie, comedy was not just a serious business. It was a grim, at times frightening one. "I was getting nowhere," he said, "just memorizing a bunch of jokes I found . . . not knowing what I was doing." In another tough dive, "I was on the stage doing my routine and I heard like a firecracker go off. This guy had fired a shot at me from the bar." The gangster came back the following night: "The guy said he was sorry about it, he had had a few drinks. Then he takes out a $100 bill and lays it on the table. 'Here, kid,' he says, 'buy yourself a tie.'"

Vernon trudged on: "I went from place to place year after year average $75 a week or something like that. . . . I was always out somewhere in the sticks. . . . My wife used to call me the Willy Loman of comedy." One night in San Francisco, facing an audience that looked as if it were auditioning for roles in *Night of the Living Dead*, Vernon called it quits. He left the silence of the club for his dressing room. But Danny Kaye had been observing him that night, recognized what was going on, and came backstage to give him an hour-long pep talk. It gave Vernon new hope.

Vernon developed two interesting identities. From his own sense of humor, and a certain jazz band hipness, he began doing surreal gags:

"Gunga Din was a great flagpole sitter. When his wife died, he sat at half mast for two weeks. . . . Remember, even if a sieve doesn't hold water, it will hold another sieve. . . . My grandfather was an optician. He fell into a lens grinding machine and made a spectacle of himself." And from his beaten-up posture of loser, he began to do self-parody: "If you don't like me, how about a nice hand for the suit."

In 1963 he hooked up with a new manager and comedy writer Danny Davis, who helped him hone his dull man character. That year he was discovered by Steve Allen. Allen wanted to book him and asked Vernon where he was staying. The comic was literally not staying anywhere. He hadn't enough money for a hotel. "The Beverly Wilshire," Vernon found himself saying. He then raced to the hotel, explained his predicament, and one of the employees let him stay.

Vernon's routines blended the bizarre with the pathetic. One of his classic routines involved his befriending a watermelon and keeping it as a pet (an idea he'd gotten from another fruit pet owner, Dean Rusk). He and his watermelon "became good buddies . . . I'd sleep with it, cuddle it, tell the watermelon my troubles . . . I'd try out new jokes on the watermelon and it would roll all over the floor . . . I'd put my ear against it and I'd hear the ocean." But while taking his watermelon for a leashed drag down the street, "a watermelon hater came out of an alley, and he shot a big hole in my watermelon. . . . Did you ever hear a watermelon scream?"

Racing to a watermelon repair man, "he asked me if I had any insurance. Blue Cross. United Fruit . . . he took one look and he says, 'Wow, that's a big hole you have in that watermelon. You gotta watch it. Those things don't grow on trees.'"

There's no hope for the watermelon, and the routine ends with black humor sadness: "A friend of mine sent me a Persian cantaloupe. They're much cleaner than watermelons, but you can't trust them. I knew a guy so lonely he befriended a grapefruit. But they're vicious. They'll attack you. They go for the eyes."

Vernon's bookings picked up, and more unusual routines gained him attention, bits on famous historical figures, a clever bit on a trip with "Guido the Guide" (done as a mock slide tour) and several talks on "What Is a Dull Man" and "How to Meet a Girl."

Vernon was unable to branch out into other areas of show business. Holding onto a prop, a broken and battered trumpet that he would sometimes pause to play (in a broken, battered way), he remained a top act in stand-up. He nearly had the role of the trumpet-playing patsy on the short-lived TV show "Run, Buddy, Run," but lost out to Jack Sheldon due to his weight.

"You have to have a bewilderment about you," Vernon remarked, describing his character. "Chaplin had it, Laurel and Hardy had it. You got to look like the kind of guy who's open, vulnerable . . . a guy who can't hurt you sitting there in the audience, the kind of guy you feel sorry for. That's always been the way I work: like life is a bewilderment to me."

Vernon correctly diagnosed that "I look as lonely and shy as anyone could possibly be without being put away." In real life married and the father of two children, Vernon keeps up his sorry front, although in recent years he's been eclipsed by other comics who also don't get respect.

"When I first came on the scene doing self-effacing material, a lot of other comedians started to copy my style, like Rodney Dangerfield." But the difference between Vernon and losers from Dangerfield to Woody Allen is Vernon's *utter* passivity. Rodney rails against his lot in life. Woody is inept but gets the girl.

Still, there is always a ready audience waiting when Vernon comes out and, like a child being thrust unwillingly onto the stage of a school play, utters a pessimistic, "Hello again, fun seekers."

Vernon's voice, sad and high pitched enough to connote questioning surprise and bafflement, has not only served him for comedy routines. He was chosen as the cartoon voice of "Frosty the Snowman" for a TV special that has become a Christmas perennial. Vernon is indeed like that character, one whom the audience feels sorry for—and loves.

CHARLEY WEAVER

"Discovered" in the 1950's by Jack Paar, and later "rediscovered" in the late 60's on "The Hollywood Squares," Charley Weaver actually had a long and prosperous career dating back to the 1930's, when he was known by his real name, Cliff Arquette.

Arquette left school when he was 14 to form a band in Cleveland called "Cliff Arquette and His Purple Derbies." It was fairly successful. He appeared with other bands over the years, then joined a comedy team called "The Three Public Enemies." From there he moved to radio, becoming one of the medium's busiest character actors.

Through the 30's Arquette specialized in rustics, lovable old codgers. Visitors to radio studios were surprised to find "Grandpaw Sneed" of the "Fred Astaire Show," and "The Oldtimer" of the "Fibber McGee and Molly Program" so youthful.

He developed the Charley Weaver character out of these older pioneering creations, and kept one of the catch-phrases he popularized on radio: "That ain't the way I heered it."

When Charley Weaver came to television, the visuals had to match the voice. The Charley Weaver uniform consisted of an upturned, beaten-up hat, a mustache, little "granny" glasses, a white shirt with an askew tie, and baggy pants held up with suspenders. Careful not to offend these same elderly hayseeds, Charley Weaver's character was not

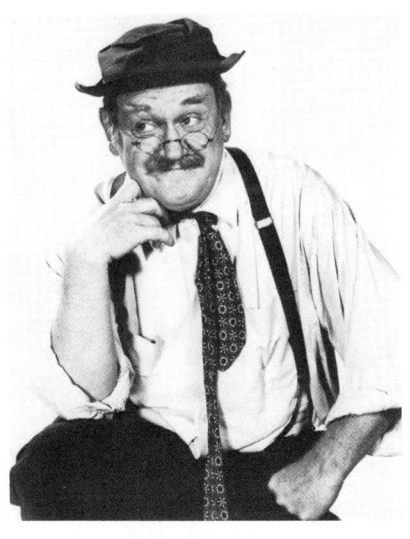

b. Cliff Arquette, December 28, 1905, Toledo, Ohio; d. September 23, 1974

Records:
Charley Weaver Sings for His People (Columbia CL 1345), Letters from Mamma (Coral 57458).

TV:
Dave and Charley (NBC 1952), The Charley Weaver Show (Hobby Lobby) (ABC 1959–60), The Hollywood Squares (NBC 1966–74).

Book:
Charley Weaver's Letters from Mamma.

a total bumbler. Charley could come up with a sly, witty remark and had a lot of country smarts.

Weaver starred with Dave Willock on the "Dave and Charley Show," and when that series ended, the character survived and became part of "The Dennis Day Show."

In 1957 Arquette retired. A history student, he planned to devote himself to creating his Civil War Museum in Gettysburg, Pennsylvania. One night he happened to be watching "The Tonight Show" when Jack Paar mused, "whatever became of Cliff Arquette." Arquette consented to a guest shot and ended up as a regular, performing monologues as Charley Weaver from the funny little town of Mt. Idy.

To cover admitted laziness and a distaste for memorizing routines, Weaver hit on the idea of reading his monologues, disguising them as "Letters from Mamma." Pulling out a letter, he would read it verbatim, filling in viewers on the latest doings of Mt. Idy's weirdly named citizens.

With humor reminiscent of old-time radio (everyone from Fred Allen's Titus Moody to Arquette's co-stars Fibber McGee and Molly and Burns and Allen) here, culled from several letters, is a sample of a Charley Weaver monologue:

"Dear Steinway, (Mamma always wanted me to be upright and grand.) Things are fine in Mt. Idy (she goes on)—except for the crops. As our corn is only an inch high, the birds have to kneel down to eat it. Our wheat is so short your father's going to have to lather it before he can mow it.

"Elsie Krack was just married, so yesterday we all pitched in and gave her a shower. It took six of us to drag her into the bathroom. She didn't mind the strong soap, but she did squawk a little about the steel wool.

"Your father and I spent Sunday with Wallace Swine and his family. My, but their oldest boy is spoiled—a steam roller ran over him. His father put a stamp on him and mailed him to the Mayo brothers. He's coming along fine now. They have to put a bookmark in bed with him, though, to find him.

"Ludlow Bean was arrested the other day for stealing a woman's change purse. He told the judge that he hadn't been feeling well, and he thought the change would do him good.

"Leonard Box was arrested for bringing his wife her breakfast in bed. She lives at the YWCA. It's too bad they've separated! They were such a lovely couple. She was so bow-legged and he was so knock-kneed that when they walked down the street they spelled OX.

"Well, son, I must close now and go help your father. He was coming up the stairs with five gallons of elderberry wine, and he slipped and fell clear down into the basement. Fortunately, he didn't spill a drop—he kept his mouth closed.

"Love, Mamma."

Weaver's popularity grew. In 1959 an eccentric album of songs about Mt. Idy residents was nominated for a Grammy. He made another record, put his monologues into a book, and was even the subject of novelties like the battery-powered "Charley Weaver Bartender" doll with his hands wrapped around a moving cocktail shaker. After amusing nighttime fans, he moved to daytime TV and "The Hollywood Squares." He was a hip old codger by now, slinging zinger answers to quiz questions:

"True or false: Doctors in Sweden report that people who get false teeth often lose their interest in sex." "True, but it's a poor substitute." "Who is more likely to grow up having speech problems, a baby boy who is breast fed or one who is bottle fed?" "Let me put it this way—Sophia Loren's two-year-old son is the #1 disc jockey in Palermo." "Your bird has a temperature of 104 degrees. Will he live?" "Gee, I hope not, my dinner guests'll be here in a couple of minutes."

Twice married and divorced, father of a son, Weaver suffered a stroke in 1972. For the first time he looked old without makeup. Partially paralyzed, the comedian was undaunted, and he courageously returned to "The Hollywood Squares." And the veteran who had once retired in 1957 remained with the program until his death. He did the show for one reason. As he put it, "Life should be a ball. If something doesn't fit my pattern of living—well, I just don't do it."

WEBER AND FIELDS

"Who is that lady I saw you with last night?"
"That ain't no lady, that's my wife!"

And that is vintage Weber and Fields. The "Dutch Comics" with the pointed goatees, German-Jewish accents and derby hats were innovators, and what seems corny now was bright and sassy coming from these two funnymen.

Both sons of Polish immigrants, the duo grew up on the Bowery. Fields's father was a tailor, struggling to feed eight children. Weber's father found work as a butcher. His family, living in a windowless basement apartment, became accustomed to seeing him hacking at the chickens while hungry rats lurked and chattered, eager for the scraps. The family had to consider the rats as "pets." Mrs. Weber was used to such adversity. On the boat to America, her baby died, and in order to avoid a burial at sea, she kept it at her breast during the last days of the voyage, pretending it was still alive.

At seven, the two boys were out busking, doing song and dance routines for pennies, peddling cookies in the street. They left P.S. 42 in the Bowery to pursue a career in show business, joining such acts as "The Standard Four," and working as a duo. Slowly they built up a repertoire of songs and jokes, and, working before German audiences, naturally used the "Dutch" dialect more than blackface or Irish accents, which they had previously adopted on occasion.

From $3 a week at the Chatham Square Museum, the duo rose through vaudeville to found their own company, and in 1896 own their own Broadway music hall, where they staged shows like *Burly Q, Hoity Toity, Pousse Cafe, Twirly Whirly* and many more. They're credited with helping to establish "music hall"–styled entertainment in America, complete with songs, beautiful chorus girls, and "ladies night" where not only were women permitted to view the proceedings, but alcohol and cigarettes were banned.

Audiences loved Weber and Fields's routines, which mixed slapstick and stand-up comedy patter. Before them, comedy teams had usually relied on one or the other. In their situation sketches, like the famous "Poolroom" routine, they would begin with comedy dialogue before moving to the game itself, where their trademarked knockabout comedy included many a bop on the head with a cue-stick.

Weber, short and fat (actually padded out with pillows), was the simple dupe. As far as he was concerned, "All the public wanted to see was Fields knock the hell out of me." His tall, bossy partner did just that,

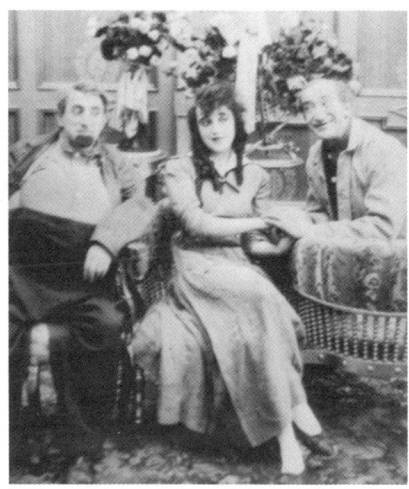

JOE WEBER b. Moisha (Morris) Weber, August 11, 1867, New York, New York; d. May 10, 1942
LEW FIELDS b. Moisha (Moses) Schanfield, January 1, 1867, New York, New York; d. July 20, 1941

Compilations:
They Stopped the Show (includes "The Drinking Routine"; Audio Rarities LPA 2290), Golden Age of Comedy (includes "The Football Game"; RCA Victor LPV 580).

Films:
Blossoms on Broadway, Lillian Russell.

Video:
"Oyster Routine" (on Tape #760, a compilation of old movie shorts and outtakes, Video Yesteryear).

with the famous "Choking Scene" where Fields almost murders his partner with "friendly" slaps on the back and fervent hands to the throat. The comedy team was also famous for staged pie-fights (well before Mack Sennett's films, obviously) and for eye-gouging, which later became a favorite routine of The Three Stooges.

Their material often came from real life. The pool routine developed after the duo witnessed a brawl between two immigrants at a neighborhood pool hall. The eye gouging began innocently enough when, in the midst of a routine, Weber winced from a bit of dust in his eye and Fields, keeping the show going, did his humorous best to get it out. Their violence became even more outrageous when Weber would retaliate, kicking Fields in the shins, only to have Fields literally plant a hatchet in his partner's head. Weber needed a cork cushion and a steel-plated wig for that one.

They utilized routines based on confusion and the kind of tinhorn misunderstanding that immigrants at the turn of the century recognized and enjoyed. In perfect imitation of the types they knew in the Bowery, Weber would come up and say,

"I am delightfulness to meet you."
"Der disgust is all mine," Fields answered.
"I received a letter from mein goil, but I don't know how to writtenin her back."
"Writtenin her back?" Fields scolded. "Such an edumunication you got it? You mean rottenin her back. How can you answer her ven you don't know how to write?"
"Dot makes no nefer mind. She don't know how to read."

Another popular routine of theirs, which still amuses fans of Laurel & Hardy and Abbott & Costello, is the "Drinking Routine." At the time people bought Edison cylinders to hear Joe and Lew's dilemma:
"I only have five cents," Fields tells his partner. "Remember, when we go into the saloon, I'll have a beer and you say you don't want any."
The comedy of this very human predicament proceeds as Fields hopes to preserve their dignity in being short of money, while Weber dim-wittedly succumbs to Fields's mock-prodding.

"Say in a sort of careless way, 'Oooh, I don't care for anything,'" Fields says before they enter the saloon. "Now, let's try it. What are you gonna have?"
"I don't care for anything."
"Something in my heart tells me you're not gonna do this right . . . come on, be a sport."
"No, no."
"Take something small."
"Well, I'll take a small bottle!"
"What!" Fields erupts. "A small bottle with my poor five cents?"
"Well, what do you wanna coax me for?"
"I wasn't coaxing, I was only making a bluff."
"Well, I don't take any bluffs!"

And on it goes, done with the Dutch accents, and the slow, steady, laugh-building pace later used by Laurel & Hardy. Fields finally makes Weber understand not to order a beer after the single bottle is ordered.

"Come on, take something."
"No, I don't wanna."

"Come on, take something."
"Okay, I'll take a cigar."
"A cigar! Are you trying to burn up my five cents?"
"Do I got to give up smoking too?"
"If you don't give up smoking I'll have to give up drinking! Please, I beg of you, use your brain!"

As the cylinder scratches to the finale, Weber and Fields are back on the street.

"What did you say in there?" Fields asks testily.
"Oh, I don't care if I do."
"So the bartender gave *you* the glass, and I had to say I don't care for any, and I have a thirst that would sink a battleship!"

The comedy team got a lot of mileage from their old standards, and enjoyed success with their music hall and their fresh revues loaded with music and mirth. They booked Lillian Russell for their show at $1250 a week, and as Fields recalled, those were really the good old days:

"Stanford White once gave a dinner and hired Joe and me to read Willie Collier's contract at a party. And for a stunt—it was a gag—it took us about eight minutes. For this he paid us $1,000."

The comedy team prospered until 1904, when, to the consternation of their fans, they began feuding and broke up the team. They reteamed again for a while, around 1912, broke up, and then reteamed again in 1921.

"Every time I saw Fields's name on a show poster after our separation I thought of a one-legged man," Weber recalled. "Lew and I have answered either to Weber or to Fields for forty years. 'Glad to meet you, Mr. Weber,' a man says on shaking my hand, and 'Goodbye, Mr. Fields,' when he leaves. Lew and I sometimes wonder if they'll get our names straight on our tombstones."

Weber and Fields still regaled audiences into the 1930's, although Weber was more inclined toward retirement.

Periodically they would accept work, and nostalgic dates on variety show bills, and even had a kind of "comeback" in movies, appearing in *Blossoms on Broadway* and playing themselves in an Alice Faye musical about Lillian Russell. They turned up on radio occasionally, and in 1940 celebrated "The Gay Nineties" on a WCBS special.

But there would be no more shows after that. In 1941, Lew Fields's passing meant the permanent end of Weber and Fields. Fields was survived by a son, and daughter Dorothy Fields, who went on to become an Oscar-winning lyricist. Joe Weber died the following year. He had been married since 1897, but had no children.

Today there are few recordings and films to preserve the legend of Weber and Fields, who in so many theatrical revues entertained thousands as "Krautnuckle and Bungstarter" or "Mack and Myer" or some other oddly named duo of wisecrackers and slapstickers. But a look at the comedy teams that followed, from the carefully timed Laurel & Hardy to the frantic Abbott & Costello, shows some of the influence of one of America's first comedy teams, legends in their own time.

PEARL WILLIAMS

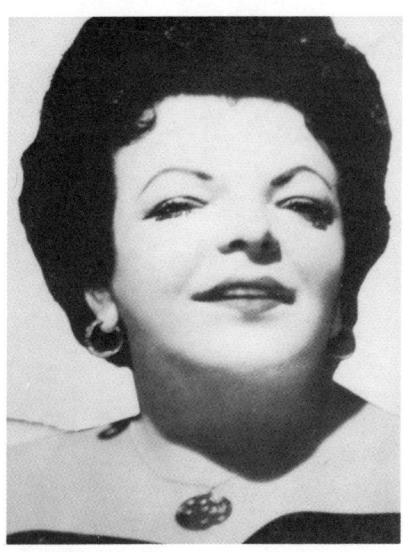

b. Pearl Wolfe, September 10, 1914, New York, New York

Records:
A Trip Around the World Is Not a Cruise (After Hours LAH 70), 2nd Trip Around the World (Surprise SUR 75), All the Way (Riot R-307), At Las Vegas (Riot 303), You'll Never Remember It, Write It Down (Laff A 128), Bagels and Lox (Laff A 127).

"I've never heard a woman comedian with your pace and timing and delivery," Jack Benny told Pearl Williams. "You're the best I've ever heard." The first and foremost of the red-hot risque raconteurs, Pearl was a natural. Her voice and cadence, which sounded like Mae West combined with Leo Gorcey, were enticing and appealing.

"When I work on stage I'm so relaxed I let my audience relax. I stand up there real cool and I can deliver a line and all of a sudden they're screaming, hollering, and I'm standing there real cool while they're screaming. It's almost like a Jack Benny, but not quite. Remember how he used to stand there, not a smile on his face, and everybody screaming all around? I'm that kind of comedian, but with a smile. Sometimes they laugh so hard I start laughing with them."

Confidence was her secret weapon: "I wasn't an amateur from the day I started. I never was afraid of an audience. That's the secret of show business, not to be afraid of the audience, to know they'll like it. So you get up on the stage very casually, very nonchalantly. . . . Most comedians are nervous wrecks: will they like me, will I bomb, what will happen. These things don't enter my mind. I go onstage knowing they're gonna like me. From my opening song on."

Pearl entered show business on the strength of one song. She was a 24-year-old legal stenographer with aspirations to become a lawyer. At a friend's singing audition, she played the piano. The agent, Feet Edson, asked her to sing a song, too. After she finished the tune, "Margie," he said, "You're hired." The shocked Pearl had never been in a nightclub, but she decided to give it a shot: "So my very first job in show business was working with Louis Prima at The Famous Door. That goes back to 1938, honey."

She discovered she could make $35 a night, which was much better than the $15 a week she had been making. She also discovered that audiences responded to risque songs, things like Joe E. Lewis's "No Room for the Groom." She began to work with more and more raunchy lines: "The other comedians were doing dull stuff. Most of them were bombing. Their material stunk to high heaven. So I figured I'll do something where everybody'll react. And you know who started my reputation in New York very big? Dorothy Kilgallen. She used to knock me in her column every day. She never saw my act, just heard about me, and the more she knocked me, the more jammed the club was, because nobody was doing what I was doing."

Her act evolved to 30 minutes of stand-up, 15 minutes behind the piano singing songs, and then another barrage of stories, heckler squelches and ad-libs. Sophie Tucker told her, "You're me at your age, only better." Shelley Winters was so impressed by Pearl she once asked if she could come on stage and try belting out a few dirty ditties: "So she got up and did two dirty Jewish songs and everyone was screaming and applauding, and she sent me two dozen roses the next day to thank me."

Asked if members of the audience thought her offstage personality was similar to the raunchy character on stage, she said, "Well, if they're stupid they'll believe that. Idiots will believe that. Think I walk around the house saying four-letter words all the time? I only say that when I'm getting paid, honey."

From the stage, she'd tell throw-away lines: "Well, as the fly said when he walked on the mirror, that's another way of looking at it." She did definitions: "Definition of a cotton picker: a girl who loses the string on her Tampax!" And with her tough New York accent, she got a lot of mileage with quick, punchy little stories:

"Two broads are passing a beauty parlor. And one says 'Gee, I smell hair burning.' The other says, 'Maybe we're walking a little too fast?'"

"Hear about the guy who takes a broad out, and he's playing with her knish. She says, 'This I like, this I love. Put in another finger.' He says, 'Waddya wanna do? Whistle?'"

"A woman goes to an optometrist to get her eyes examined. He shows her a chart, she can't see the letters. He shows her a bigger chart—she can't see the letters. He shows her a real big chart, she still can't see the letters. What's he gonna do with this bitch? He backs up, opens his fly and says, 'Lady, this you see?' She says, 'Yeah.' He says, 'I figured. Yer cock-eyed!'"

Pearl would accompany these stories with punctuation, chords on the piano. "Hear about the guy who bought his wife a gold diaphragm? He wanted to see how it feels to come into money. . . ." She would break into a familiar song: "By the sea, by the sea, by the sea -U-N-T." And to ringsiders, she would maintain a running commentary of wisecracks and insults. She'd encourage shocked, laughing women to try the sex acts she joked about, and she'd tell the men to try new sexual avenues, too.

She recalled that her audience loved "true stories, human situations, not necessarily jokes, jokes, jokes. Women were the ones that dragged their husbands in. I had grandmothers, 90 years old for crying out loud, saying 'we love you, you're wonderful.'"

Others came along to make a name for themselves in risque comedy, and Pearl knew them well: Belle Barth, B.S. Pully and Rusty Warren. And there was Lenny Bruce: "Oh, I loved him, he was brilliant. Before he went on the dope, honey, this was one of the most brilliant minds. I have all his records myself. I loved that boy . . . what a darling boy he was. I was friendly with him right to the end."

Unlike Bruce, who strayed into religious humor, or Barth who sometimes used too many four-letter words, Williams always maintained control: "I only used certain words in my act that the audience would accept. I can see people using bad language if it's the punchline of a story and it enhances the story and it gets a scream from the audience. But just to stand around and say motherfucker for no reason, I can't see it. I'm not as dirty as they are on cable now. I heard Richard Pryor and Eddie Murphy on cable and I didn't believe my ears. I think it's horrible. They use filthy language. There are words that I just can't say, that I could never think of using."

In 1962 she recorded her first album, "A Trip Around the World Is Not a Cruise," which had worldwide distribution and sold more than a million copies. She worked Las Vegas regularly until 1967, but never "toned down" to get on television.

"I'll tell you what happened. I had a great manager, Joe Glazer, and after he died I didn't bother getting a new manager, I just settled down in Florida, bought a house, and stayed here. I've traveled, honey, all over the country, so I decided this is it. Had I gotten another manager, I probably would've gone on to bigger and better things. With the way I deliver comedy, maybe a television series."

Pearl became a fixture at the Place Pigalle in Miami, ending an 18-year run in April of 1984 when she retired. She acknowledged that over the last few years she actually found herself doing milder routines, to an audience no longer interested in hearing hardcore comedy. Actually, the jokes were never as important as the flair with which she worked, and the talent she had for wringing laughs out of long dialect stories. She feels she's not egotistical—just truthful—when she says, "I have a better delivery than any female comedian you know or have heard of . . . it may sound very conceited, but again I tell you I'm the most brilliant of them all when it comes to presenting comedy." Few would deny that the pure "sound" of Williams is wonderfully comic, and, risque or not, she was a star of stand-up with a strong, distinctive style.

She never watches today's X-rated films: "I hate them. You know I'm really a prude at heart. I don't like sex on a screen. To me sex belongs in a bedroom, just four walls and two people. The two people could be of any sex—that doesn't bother me at all, who's doing it, but I believe it should be done very privately. I think X-rated films are disgusting, in spite of the fact that I work dirty. Talking is one thing but actually showing it—oh my god—I think that's horrible."

In retirement, she plans to do "nothing. Knit and crochet and read and watch television and tape my favorite shows and watch them over and over again and just do nothing. Don't you think it's time after 46 years?"

ROBIN WILLIAMS

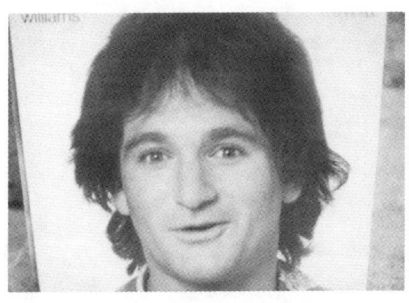

b. July 21, 1952, Chicago, Illinois

Records:
Reality, What a Concept (Casablanca NBLP 7162), Throbbing Python of Love (Casablanca 811 150-1 M1).

TV:
Mork and Mindy (ABC 1978–82).

Films:
Popeye, The World According to Garp, The Survivors, Moscow on the Hudson.

Video:
Comedy Tonight (Vestron), The Frog Prince (CBS-Fox), An Evening with Robin Williams (Paramount).

Described as Jonathan Winters on speed, Robin Williams began his comedy career as a child when he would memorize and then perform Winters's routines. His audience was usually himself.

The son of a Ford Motor executive, he grew up in a Detroit suburb where he had the entire third floor to himself in a 30-room mansion on a 40-acre estate. He had two half brothers who were much older, so he was actually an "only child," living in solitude.

"I used to spend hours in the basement playing with my collection of two thousand toy soldiers," Williams says. "I had all these voices I would use, and sound effects, and I would entertain myself. I was fat, too, and wore a blazer and carried a briefcase to school. The other kids called me dwarf and leprechaun so I took up wrestling to get rid of my hostility and anger—and lost 30 pounds."

The Williams family eventually moved to Tiburon, California, and Robin's fantasy world began to include others. "I went from a very disciplined all boys school to a school where the teachers said things like, 'You can graduate if you have reasonable energy.'"

Williams had more than reasonable energy, and he was voted "Funniest" student in class. By the time he reached Claremont Men's College he had switched from a career in business to the theater. He won a scholarship to Juilliard and trained with John Houseman for three years alongside classmates William Hurt and Christopher Reeve.

Back in California, Williams found an outlet for his creativity in the burgeoning comedy clubs where young comics could try out new material. Audiences immediately responded to the nervous, fast-paced cartoon-like characters Williams hid behind. With bewildering quickness he could seize on almost anything to use as a comic prop, and his manic charm helped him quickly ditch a failing routine and move on to something else.

He was picked for the ill-fated return of "Laugh-In," but soon found more work, turning up as a wacky alien in an episode of "Happy Days." His work was so well received he ended up with a spin-off show, the phenomenally successful "Mork and Mindy," which delighted youngsters and also appealed to elder space cadets into off-the-wall humor and fantasy.

Despite the seeming ease with which Williams could rearrange reality, the pressures were tremendous and there was real nervousness behind his nervous energy. A newlywed of three months, and new to full-blown success, Williams suffered through the unpleasantness of anxiety attacks as he dealt with his first season on television. Perhaps more than ever before, his frenzied comedy was his greatest escape.

One of the "new breed" of 1980's comics, he took his stance more from the rock field than stand-up. Audiences loved to watch him sweat, strain and bust a gut going "full-tilt bozo." They encouraged zaniness: pantomime, face-making, quirky voices, anything for a laugh. Williams thrived on stream-of-consciousness comedy and even unconsciousness when he'd take his audience for a trip inside his brain where, to the point of all-out panic, he was trying to manufacture fresh material.

Jonathan Winters had found that there was a limit to the number of "routines" he could do, but not the number of things he could "wing." Williams too discovered that audiences responded to the magic of "winging it" as well as to simple jokes. But only a few comics, like Winters and Williams, could manage enough zany improvisation to keep the audience involved. In the 80's, Williams has more of an arsenal than Winters: blue humor (a grab for the pants and what he has called "Mr. Happy" and/or his "Throbbing Python of Love") and drug humor (the distorted speech of downer and speed freaks are among his favorites).

In a live performance, Williams is bewilderingly fast, the audience always off-balance, never sure when the comic will suddenly "attack," diving offstage to rummage around for props to play with and ringsiders to spin jokes off. No one can be sure if this will be the night Williams exposes "Mr. Happy" or literally takes off into space. In a club, the infectious hysteria is impossible to resist. On TV and videotape, the effect lessens. On record, despite having won a Grammy award, Williams loses a great deal of his charm.

On wax, sans the flashy visuals and pantomime, the spur of the moment ad-libs don't endure, and the standard jokes that form a loose net for his ad-lib gymnastics are sometimes the kind that would make Henny Youngman cringe:

"A drunk says to a parking meter, 'Fuck it if you're expired, I still love you'.... In San Francisco 'God Save the Queen' has a different meaning...." He tells of people who are "so damn wealthy they don't get crabs, they get lobsters." And throw-away puns can be thrown away, like his remarks in a "child in the womb" routine, "Fetus don't fail me now" and "womb with a view." His audience also accepts as original some tried and true remarks like "We men spend nine months trying to get out of the womb and the rest of our life trying to get back in there." And, like a hangover, there's a question as to how profound his "think" lines the night before really were: "What's right is what's left if you do everything else wrong." Still, if his genius is best seen live, it's still a genius for getting laughs.

Many of today's comics, from Steve Martin through to Eddie Murphy, have been accused of getting easy laughs from their drunk/high adoring audiences. But Jack Benny, Don Rickles and other old-timers proved long ago that audiences *can* be conditioned to laugh at the sight of a famous comic face, or over a line that is intellectually weak but delivered with strength. The important thing is to be able to condition the audience. Robin Williams has certainly done that with his vast, infectious arsenal of comic weapons.

Williams's stand-up comedy has progressed over the years. Aside from monetary gain ($25,000 for his 1978 HBO special, $750,000 for the one he did in 1983) he's gained depth and more ironic self-satire to go with the airy, good-natured hysteria. He's been through a lot since he was an overnight star making $40,000 a week as "Mork from Ork." The unpredictable comic wandered through such predictable star crises as drinking and the pursuit of too many medical and sexual highs. Much of the excess ended around the time his friend John Belushi died of a drug overdose.

"I was being an asshole," says Williams. "I wasn't being considerate. I leave it at that and let people make their own conclusions."

Living on a country ranch with his wife, relaxing through yoga, jogging and swimming, observing a vegetarian diet, the older and wiser Williams can say, "What's fame like? It's like jerking off with sandpaper."

If his stand-up model is Winters, on the screen Williams's image is more like that of Danny Kaye: manic, handsome, silly, warm and fun. He continues to bring his love of fantasy to children (the made-for-video "The Frog Prince") as well as earning solid notices for his feature films for adults. Following courageous choices in his first films, he scored almost unanimous raves for the sappy *Moscow on the Hudson*.

FLIP WILSON

Some comedians are serious by nature. Flip Wilson is serious and studious. Deciding at an early age that he wanted to be a comic, he "spent years studying all the funnymen. I always wanted to find out what makes an individual funny . . . what is the one unique thing they have that no one else has. I studied those qualities."

While he toiled for more than a decade for a salary just about at poverty level, he "evaluated Jerry Lewis, his antics, his mobility . . . Bob Hope, his timing, the best in the business . . . the attitude of George Burns, that's his claim to immortality . . . I set about trying to utilize all these qualities, all these different aspects of their characters to create something totally unique. I figured if they used one quality to come across, then my using two more should let me slide by."

Wilson developed as a monologist, dead-panning jokes without cracking a smile, dragging on a cigarette while waiting for the laugh. But he also developed character comedy, and it was as "Geraldine Jones" or "The Reverend Leroy" that he could perform the most manic routines. But even as he rose to stardom through appearances on "The Tonight Show" in 1965, Wilson was still careful with his craft. Although his "Geraldine" blossomed into a joyful, funky free-spirited and sassy character with her own catch-phrases ("What you say! You devil, you!") Wilson brought across the uniqueness of black speech and mannerisms without getting caught up in racial humor:

"I'm involved in the civil rights movement," he said in 1967, "but in the manner Dick [Gregory] is, I'd have to say no. If you are a comic, your first obligation is to be funny. The message has to be secondary to the humor. This is a thing that might have had a large bearing on Dick's decline in popularity. You see, he went against the laws of humor."

Wilson has actually written a book of "laws" that he follows, theorizing on "How to Tell a Funny Story," and, as he says, "formulas on how to approach situations and how to ad-lib. I even use formulas on hecklers."

b. Clerow Wilson, December 8, 1933, Jersey City, New Jersey

Records:
Flip Wilson's Pot Luck (Sceptor 502; reissued as "Funny and Live at the Village Gate," Springboard SP-4004), Flippin (Minit 24012), Cowboys and Colored People (Atlantic ATS 8149), You Devil You (Little David SC 8179), The Devil Made Me Buy This Dress (Little David LD 1000), The Flip Wilson Show (Little David LD 2000), Geraldine: Don't Fight the Feeling (Little David LD 1001).

He even feels that one of the laws of comedy is not to be *too* funny:

"I would never be as outright funny as I think I could be, because I don't believe in constant hysterics. That's painful to me . . . someone said laughing is a strain on the heart and it's true. To me, great comedy is like a fine musical performance, it flows, it goes up and down, it has different moods, expresses different feelings. My goal is to hit all of those various levels during a performance, not just plain laughter.

"There's a smile, for instance, and a wink and even a subtle chuckle. I don't think they should be overlooked. And there are all kinds of laughs, laughs from the heart and belly laughs too . . . it's important to have all those elements." Wilson even believes bad jokes have their place: "I've built bad jokes into my act just to let people know I'm not perfect. People don't relate to people who are perfect. I think the audience must know you as a person."

Those who know Wilson recall that he had a tough childhood. One of 18 children, his parents separated when he was eight. He ended up in foster homes, and in reform school where he was befriended by a teacher who gave him his first taste of personal attention. "This teacher took an interest in me. In fact, he gave me the first birthday presents I ever got—a box of Crackerjacks and a can of ABC shoe polish."

His escape route was the Air Force. His commanding officer encouraged him to continue his education. In the barracks, he was encouraged by his bunkmates, who laughed at his improvised routines.

One of his routines was a zany bit of Shakespearean double-talk. When he'd start in with it, his buddies would be amazed at the way "he flippith his lid," and before long, the flipped-out comic had his nickname.

In 1954, the young man, evidently taking a cue from the "toomlers" of the Catskills who got their start entertaining guests, worked as a bellhop at the Manor Plaza Hotel in San Francisco, ad-libbing, even doing a comic drunk act to liven things up between shows. Many long years of struggling saw Wilson slowly earn bookings, building routines, doing risque comedy, appearing before all types of audiences until he managed to get his "Tonight Show" break with the help of Redd Foxx.

He told jokes about ugly women ("a peeping tom looked in her window and closed his eyes"), about funky characters from history (Queen Isabella finances Columbus's trip because "Chris gonna find Ray Charles! Ray Charles in America! What you say!") and sheer silliness (a shaggy dog story about an Ancient Roman named Herman, who owned a beautiful berry that everyone admired. Until soldiers came to take it away from his girl: "We've come to seize her berry, not to praise it.").

Wilson's first major-label release, "Cowboys and Colored People," won excellent reviews and was nominated for a Grammy in 1967. He was nominated the following year for "You Devil You." The same year, he signed an exclusive contract with NBC and made numerous variety show guest appearances.

"The Devil Made Me Buy This Dress" won a Grammy for Flip in 1970. That was the year he got his own TV show, which popularized not only that routine about a woman's comical attempt to rationalize an expensive purchase, but also led to the fame of "Geraldine," the ultimate conception in Wilson's portrayal of female characters.

On the Emmy-winning program Wilson was often decked out in complete drag, conducting skits as Geraldine, strutting out and saying, "What you see is what you get!" and coming up with statements like this:

"Honey, lemme tell you, nobody can tell Geraldine what to say. I

TV:
The Flip Wilson Show (NBC 1970-74), People Are Funny (NBC 1983-84), Charlie & Co. (CBS 1985-).

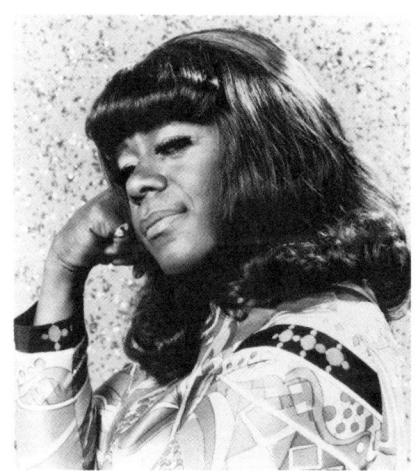

listen to what everybody has to say about everything, but Geraldine'll say what she want to say. And it's my opinion that the cost of living's goin' up, and the chance of living's goin' down!"

While Wilson worked tirelessly on his career, and providing for his four children, he also took the time to work for charity. Given a humanitarian award by the American Cancer Society, Wilson made regular appearances at charity golf tournaments and in 1975 was invited to the White House to be applauded by President Gerald Ford for his generosity. For relaxation from his busy schedule, Flip enjoys piloting hot-air balloons.

Wilson continues to delight audiences on stage and on television. In 1984 the durable comic starred in an updated version of "People Are Funny," where the jokes were on average people, asked questions of great importance ("Who would you least like to see naked?") and near-great importance ("Should the U.S. withdraw its troops from Provolone?").

With the huge success of Bill Cosby's sit-com in 1984, CBS began preparations for a new show for Wilson, "Charley and Company," co-starring Gladys Knight. It's obvious Wilson still has many comic surprises awaiting audiences, and he also has one for comedy scholars: plans to eventually publish his "Laws" of comedy. But only after he retires from practicing law.

JONATHAN WINTERS

An offbeat original, Jonathan Winters is a stand-up comic with a strong cult following. He'd have more universal acclaim except that his inventive material is matched by a paradoxical persona too complex to pigeonhole. Most comics define themselves easily for their audience, or become identified as clown (Skelton), insulter (Rickles), loser (Dangerfield), jerk (Martin), etc.

Winters operates from outer space, down to earth, and in several conflicting levels in between. He's considered sick for doing bits on funerals, undressing in front of a dog, and talking about used pet shops. Yet he's also an old-fashioned right-wing mid-American. He's the "wild man" who does dozens of bizarre sound effects, but few comics look or dress more subdued and normal. He's a fun guy who does silly "stuff and nonsense," but he's also a deadly satirist with undertones of hostility.

Had he the overt anger and iconoclastic streak of a Sahl, he would have been lauded as a premiere satirist. Had he lost the spacey sick stuff and kept his sillier characters, he might have been hailed as a beloved clown, his Maude Frickert more popular than the Johnny Carson copy Aunt Blabby, his Elwood P. Suggins another Gomer Pyle. But Winters instead combines both worlds, mid-America and the big city. He seems to both love and loath his characters, and by breaking some logical rules of comedy and following his own instincts, he has come to be considered by critics and other comics to be one of the most inventive, influential and important stand-up artists of all time.

Winters was an only child whose parents separated when he was 7. Of his school days, he said, "You could never say that I was one of those class cut-ups. I was too busy worrying about my studies. I was frightened to death of failing." At 17 he enlisted in the Marines, and after World War II held a bewildering variety of odd jobs before marrying his wife, Eileen, in 1948 and settling down. Both studied at the Dayton Art Institute, but everyone noticed Winters's flair for comedy.

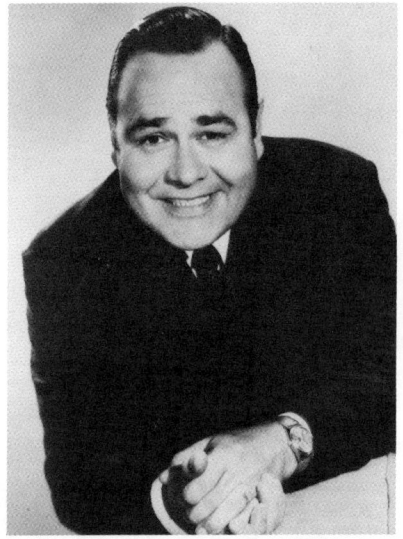

b. November 11, 1925, Dayton, Ohio

Records:
Wonderful World of Jonathan Winters (Verve V/V6 15009), Down to Earth (Verve V 15011), Here's Jonathan (Verve V/V6 15025), Another Day Another World (Verve V 15032), Humor Seen Through the Eyes of Jonathan Winters (Verve V 15035), Whistle Stopping (Verve 15057), Wings it! (Columbia CS 9611), Stuff 'n' Nonsense (Columbia CS 9799), Laugh Live (a rerelease of "Wings It" and "Stuff 'n' Nonsense";

"One afternoon when I came home from art school, Eileen had a strange look on her face and I knew she was about to ask for a big favor. She said, 'Darling, there's going to be a talent contest at the local theater tonight . . . they're going to give a wrist watch to the winner and I don't have a wrist watch. . . .'" She urged him to go, claiming he was always "the life of the party." And besides, she told him, "I think your art stinks."

Winters was a hit, and later landed a job as a disc jockey for WING in Dayton. By 1950 he was at WBNS-TV in Columbus and in 1953 went to New York, pushing himself against closed doors and a discouraging reality that threatened his comic fantasy. He lost on "Arthur Godfrey's Talent Scouts," but eventually got some club work.

Many recall Winters in New York as a man who enjoyed a drink, a guy who was always "on" with dazzling ad-libs and comic characters. "For a number of years I *was* on," he recalled. "Because a fella just doesn't know how to get off. Or because when he gets off, he's very much alone. He doesn't know what to do or be . . . it's a disease and I've learned to get over it."

Winters made his first TV appearance with the help of acquaintance Mickey Spillane. Billed as the "John O'Hara of Sound" Winters did sound effects while Spillane read from his novel *I, the Jury*. Jack Paar featured Winters often in 1954 and later the comic replaced Orson Bean on Broadway in *Almanac*. In 1957 he had his own 15-minute TV series where he was pressured by a tight format and "always watching the clock." Critics complained that the show wasn't spontaneous. Critics would make a habit of complaining that Winters's TV shows or movies didn't use his full potential. The problem was largely that most screenwriters and gag men couldn't possibly write the kind of stuff Winters ad-libbed in clubs or on talk shows.

Winters continued to journey around the grinding nightclub circuit and made records. General audiences admired his quick, crazy impressions and kids enjoyed his spirit of fantasy. But there was always a darker inspiration.

He never called it revenge, but when asked how he came up with characters, Winters said he observed. Like the irritating and boastful Texan he once met: "This Texan who tried to impress me with the fact that he was worth 64 million dollars is going to be part of my show some day. Just like the characters I met when I worked at a gas station, as a dishwasher in a gin mill, and when I picked apricots in California and when I was a fry cook at a lumber camp in the Yellowstone." Offstage, Winters did a slow burn, and on stage, he blazed, becoming these characters and destroying them, the "hip rubes, the Babbitts, the pseudo-intellectuals, the little politicians" who got under his skin.

Winters was often a step beyond his fellow comics: Lenny Bruce did a prison satire in which a priest and warden let the prisoners open a gay bar. In Winters's version, the priest ends up shooting the prisoner. Red Skelton touched hearts with a pantomime of an old man watching a parade. Winters offered "Thoughts on a Turtle Crossing the Road," desperate to meet his girlfriend, anxious, afraid of being crushed by an oncoming car. Other comics, hip or straight, were awed by the Winters technique.

Even his most popular characters had a message beneath the surface. Of Maude Frickert, Winters said, "She's putting down a weaker generation . . . what she's saying to people in essence is: 'What's happening here? What's happened to the Spirit of '76?'"

At his best, Winters was a modern-day Daumier, etching his characters to hint subtly at the grotesque, the absurd, the pathetic and the silly in average people. "Aren't most men little boys?" he had one character say. "They're just playing with bigger toys."

He extended his fantasy to real life, when he'd put off pesty cab drivers

Columbia PG 31985). Reissues include: Best of Maude Frickert and Elwood P. Suggins (Verve), Movies Are Better Than Ever (Verve), Great Moments of Comedy (Verve), Mad Mad World (Verve); Rhapsody for Bar Users (promo for Republic Steel), Jest of Flair (promo for Flair Radio, ABC).

TV:
The Jonathan Winters Show (NBC 1956–57; CBS 1967–69).

Films on Video:
The Russians Are Coming, the Russians Are Coming (CBS/Fox), It's a Mad, Mad, Mad, Mad World (CBS/Fox); Pogo for President (WD), Oh Dad, Poor Dad, Mama's Hung You in the Closet and I'm Feeling So Sad (Paramount).

Video:
The Jonathan Winters Show 1957 (Video Yesteryear), NBC Comedy

Book:
Mouse Breath and Other Social Ills (cartoons and drawings).

by laughing insanely, patting his briefcase and saying, "It's too bad about the mad bomber, isn't it?" He'd silence talkative train companions by hollowly intoning, "When I get off, I'm taking a cab to the sanitarium." And calling up an old girlfriend's mortician husband, he said he was a customer with a week-old corpse to deliver, one that had had its eyes removed by some playful children. He could be blunt, too. "Why do you wear dark glasses at 10 o'clock at night?" he asked one movie star. "You ain't got pink eye or anything. You're a phony. You're asking for recognition."

Winters was brilliant, but he was drinking too much, pushing himself, playing too many club dates on the road. He swore off drink, and that put pressure on him, too. He switched to coffee, downing cup after cup to do his three shows nightly.

In May of 1959, Winters's ad-libs on the stage of the Hungry i came out as a long ramble about an organization he belonged to: Alcoholics Anonymous. The next show also went serious. Patrons walked out. Some heckled. The comedian left the stage in tears. He called his wife long distance.

His next public performance was aboard the *Balclutha*, an old sailing ship moored at Fisherman's Wharf. He'd asked the ticket-taker if he could climb the rigging. Before long he was atop the ship, shouting things like "This boat's a fake. It's got an outboard motor on it!" Someone called out, "You're Jonathan Winters," and he said, "I'm the cat man, I'm in orbit, man, I'm a moon cat."

Officer Anthony Trianchero was at the scene: "You ask him his name and he says he is John Q from Outer Space and had been here for light years. He started to resist us and we had to use handcuffs."

Some thought it was an act. A few cruelly considered it madness from a sick comic. It was probably Winters taking the exhaustion, the frustration, the loneliness, and the pressure to be constantly "on," crazy and funny to its logical/illogical extreme. The comedian's wife flew in to be with him. The Hungry i management vowed to rehire him. Winters took a two-week rest, far removed from the public's eye.

Earning $4,500 a week, Winters eventually had the financial security to leave the road. He slowed down his harsh touring schedule after 1961 to spend more time with his two children. When he appeared on TV or in the movies, his fans saw the same incredibly talented and funny performer as before. In the mid-60's he came back to TV for his own series.

The variety show wasn't given a chance, but Winters took it all philosophically. "To me it's a miracle I've come as far as I have. I quit complaining because I found too many people could top me. Everybody's got tragedies and skeletons in the closet. But you've got to have fun. If you don't, you're a fool." On an album jacket (under a drawing of a frayed-nerve comic) he once wrote, "I've tried being a lot of things, assuming all kinds of roles, but I've come to the conclusion that in the long run, 'being down to Earth' is the answer for me . . . it makes living with yourself a hell of a lot easier."

Mellowing a bit, Winters began to prefer "winging it" to performing monologues. Audiences loved the way he invented comedy out of odd props and demented suggestions from ringsiders. His last albums didn't have the sharpness or satire of his Grammy-nominated Verve discs, but they were relaxed, light and amusing, the characters now softer cartoons.

An accomplished artist and wood sculptor, Winters spends more time in these pursuits. He's repeatedly voiced displeasure at the "scale" wages offered by "The Tonight Show" and similar venues. Accordingly, he hasn't been seen often on talk shows, and with the lack of variety programs on TV over the past decade, he adds, "it's frustrating not to be able to use what you've got. I've got more tools than some guys. I'm on the bench a lot, but how many people are playing?"

Fans were delirious when Winters appeared on "Mork and Mindy" with Robin Williams. "Reality, what a concept," was a Williams catchphrase. Says Williams's mentor, "Reality can be both frightening and funny. I take situations from life and exaggerate them, but not too much. You don't have to go too far out to make it funny." He insists "reality is where it's at," even if it's painful. He's said his autobiography will be dedicated to "all people who are overly sensitive. It beats being overly bitter. Never be ashamed of this. If there were more overly sensitive people in the world we wouldn't be in the position we're in as a people and as a world."

HENNY YOUNGMAN

"A fellow walked up to me, he said, 'You see a cop around here?' I said, 'No.' He said, 'Stick 'em up.'"

"I've been married for 49 years and I'm still in love with the same woman. If my wife ever finds out, she'll kill me."

"A drunk walked up to a parking meter and put a dime in. The dial went to 60. He said, 'How about that. I lost 100 pounds.'"

"Things were rough when I was a baby. No talcum powder!"

"Take my wife—please!"

Joke joke joke. Make that old joke old joke old joke. Who stands up and fires a ceaseless staccato of comic jabs? "Oh, *that* Henny Youngman." But for 50 years the man has persevered with old jokes that are now "classics," and he's become a kind of comic icon, the crowd roaring when he delivers one of his familiar lines in his unflappable, faintly smiling style.

The Youngman legend, according to comic and writer Joey Adams, began in the Borscht Belt: "Henny, who played the violin only because his mother made him take lessons, had a small combo at the Swan Lake Inn. His violin playing was funny enough, but one day in 1932 the Social Director was taken suddenly drunk and didn't show up. A frustrated comic who had been thrown out of Manual Training High School for clowning, Henny stepped out of the band into the spotlight and nobody has been able to shove him back since."

"I didn't figure to be a comedian," Youngman admits. "It sort of happened. I was always in trouble, the teacher'd ask a question and I'd make a funny reply and nobody would laugh. . . . I took fiddle lessons, but I wasn't great. To hide my bad playing I kept cracking jokes."

Youngman's father was a hat maker who fled from Russia to Brooklyn by way of London: "My father made $13 a week working 12-hour days. I used to pick coal on the street and sell it." He also found he could make money by busking, telling jokes and playing lively pop standards. In his teens he was part of a band, "Hen Youngman and His Syncopaters." He also had a sidelight, working odd jobs as a summons server and as the owner of a business card printing machine.

It was in the Catskills that he learned "the value of one-liners. Up there, when you're toomling, you have to have something funny to say to everyone when you meet them." Although known for jokes, Young-

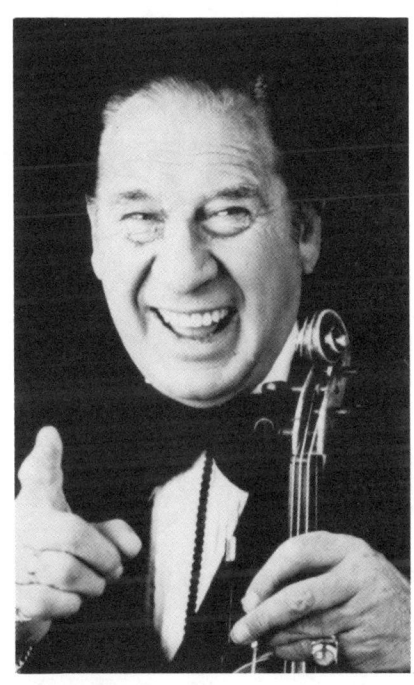

b. Henry Youngman, January 12, 1906, Liverpool, England

Records:
Sol Hurok Does Not Present The Best and Worst of Henny Youngman (Certron CS 7009), Primitive Sounds (National Recording Corp. LPA 10), Take My Album Please (Waterhouse 4), 126 Greatest Jokes (Rhino 011), Take My Project, Please (promo for Ryerson & Haynes Real Estate).

Compilations:
Golden Age of Comedy (RCA Victor LPV 580), Fun Time (Coral CRL 57072), Laugh of the Party (Coral CRL 57017).

Books:
Take My Wife, Please, How Do You Like Me So Far, 400 Travelling Salesman's Jokes, Don't Put My Name on This Book, Henny Youngman's Giant Book of Jokes.

man was a zany slapstick comic as well in the Catskills. At Cohen's Hillside Inn, he started a fire indoors because it was raining outside, and some campfire fans were disappointed.

It was a series of performances on "The Kate Smith Show" in 1936 that established Youngman as a star. He stayed on the show until 1938, when Abbott & Costello replaced him. While other comics worried over phrasing, the perfect character to build routines with, and fresh material, Youngman scored as the forerunner of the "No Frills" system for consumers. He just gave jokes, nothing but jokes, firing off a one-liner every eight seconds on the average. Audiences had only to wait a moment or two before hearing one they liked.

Other comics couldn't believe what Youngman was getting away with: a fast, artless delivery and a barrage of old wheezes. Milton Berle wrote, "Youngman's secret is in his delivery and his masterful ability to segue from one topic to another with such subtle-like blends as 'I love California . . . Say, didja hear about Mayor Wagner. . . .' Youngman hasn't got a routine, he has a master code. . . . I kid a lot about Henny, but actually he is one of the fastest comedians around. He has to be, with his act."

On stage the big (6'2"), affable man projects an easy-going likability. It's matched by hard-headed tenacity offstage. He memorizes thousands of gags and buys bunches of them ("Do you realize what a comedian like me has to pay to writers? One of them hands me 3 or 4 typewritten pages of jokes and I'll pay $1,000 to $1,500 for them"). He acts as his own agent, listed in the telephone book to assure availability, booking himself for TV, nightclubs, conventions and banquets. "I'm only funny when I get paid," he adds. He's dodged photographers trying to get a picture—expecting to be paid for a pose. For friends, or for expectant fans or reporters, he may indulge in his penchant for novelty card and joke-shop gags. With someone watching, he'll hail a cab and when one pulls up, he'll flash a card that says "Off Duty" and walk away.

Fast working and inoffensive, Youngman gets big laughs before almost any audience: "You have to keep jokes simple so the people in Omaha can understand. Every joke is a picture. A guy walks up and says, 'Do you know where Central Park is? No? Then I'll mug you here.' You see, it's a picture, everything is a picture."

Over the years Youngman's become an institution and each generation rediscovers his classic jokes, relentlessly delivered one after another, the good, the bad, the corny. "No joke is an old joke to people who haven't heard it," he says. "And most people who have heard jokes don't take the trouble to remember them."

"The King of the One-Liners," when "Laugh-In" began to use old jokes on the show, someone would say, "Oh, *that* Henny Youngman," as a semi-tribute. Youngman seems to tolerate gags other comics make about his old material, and over the years, there's almost self-parody in his stand-up. In hip nightclubs, he's the rage, audiences waiting to cheer for sweetly worn gems like "Take my wife—please." They enjoy his rhythmic tenor cadence and the surrealism of seeing him play a piercing rendition of "Smoke Gets in Your Eyes" while interrupting himself with non sequitur gags.

His most recent records have been for labels that offer mostly rock albums, owned by people who find Henny "campy" and cool. His album for Rhino Records was pressed using a "trick track" system. One side has four different routines stamped into the vinyl. Each time the needle comes down, it hits a different one.

Into the 70's, Youngman updated some of his material, adding lines like these:

"They sent a Polish terrorist to blow up a car. He burned his lips on the exhaust pipe. . . . A Polish man buys a zebra for a pet—know what he calls it? Spot. . . . On Halloween two Polish guys got burned faces. They were bobbing for french fries. . . . Are you Polish? I'll talk slower. . . ."

Youngman's mechanical approach to comedy netted him fame as the star of the "Dial-a-Joke" telephone lines, where 250,000 callers a day waited to hear a minute of jokes. Youngman offered a bargain, clocking an easy half-dozen before the click-off.

The blizzard of telephone calls proved his contention: "I play for the masses. I tell easy jokes. You don't have to think. My jokes happen to everybody. Some people get embarrassed because my jokes are corn. They're plain. They make people laugh."

Using his simple formula, Youngman continues to work, getting $2,500 minimum a performance, not for himself, "for my family. I don't want it for me. . . . I'm busier now than I've ever been. Twenty dates a month. I get sales meetings, trade shows, conventions, roasts. . . ." A classic story on Youngman is the time he played a convention, met a man at the same hotel whose son was getting bar mitzvahed, struck up a deal, and for a quick $150 did 15 minutes at the party.

Whether it's at The Bitter End before roaring fans of old comedy, or conventions, the Catskills, or even sun-fans at a Miss Nude U.S.A. Pageant, Youngman endures, living proof that if something's a classic, "once is never enough."

R
792.7
SMI

17665